History of the Medical Profession of Philadelphia

Standard History
of the
Medical Profession of Philadelphia

Edited by

Frederick P. Henry, A. M., M.D.

Fellow and Honorary Librarian of the College of Physicians of Philadelphia;
Member of the American Medical Association: of American Physicians:
of the Philadelphia County Medical Society, and of the Pathological Society of
Philadelphia: Corresponding Member of the Royal Academy of Medicine of Rome;
Professor of the Principles and Practice of Medicine, and of Clinical Medicine, in the
Woman's Medical College of Pennsylvania;
Physician to the Philadelphia Hospital, Etc.

With the collaboration of
**James M. Anders, M.D., Richard J. Dunglison, M.D.,
Charles K. Mills, M.D., Francis R. Packard, M.D.,
William H. Ford, M. D., and others.**

Illustrated

Ross & Perry, Inc.
Washington, D.C.

Reprinted by Ross & Perry, Inc. 2003
© Ross & Perry, Inc. 2003 on new material. All rights reserved.

Protected under the Berne Convention.

Printed in The United States of America

Ross & Perry, Inc. Publishers
216 G St., N.E.
Washington, D.C. 20002
Telephone (202) 675-8300
Facsimile (202) 675-8400
info@RossPerry.com

SAN 253-8555

Library of Congress Control Number: 2003106583
http://www.rossperry.com

ISBN 1-932109-36-6

Cover photo provided by Annenberg Rare Book & Manuscript Library, University of Pennsylvania

Book Cover designed by Sapna. sapna@rossperry.com

♾ The paper used in this publication meets the requirements for permanence established by the American National Standard for Information Sciences "Permanence of Paper for Printed Library Materials" (ANSI Z39.48-1984).

All rights reserved. No copyrighted part of this publication may be reproduced, stored in a retrieval system, or transmitted, in any form or by any means, electronic, photocopying, recording, or otherwise, without the prior written permission of the publisher.

PREFACE.

The object of this work is to describe the evolution of medicine in Philadelphia, from the time of Jan Petersen, the earliest practitioner on record, to the present day. It is, as all history must necessarily be, a description of events and of institutions, and, incidentally, a biographical record of those who have been most prominent in both. Estimates of the character of the distinguished men whose names appear on almost every page, and comparisons of institutions, have been sedulously avoided. The facts are left to speak for themselves, the true office of history being, in the words of Lord Bacon, "to represent the events themselves . . . . and to leave the observations and conclusions thereupon to the liberty and faculty of every man's judgment."

In dealing with such a multiplicity of names, dates and events, mistakes may have crept in, in spite of the most careful supervision; but, if this be so, it is a consolation to know that many errors of previous writers have been corrected.

A work of this sort has never before been attempted. The nearest approach to it is the admirable Early History of Medicine in Philadelphia, by the late Prof. George W. Norris, M. D., but this was, "for the most part, written in 1845," and was unfinished at the time of the distinguished author's death, in 1875. Chapters of the medical history of Philadelphia have been written by others, notably by the late Drs. Joseph Carson and W. S. W. Ruschenberger, but the work of the former is limited to the University of Pennsylvania, and that of the latter to the College of Physicians.

The authorship of this history is compound. The materials of the first five chapters were collected by an experienced historian in the employ of the publishers, and then subjected to careful editorial revision. That portion of Chapter V containing the history of the Medico-Chirurgical College was written by Dr. James M. Anders. The chapter on the Public Medical Libraries of Philadelphia was written by Dr. Richard J. Dunglison; that on Medical Jurisprudence, by Dr. Charles K. Mills; that on Medical and Surgical Appliances, by Dr. Francis R. Packard; and that on Medical Literature and Journals, by the editor. The History of the Board of Health, contained in Chapter IV, was contributed by the late Dr. William H. Ford. Among others who have been helpful in the preparation of the work, either by their advice or more active coöperation, may be mentioned Drs. Theophilus Parvin, John Ashhurst, Alfred Stillé, William F. Norris, John H. Brinton, William Pepper, James C. Wilson, William M. Welch, John H. Packard, Charles E. Cadwalader, Roland G. Curtin, Henry Leffmann, William B. Atkinson, J. Ross Gordon, I. T. Strittmatter, Samuel Wolfe, Clara Marshall, Anna M. Fullerton, Frances Emily White and Pemberton Dudley.

The work of examining the books and manuscripts of the College of Physicians was greatly facilitated by the cordial coöperation of Mr. Charles Perry Fisher, the librarian, and Miss M. C. Rutherford, the assistant librarian, of that institution. Thanks are due Mr. F. Gutekunst for the use of photographs for illustrations, and the editor is under special obligation to Dr. Anna M. Fullerton for assistance in the arduous work of revision.

THE EDITOR.

CONTENTS.

CHAPTER I.

	PAGE.
Reference to the First Book on American Surgery	17
Jan Petersen, Barber, a Salaried Surgeon	18
First Medical Representative on the Delaware	18
Early Settlement of the Dutch and Swedes	19
"Jan Oosting, the Surgeon"	19
William van Rasenberg	19
Peter Tyneman, Volunteer Surgeon	20
Olaf Person Stillé	20
John Goodson, Chirurgeon	21
First Pennsylvania Practicing Physician	21
Dr. Nicholas Moore	21
Names of Many Early Physicians	21
First Recorded Amputation	23
First Quarantine Law Passed	23
Advent of Early English Episcopalians	24
Duties of "Apprentices"	24
John Redman, the Preceptor of Rush	24
Thomas Cadwalader, William Shippen, Thomas and Phineas Bond and Cadwalader Evans	25
Drs. Thomas Graeme and John Bartram	26
Early Medical Lectures in Philadelphia	28
Autopsy in a Case of Mollities Ossium	29
Lazaretto Buildings at the Mouth of the Schuylkill	32
Dr. Thomas Bond and Founding of the First Permanent Hospital	32
Extract from the First Regular Clinical Lectures	34
Dr. William Shippen, Sr.	38
Proceedings of Hospitals Managers	38
Dr. John Fothergill	40

CONTENTS.

	PAGE.
Early Medical Schools of Dr. Shippen	42
Dr. Morgan, "Shippen's Assistant"	48
College of Philadelphia	61
Portrait of Dr. Benjamin Rush	67
Hospital Ward of the Almshouse, or "Bettering House"	71
Drs. Gerardus Clarkson and Thomas Parke	72

CHAPTER II.

Revolutionary War Physicians	73
The Hospital Department	74
Conflict of Authority Between Drs. Morgan and Stringer	76
Transfer of the General Hospital to New York	77
Appointment of Dr. William Shippen, Jr	78
Removal of the Sick to Philadelphia	81
Dismissal, by Congress, of Drs. Morgan and Stringer	83
Elevation of Rush to the Office of Surgeon-General	84
"Single Brethren's House" as a Hospital	86
Forcible Occupancy of the Almshouse Hospital	87
Congress Endorses the Action of Dr. Morgan	88
Philadelphia Occupied by the British in 1777	91
Partial List of Philadelphia Revolutionary War Physicians	95
Philadelphia Physicians According to the Directory of 1785	96
Dr. Samuel Powel Griffitts	98
Establishment of the Philadelphia Dispensary	98
Founding of the College of Physicians of Philadelphia	99
Drs. George Glentworth and Abraham Chovet	103
Union of the Two Medical Schools as Advocated by Dr Rush	105
Medical Department of the University of Pennsylvania	105
Yellow Fever in Philadelphia	108
Dr. Benjamin Duffield	111
Rush Hill as a Hospital	112
Treatment of Yellow Fever by Dr. Rush	114
Dr. William Currie	116
Resignation of Dr. Rush from the College of Physicians	117

CONTENTS.

	PAGE.
The Academy of Medicine of Philadelphia	119
Recurrence of Yellow Fever in 1798	120
Example of Heroic Fortitude	121
Estimates of the Life and Character of Dr. Rush	122
History of Dr. Rush	122 to 138
Dr. John Redman Coxe	139
Introduction of Vaccination in Philadelphia	141
Dr. Thomas C. James	142
Dr. Caspar Wistar	143
Dr. Philip Syng Physick	145
The Philadelphia Medical Institute	148

CHAPTER III.

Location of Many Physicians	150
The University Faculty	152
Methods of Dr. Nathaniel Chapman	153
Dr. Charles Caldwell	155
Dr. Joseph Parrish	156
The Philadelphia Anatomical Rooms and Dr. J. V. O. Lawrence	157
Dr. T. T. Hewson	159
Dr. George McClellan	159
Dr. John Eberle	160
Cause of Establishing a New Medical School in Philadelphia	159
Commencement of the Jefferson Medical College	164
Dr. Benjamin Rush Rhees	164
Dr. Jacob Green	165
An Incident in the Career of Dr. McClellan	167
Dr. Samuel McClellan	171
Dr. Granville Sharpe Pattison	171
Dr. Samuel Colhoun	171
Dr. Robley Dunglison	173
Independent Charter Secured by Jefferson Medical College	174
Early Disagreement in the New College Faculty	175
A New School Founded by Dr. McClellan	175
Dr. Samuel G. Morton	176

CONTENTS.

	PAGE.
Philadelphia College of Medicine	178
Franklin Medical College Chartered	179
Establishment of the Homeopathic Medical College	180
Washington Medical College	180
Eclectic Medical College of Philadelphia	180
Female Medical College	181
First Graduates from the Female Medical College	181
First Woman Professor in a Medical College	182
Dr. Elizabeth Horton Cleveland	182
Penn Medical University	182
National Convention of 1844	183
Organization of the Philadelphia County Medical Society	184
Woman's Medical College Founded	186
Dr. William P. Dewees	188
Dr. William E. Horner	189
Dr. William Gibson, LL. D.	190
Dr. Robert Hare	192
Dr. George B. Wood	193
Dr. Hugh L. Hodge	194
Dr. Samuel Jackson	195
Dr. William W. Gerhard	197
The New Jefferson Medical College	199
Dr. Joseph Pancoast	201
Dr. Thomas D. Mütter	202
Dr. John Kearsley Mitchell	203
Dr. Charles D. Meigs	205
Dr. Franklin Bache	208
Dr. René La Roche	209
Dr. Isaac Hays	210
Extract from Address of Dr. Alfred Stillé, in 1863	211

CHAPTER IV.

Extract from the Directory of 1860	213
Effect of the War on Jefferson Medical College	219
Effect of the War on Other Philadelphia Medical Schools	223

CONTENTS.

	PAGE.
Dr. James B. Rogers	223
Dr. Robert E. Rogers	224
Dr. Joseph Carson	226
Dr. Joseph Leidy	227
Dr. D. Hayes Agnew	234
Portrait of Dr. D. Hayes Agnew	237
Dr. William Pepper, Sr	241
Dr. Francis Gurney Smith	243
Portrait of Dr. Alfred Stillé	246
Dr. Alfred Stillé	247
Dr. S. D. Gross	250
Dr. Thomas Mitchell	256
Dr. Samuel H. Dickson	257
Dr. Ellerslie Wallace	258
Dr. B. Howard Rand	259
Dr. John B. Biddle	259
Dr. James Aitkin Meigs	260
First Military Hospital	263
List of Philadelphia Volunteer Surgeons	264
Satterlee Hospital	267
Mower Hospital	269
McClellan Hospital	269
Hospital Statistics	270
Founding of New Colleges	271
"Bogus Diploma" Schools	272
Woman's Medical College, and Women in Medicine	272
Resolutions, in 1858, of the County Medical Society	274
Epidemics	276
Dr. William H. Ford	280
Sanitary Conditions	281
Quarantine Station on Little Tinicum Island	286
Statistics	287
Hygienic Conditions in 1869	290
Important Changes in 1885	292
Influenza Epidemic of 1889-90	294
"Wigwam Hospital"	296
Hospitals for Contagious Diseases	296

CONTENTS.

	PAGE.
Present Sanitary Conditions	298
Philadelphia as a "City of Homes"	302
Physician Presidents of the Board of Health	304
Centennial Anniversary, 1876	307

CHAPTER V.

Hospitals and Societies in 1868	314
Dr. John Neill	316
Dr. Theodore G. Wormley	318
Present Faculty of the Medical Department of the University	320
Portrait of Dr. William Pepper	325
Samuel W. Gross, M. D., LL. D	327
Portrait of Dr. J. M. Da Costa	330
Present Faculty of Jefferson Medical College	332
Recognition of Women as Physicians	335
Jefferson Medical College of To-day	332
Present Faculty of the Woman's Medical College	339
The Medico-Chirurgical College	340
Dr. George P. Oliver	345
Dr. James E. Garretson, A. M., M. D., D. D. S	349
Dr. William H. Pancoast, A. M	350
Dr. Henry Ernest Goodman	351
Professors of the Medico-Chirurgical College	353
Philadelphia Polyclinic and College for Graduates in Medicine	360
Dr. Richard J. Levis	361
Philadelphia Post-Graduate School of Homeopathics	369
Medical Societies	370
Dr. W. S. W. Ruschenberger	372
Dr. Samuel Lewis	372
Presidents of the College of Physicians	372
Lewis Library	372
Portrait of Dr. S. Weir Mitchell	373
Philadelphia County Medical Society	379
International Medical College of 1887	382

CONTENTS.

	PAGE.
American Medical Association of 1886	386
Resolutions of the Philadelphia County Medical Society	388
Presidents of the County Medical Society	389
Pathological Society	391
Northern Medical Association	394
Medical Jurisprudence Society	396
Early Clinical Instruction in the Philadelphia Hospital	400
Revival of Clinical Instruction of Philadelphia Hospital in 1854	402
Pennsylvania Hospital Staff	403
Philadelphia Hospital Staff	405
Other Hospitals	408
Philadelphia Lying-in Charity	420
West Philadelphia Hospital for Women	423
Training School for Nurses	424
Orthopædic Hospital	428
Home for Incurables	429
Recapitulation	430

CHAPTER VI.

Earliest Inventions by Philadelphia Physicians	434
Inventions by Dr. Thomas Bond	434
Inventions by Dr. Philip Syng Physick	434
Inventions by Dr. Joseph Hartshorne	438
Inventions by Drs. Parrish, Syng, Dorsey, Gibson, Meigs, Barton, and Horner	439
Inventions by Drs. Hodge, S. D. Gross, Pancoast, and Fox	440
Inventions by Drs. Henry Horner Smith, D. Hayes Agnew, and John Neill	441
Inventions by Drs. Levis, Hewson and others	442

CHAPTER VII.

Medical Library of the Pennsylvania Hospital	445
Library of the College of Physicians	450
Portrait of Dr. J. C. Wilson	455
Medical Library of the Philadelphia Hospital	466

CHAPTER VIII.

	PAGE.
Medical Jurisprudence in Philadelphia	467
Lecture by Dr. Rush in 1810	467
Publications by Drs. Thomas Cooper, J. Bell and by Michael Ryan	468
"Medical Jurisprudence of Insanity"	469
Dr. John James Reese	469
Auxiliary Department of Medicine of the University of Pennsylvania	470
Medical Lectures on Medical Jurisprudence by Dr. Charles K. Mills	471
Dr. Henry C. Chapman as a Teacher on Medical Jurisprudence	471
Medical Jurisprudence in the Woman's and the Medico-Chirurgical Colleges.	472
"A Monograph on Mental Unsoundness"	473
Wharton and Stillé's Medical Jurisprudence	473
Hamilton's System of Legal Medicine	474
Medico-Legal Society of Philadelphia	474
The Medical Jurisprudence Society of Philadelphia	475
Professor Theodore G. Wormley, M. D., Ph. D., LL. D.	476
Dr. Henry Leffmann, A. M., M. D., Ph. D.	477
H. C. Wood, M. D., LL. D.	477
Other Experts on Medical Jurisprudence	478

CHAPTER IX.

Medical Literature of Philadelphia	479
Early Publications	480
Publications Between Cadwalder's Treatise and the Writings of Rush	481
"A Relation of a Cure Performed by Electricity"	482
Thesis and Writings of Dr. John Morgan	483
Principal Contributions to Literature by Dr. Rush	487
Dr. William Currie on Yellow Fever	490
Principal Works by Dr. William Currie	491
Dr. Charles Caldwell as an Author	492
Prof. Caspar Wistar's Publications	493
"Elements of Surgery," by John Syng Dorsey	493
John Redman Coxe's Contributions	494
Contributions of Dr. John C. Otto and Philip Syng Physick	495
Writings of Dr. William Potts Dewees	496
Nathaniel Chapman's Contributions	497
Samuel Jackson's Articles in the Various Medical Journals	498

CONTENTS.

	PAGE.
Charles D. Meigs' Notable Works	498
Contributions to Medical Literature, by Dr. William E. Horner	499
Dr. René La Roche and His Contributions	500
Joseph G. Nancrede, Reporter of the First Case of Cæsarian Section in Philadelphia	500
Dr. Hugh L. Hodge on Obstetrics	501
Principles and Practice of Surgery	501
John Kearsley Mitchell on Fevers	503
Works of John Bell	505
Contributions of Drs. David Francis Condie and George B. Wood	505
Robley Dunglison's Writings	506
Samuel David Gross as a Literator	508
Portrait of Samuel D. Gross	509
Joseph Pancoast's Contributions	512
George W. Norris' Writings	513
Puerperal Eclampsia, by Joseph Carson	514
Ovariotomy as Performed by Washington L. Atlee	514
William Wood Gerhard	515
Literary Work of William Pepper	519
"Review of the Materia Medica for the Use of Students"	520
Brochure by Thomas Dent Mütter	520
Henry Hollingsworth Smith's Contributions to Surgical Literature	521
The Surgical Literature of D. Hayes Agnew	521
"Diseases of Children," by J. Forsyth Meigs	522
Writings of John Neill	524
Contributions of Henry Hartshorne and William Hunt	525
Surgical Literature of Richard J. Levis	526
Works of William Goodell	527
Obstetrics and Gynecology, by Albert H. Smith	528
James Howell Hutchinson	528
Samuel Weissel Gross' Writings	529
Medical Literature of John S. Parry	532
Henry F. Formad and His Writings	533
Principal Works of Edward Tunis Bruen	534
Dr. John M. Keating	535
Numerous Writers of Medical Literature	536
Medical Journals of Philadelphia	537

A Standard History of Medicine in Philadelphia.

CHAPTER I.

THE COLONIAL PERIOD.

IN THE first book (a) on American surgery, whose author was a pupil of the first Philadelphia author (b) in medicine, is this interesting résumé: "At the revival of letters in Europe, when the cultivation of the languages had opened the treasures of the Greek and Latin writers, there arose a number of great men, in all the different branches of science; but what was very peculiar to the state of surgery, particularly in Italy and Germany, is, that this science was cultivated and practiced by the same men who studied and practiced physic; so that the same persons were at once admirable surgeons, and excellent physicians; and it is precisely at this era, that a crowd of celebrated men arise, whose works will forever do honor to themselves and their profession. But it was not long before the operation of some of those passions (which have so much influence in the affairs of mankind, occasioned the decline, and almost total extinction of surgery. The exterior of this science has nothing pleasing or attractive in it, but is rather disgusting to nice, timid and delicate persons. Its objects, too, except in time of war, lying chiefly among the poor and lower class of mankind, do not excite the industry of the ambitious or avaricious, who find their best account among the rich and great; for this reason, those illustrious men who were at once great physicians and surgeons, abandoned the most disagreeable and un-

---

(a) "Wounds and Fractures," by Dr. John Jones, 1775.
(b) Dr. Thomas Cadwalader, 1745.

profitable part of their profession, to follow that branch alone which at once gratified their ease, their avarice and ambition. This revelation gave rise to the second state of surgery. The medical surgeons, in quitting the exercise of the arts, retained the right of directing the barbers, to whom the operations and external applications of surgery were committed. From this separation, the surgeon was no longer one and the same individual, but a monstrous and unnatural composition of two persons; of a physician who arrogated to himself an extensive knowledge of science, and consequently the right of directing, and a surgeon operator, to whom the mere manual part was committed. The danger of this separation of the science of surgery from the art of operating was not at first perceived. The great masters who had exercised surgery as well as physic, were still alive, and the dexterity they had acquired was sufficient to direct and assist the automaton or man operator; but as soon as this Hippocratic race of men, as Fallopius justly styles them, were no more, the progress of surgery was not only retarded, but the art itself was almost extinguished, little more than the bare name remaining."

Even down to the very years of Jones' pupilage (d), there had been in London an authorized alliance of the Barber's Company and the Guild of Surgeons since the time of Columbus, so that, in the years when the Dutch and Swedes were seeking to forestall one another and the English, in the North and South Rivers on either side of peninsular Jersey, one is prepared for the statement that Jan Petersen (e), barber, from Alfendolft, was a salaried surgeon on South River (f) at ten guilders a month, beginning with July 10, 1638, the year of the first arrival of Swedish colonists. Whether he was located at Fort Nassau, an old Dutch fort near the site of Gloucester, or at that made by the colonists at Fort Christina, now Wilmington, he is the first representative of the medical profession on the Delaware, of which record is known,

(d) 1745.
(e) Dutch archives of the Albany Records of 1841, by Broadhead.
(f) The Delaware.

and his second year of practice was characterized by numerous climatic diseases among the colonists.

The Dutch and Swedish colonists mingled freely together, however the authorities might fight, and when in 1654 the Dutch gained the Delaware and founded the first permanent settlement, New Amstel, near New Castle, there were only 368 souls of both tongues. Nothing indicates that those Swedes, who began to turn their eyes toward the Schuylkill, took a physician with them, and "Mr. Jan Oosting, the Surgeon," at New Amstel, of whom the vice-director (g) writes on May 5, 1657, may have served for the whole region. A letter of the following year (h) also refers to "Master Jan," and gives a quaint picture of the situation, politically and medically: "In respect to the Swedish nation and their lands, which are now partly vacant and partly occupied and cultivated by them," he writes, "there are two parcels of the best land on the river on the west bank; the first of which is above Marietiens hook about two leagues along the river and four leagues into the interior; the second, on a guess, about three leagues along the same, including Schuylkill, Passajonck, Quinsessingh, right excellent land, the grants and deeds whereof, signed in the original by Queen Christina, I have seen; they remain here. I believe the proprietors, as they style themselves, or those who hold the ground briefs, would willingly dispose of them for a trifle, according to their value and worth. In like manner there are some old inhabitants here, sworn subjects of this province, who, in the years 1652 and 1653, purchased, with the consent of the General, from the Indian nation, about two leagues on the east bank of this river, with convenient kills, woods and fine land, which it would also be well to obtain." He also says: "William van Rasenberg, who came over as Surgeon, puts forth sundry claims against people whom he attended on the passage," the earliest record of this kind, "inasmuch as his wages did not run at the time and on the voyage, and he used his own provisions. There were on board the ship consider-

---

(g) Albany Records of 1841. Jan Petersen's will, dated April 10, 1640, is said to be still on file at Albany, N. Y.

(h) October 10, 1658.

able sickness, accidents and hardships in consequence of a tedious voyage. One hundred souls required at least a hogshead or two of French wine and one of brandy, and a tub of prunes had also to be furnished for refreshment and comfort to those sick of scurvy and suffering from other troubles, thro' the protracted voyage; for, from want thereof the people became so low that death followed, which is a pretty serious matter. Here, on shore, I see clearly that the poor, weak, sick or indigent, sometimes have need necessarily of this and that to support them, which one can not easily, or will not, refuse; though it be sometimes but a spoonful, frequently repeated, it amounts to more than is supposed. The barber also speaks of a house which Master Jan occupied being too small for him; he hath a wife, servant and child or children also. If he hire, as he says, at the expense of the city, he shall be obliged to show a paper to that effect." He had occasion also to say in another letter that "our barber surgeon" died and "another well acquainted with his profession is very sick." In 1660 a surgeon is called for and Peter Tyneman volunteers.

From these quaint pictures of the Swedish and Dutch settlers it will be seen how low was the standard of medicine among them. One barber-surgeon, too, covered a wide field among these pioneers, so that scarcely more than one at a time was necessary for the "South River" settlements for the next score of years. The Swedes on the Schuylkill were a simple pastoral people and the illness that did not respond to their own simple remedies, or to those they obtained from the friendly Indians, could await the New Amstel barber-surgeon's arrival. Little as they left of medical record, it is interesting to note that one family among them is linked to the present in having as a representative the Nestor of Philadelphia medicine, Dr. Alfred Stillé. On Lindstrom's map of what is now called "the neck" is Stillé's Land," the property of Olaf Person Stillé, said to be one of the colonists of 1638, and which, says a biographer of the family (i) "is the only homestead, Mr. Watson informs us, now known of any of the Swedish families whose names

(i) Hollingsworth on Moreton Stillé, 1856.

are on the list taken in the year 1693 for the information of William Penn," over ten years after he established the city.

In the van of Penn came some agents of the Free Society of Traders, and among them was John Goodson of London, chirurgeon to that organization, who first stopped at Upland, now Chester, and then removed to Philadelphia. Little else seems to be known of him, except that "he was a man of merit, and was probably the first practicing physician in Pennsylvania" (j), the barbers all residing at New Amstel. Dr. Nicholas Moore, the president of the society, was also a physician, but little is known of him.

With the arrival of Penn in 1682, the barber-surgeons were overshadowed, tho' not displaced, by an entirely different class of practitioners. The Swedes were simple pioneers, while the colony brought by Penn was made up largely of choice British stock come to found a British "Brook Farm," destined to a success not usually accorded to Utopias. The Welsh Quaker medical men were of this fine grade, and to the standard set by them is in no small degree due the high professional position taken by Philadelphia at so early a date. Their names were enrolled, with some others, among the list (k) of first purchasers of land on the new plat: Thomas Wynne of Cajerwit, in the County of Flint, Chirurgeon; Hugh Chamberlain of the City of London, Doctor of Physic; Robert Dimsdale of Edmonton, in the County of Middlesex, Chirurgeon; John Goodson of London, Chirurgeon; Edward Jones of Bala, in the County of Merioneth, Chirurgeon; Charles Marshall of the City of Bristol, Physician, and William Russell of London, Physician. Griffith Owen and Thomas Lloyd, who were among them, seem not to have been among the first purchasers. Of all these, however, only Dr. Edward Jones, who had direct charge of the Welsh section and came first in August, 1682, Dr. Thomas Wynne, his father-in-law, and Dr. Griffith Owen, both of whom came on the Welcome with Penn two months later, and Thomas Lloyd, seem to have become colonists, for little is known of John Goodson's residence. These

---

(j) Dr. George W. Norris—"Early History of Medicine in Philadelphia."
(k) Published by John Reed, 1774.

were personal friends and admirers of Penn, men of eminent practice in Britain and of the highest professional training of London. Medicine was the only one of the learned professions of much esteem among the Friends, so that it is perfectly natural that these chirurgeons should become leaders of the colonial government. To such an extent was this carried that Thomas Lloyd, an Oxford man, became the first deputy-governor, and did not practice at all, while Dr. Wynne organized and became president of the first Assembly held in Philadelphia, as well as Judge of the Principal Supreme Court, practicing but little in the nine years of his residence, for his death occurred in March, 1691. Dr. Edward Jones and Dr. Owen were also members respectively of the Assembly and the Governor's Council, and held other offices, and the former seems to have led the life of a planter and public man with but little attention to medicine during his long life (l), except what was required for the training of his son, Dr. Evan Jones, who spent a portion of his career in Philadelphia and is chiefly known by his being the father of the eminent New York surgeon, Dr. John Jones, and the preceptor of Dr. Thomas Cadwalader.

Indeed, "tender Griffith Owen, who both sees and feels" (m), was the first well-known, permanent, practicing physician in Pennsylvania, where he spent the last half of his three-score-and-ten years in by far the widest and most valuable practice in the colony during his time. This was of course not confined to the town of about seventy houses (n), mostly along the deep Delaware dock, but extended into the surrounding country and settlements, where he was always welcomed as one of the favorite preachers among the Friends. It is not probable that it was very exacting, if a letter (o) from New Jersey, dated in 1685, in any measure describes medical conditions in Penn's colony. "If you desire to come hither yourself you may come as a Planter or Merchant, but as a Doctor of Medicine I cannot advise you; for I hear of no diseases here to cure but

(l) He died in 1737.
(m) Letter of William Penn.
(n) "Picture of Philadelphia," by Dr. James Mease.
(o) From Charles Gordon of New Jersey to Dr. John Gordon of Montrose.

some Agues, and cutted legs and fingers, and there is no want of empirics for these already; I confess you could do more than any yet in America, being versed both in chirurgery and Pharmacie, for here are abundance of curious herbs, shrubs and trees, and no doubt medicinal ones for making of drugs, but there is little or no employment in this way." Even five years later a traveler (p) in the colony writes: "Of lawyers and doctors I shall say nothing, because the country is peaceable and healthy." Owen himself seems to have left no medical records and what little is known of his work is related by others. Seventeen years had passed since his coming, when it is related (q) that in honor of a second visit of Penn from England, the firing of a salute led to the accidental injury of a young man's arm, making necessary the first recorded amputation in the colony: It was "resolv'd upon by Dr. Griffith Owen (a Friend), the Surgeon, and some other skillful persons present; which accordingly was done without delay. But as the Arm was cut off, some Spirits in a Bason happened to take Fire, and being spilt upon the Surgeon's Aprin, set his Cloaths on fire; and there being a great Crowd of Spectators, some of them in the Way, and in Danger of being scalded, as the Surgeon himself was upon the Hands and Face; but running into the street, the Fire was quenched; and so quick was he that the patient lost not very much Blood, though left in that open, bleeding Condition." It was during the next year, 1700 (r), when Philadelphia had about 700 houses about the Delaware wharf, that the first quarantine law was passed, but whether he was connected with it or not is unknown. During the first seventeen years of the century, he was growing old, and, having taught his son, Dr. Griffith Owen, Jr., his profession, he withdrew more and more from practice and spent much time in attending Friends' meetings. The son seems to have been a child of his later years and did not long survive him, his

(p) Gabriel Thomas, 1689.
(q) Journal of Thomas Story. The landing was at Chester in 1699.
(r) Yellow fever or Barbadoes distemper had taken off about 220 the previous year, but Owen leaves no record of it, or of smallpox, which came on the vessel with Penn.

decease having occurred, it is said, in 1731, at an early age, so that in the elder Owen's later years his practice seems to have been divided among several, like Edward Jones and his son, Evan, who had other interests, or a few less known men, among whom are said to have been a Dr. Hodgson and John Le Pierre (s), the latter having an inclination to alchemy, according to popular report. At any rate when the gentle and lovable Friend preacher and physician died in 1717 the most prominent figure in medicine and the dominance of the Welsh chirurgeons were gone.

Their real successors were English Episcopalians, inasmuch as on one of them fell the mantle of pre-eminence as a practitioner. In 1711, six years before Owen's death and the next year after the appearance of smallpox in this port, there came a young Londoner of about twenty-six years, vigorous, talented, of liberal education and large views, fitted to become one of the typical colonial leaders. Dr. John Kearsley was born in England in 1684 and received the best medical training of his time. Six years after his arrival, the very year of Dr. Owen's death and of the arrival of another English Episcopalian, Dr. Thomas Graeme, he had become so eminent and successful that, in addition to an extensive practice, he had begun, with the gentle young Zachary, a career as preceptor of young native Americans so remarkable as almost to entitle his office "the first American medical college." Out of it came some of the most notable men of the next generation. Quaint John Bard, who became famous in New York, and whose son, Samuel, was the founder of the first medical school there, was one of them, and, according to Thatcher, found Dr. Kearsley's interpretation of the seven-year apprentice system of England both onerous and exacting, as it seemed to include the duties of a servant, coachman, messenger-boy, prescription clerk, nurse and assistant surgeon. Young John Redman, who afterwards became the preceptor of Rush, was another "apprentice," and among others who are said (t) to have listened to his teachings, though not as apprentices, probably,

---

(s) Scharf and Wescott, 1884.
(t) Dr. S. Weir Mitchell's Commemorative Address of 1887.

are young Thomas Cadwalader, who was born a short time before Kearsley arrived, William Shippen and Thomas Bond, both born in 1712, and Phineas Bond and Cadwalader Evans, slightly younger, nearly all of whom were friends of the inspiring young printer, Franklin. Among them also was his nephew, John Kearsley, Jr., who became prominent and contributed one of the first articles (u) to a foreign journal by an American physician, and whose sad ending in insanity furnishes the first tragedy in Philadelphia's medical history and one of the first of the Revolution. But important as was Dr. Kearsley's teaching in its extent and consequent influence on the city's medical development, it was incidental to a long and vigorous life in a large practice in both city and country, contemporary with that of his students almost down to the Revolution, and was mingled with civic and provincial activities of the first order. "He was long one of the representatives for the city in the House of Assembly," says a writer of the time (v), "and distinguished himself so much in every debate when the liberty or interest of the province was concerned, that he has often been borne from the Assembly to his own house on the shoulders of the people." Talented as an architect, he left two noble monuments of his activities in church and state, one none other than Independence Hall itself, and the second, Christ Church, to which he gave both substance and care during its twenty years of building, for the latter was designed to be, and was for long years after, "equal to anything of the kind in America." It was natural, then, that as a hale old man of eighty-five, when making his will, his three great interests should crystallize into a public institution so characteristic as Christ Church Hospital (w), now one of the oldest in the city, which was established accordingly at 111 Arch street, soon after his decease, three years later, early in January, 1772.

(u) 1769, on angina maligna which prevailed in 1746 and 1760.
(v) "The Pennsylvania Packet," 13 January, 1772.
(w) Neither this nor that of the Friends' Almshouse were hospitals in the recent sense.

Spanning almost the same period as that of this English preceptor's life are two careers of medical interest, one that of Dr. Thomas Graeme, 1684 to 1772, and the other that of John Bartram, 1701 to 1777, the former most notable in the early quarantine service and the latter the first American botanist. Dr. Graeme was to Deputy-Governor Keith much what Jones and Wynne were to William Penn. He was of an ancient Perthshire family, had a large estate in Montgomery County, well-known as "Graeme Park," held many prominent positions, but the most distinctive thing known of him in medicine, aside from his being on the hospital staff, is his occupation of a position corresponding to Port Physician. The act of 1700 seems to have been spasmodically effective until about 1720, in which year the Governor gave notice that he had appointed Patrick Baird, chirurgeon, to carry out its provisions. This is about all that is known of Dr. Baird, but Dr. Graeme seems to have been in office the year after his arrival in 1717, and in 1728 was commissioned together with Dr. Lloyd Zachary. He was serving as late as 1740, and seems to have been occasionally somewhat of a bone of contention in the struggles between the people and the deputy-governor. Wholly unlike the port physician, however, and far more widely known as a scientist, John Bartram, through his self-taught acquaintance with materia medica and surgery, became, to quote the words of Linnæus himself, "the greatest natural botanist in the world." His well-known Botanical Garden on the Schuylkill was the first of the kind in America, and his contributions to that science led to his being under salary from the British Royal Family previous to the Revolution.

Philadelphia was growing rapidly and by the end of ten years after Dr. Baird was appointed port physician, it was spreading north and south along the wharf, with a population estimated at 12,000. There was also great activity in medicine abroad, the Monros having returned from Leyden, founded the medical school of Edinburgh the very year the port physician was appointed, and the time was now coming when the colony should no longer depend upon imported physicians nor be content with the meager advantages of the practitioner's apprenticeship system. Rising about Dr. Kearsley already were those native American students, some of whom were to afford themselves additional training in Europe, especially in London, and to receive a stimulus that destined them to overshadow their preceptors and dominate the whole medical atmosphere of Philadelphia. The oldest and first of these favored ones to begin practice was the gentle and gifted Lloyd Zachary, a native of Boston, born in 1701, though reared in the Quaker City, grandson of the one-time Deputy-Governor Thomas Lloyd. Having gone to Europe in 1723, the year after he attained his majority, he spent three years in study and returned the same year that young Franklin came back a master printer, even then with some of the power that, sixty years after, led Dr. John C. Lettsom of London to write of him: "When that legion of science, Dr. Franklin, arrives, which, may heaven permit, I hope he will spread an intellectual shock throughout your continent." Dr. Zachary assumed a successful practice and received a degree of consideration that gave him position among the older men and a worthy seniority among the younger. Within two years, 1728, he and Dr. Graeme became port physicians, and when, in 1751, the first hospital was organized, he and two younger confrères were the first appointees and secured the Assembly's final action in its favor by offering their services free. Although during three of his remaining five years he was crippled by paralysis, he devoted them warmly to this institution until his death in 1756, at the age of fifty-five years.

Four years after Zachary began practice another of these young men, the first native of Pennsylvania to receive his medical education abroad, returned from London, where he had been under the tuition of the celebrated surgeon, William Cheselden, and had witnessed that revival of surgery which was to result, fifteen years later, in a rupture of the ancient alliance of the Associations of Barbers and Surgeons. This was young Dr. Thomas Cadwalader, who was only twenty-three, born in 1707, in Philadelphia, and yet so proficient in dissection, at that time "rare in Europe and unknown in America," that students and physicians alike urged him to give a public course of lectures on the cadaver. In this, William Shippen, who was but five years older, and without European advantages, took the initiative. "According to correct information," says Dr. Caspar Wistar in 1818, "I find that on his return (x) to Philadelphia he made dissections and demonstrations for the instruction of the elder Dr. Shippen and some others who had not been abroad." These were given in Second street above Walnut on the site of the old Bank of Philadelphia (y), and were the first public medical lectures and dissections in America (z). Other innovations followed. In 1731 he was one of several to introduce inoculation for smallpox (a) and is said to have written on the subject; eleven years later,

(x) 1730. Through some error the dates 1750 and 1751 have gained a good deal of currency.

(y) Watson's Annals.

(z) The earliest known efforts at the institution of medical lectures in Philadelphia was in 1717, the term "physical lectures," derived from physic, being applied to them. The effort was made by Dr. Cadwalader Colden, 1688-1776, who was a Scotchman living in Philadelphia from 1708 to 1718, when he removed to New York, the seat of his greatest activity. He was a physician, botanist and natural philosopher, and it was he who suggested the American Philosophical Society to Franklin. He became Lieutenant-Governor of New York. It was between his twentieth and thirtieth year that he was in Philadelphia, and a letter of James Logan, dated "5th month 1st, 1717-18," and quoted by Librarian F. D. Stone, refers to it thus: "All I know of that bill is only this. He (Colden) came to me one day to desire my opinion of a proposal to get an Act of Assembly for an allowance to him as physician for the poor of this place. I told him I thought very well of the thing, but doubted whether it could be brought to bear in the House. Not long after, R. Hill showed me a bill for this purpose, put in his hands by the Governor, with the two farther provisions in it, which were, that a public physical lecture should be held in Philadelphia, to the support of which every unmarried man, above twenty-one years, should pay six shillings eightpence, or an English crown, yearly, and that the corpses of all persons whatever that died here should be visited by an appointed physician, who should receive for his trouble three shillings and fourpence. These things I owned very commendable, but doubted our Assembly would never go into them, that of the lecture especially." Nothing further is known of the effort.

(a) The first mention of inoculation in Philadelphia is as follows, in the Pennsylvania Gazette of March, 1731: "The practice of inoculation for the smallpox begins to grow among us. J. Growden, the first patient of note that led the way, is now upon the recovery." Dr. Franklin says in a letter that about fifty were vaccinated and but one, a child, died. Watson says that Drs. Kearsley, Zachary, Cadwalader, the elder Shippen, Thomas Bond and Dr. Sommers were the only physicians who inoculated, as Dr. Graeme was himself sick during the whole epidemic. In 1750 Dr. Adam Thompson, of whom little is known, gave a public lecture in the Academy on a method of preparing for inoculation by using

1742, in a most interesting case of mollities ossium, he made the first autopsy for purely scientific purposes in America (b). During this period a very prevalent disorder, due to the general use of punch made from Jamaica rum distilled in leaden vessels, drew from him studies that revolutionized the treatment of the "iliac passion," or colica pictonum, as it is now called. The original draft of a manuscript on this subject may be seen in the archives of the College of Physicians, as well as the only extant copy of the double-preface print of 1745. This was the first medical work published in the province and one of the first in America, said, indeed, to be the earliest extant. Its title, with the popular name then used, is "An Essay on the West India Dry-Gripes; with the Method of Preventing and Curing that Cruel Distemper. To Which is added An Extraordinary Case in Physic" (c), "Printed and Sold by B. Franklin." That he was apprehensive of its public reception among physicians is curiously illustrated by two prefaces of the same date, March 25, 1745 (d), the first treating chiefly of the Horatian distinction of "a critic from a caviller;" but whether this was suppressed as unwise, in the midst of the printing, and another substituted, it is certain that the second is the only one that appears in most copies. In this he says: "I have long been of opinion that 'tis the duty of Physicians to frankly communicate to the world any

---

mercury and antimony, which, according to Dr. J. M. Toner, was widely influential. In 1756 Dr. Lauchlin Maclean published a pamphlet on the subject, which was printed by Bradford, a copy of which is in the Toner collection. Dr. Maclean was born in Ireland about 1728, graduated in medicine at Edinburgh in 1755 and came to Philadelphia. He became a surgeon in Otway's regiment and was with Wolfe at Quebec. He was the friend of Goldsmith, Burke and Wolfe, and was believed by many to be the author of the Junius letters. He afterward became a public man in British service and died en route for home from India in 1777.

(b) A medico-legal autopsy was made in New York in 1691.

(c) An account of his autopsy case. In his "Issues of the Press of Philadelphia," Mr. Charles R. Hildeburn mentions a notice of "An Essay on the Iliac Passion, by C. Colden," in 1741; but he tells the writer he believes himself to have been misled in the matter, and that it is an error. Dr. Colden had lived in New York since 1718. The first printed notice of medicine in the province seems to have been in Atkin's Almanac, 1685, in which the publisher advertises a small stock of remedies, thus: "Some Experienced Medicines, sold by William Bradford at Philadelphia."

(d) He was temporarily at Trenton at this time.

particular Method of treating diseases, which they have found to be successful in the course of their experience, and not generally known or practiced by others. By this the medical art has been and may still be improved. Many are the advantages the present age reaps from such disinterested conduct in our predecessors; and where we have freely received, surely we should freely give." He also adds: "And tho' the method here laid down may be new to the generality of the profession, it has been practiced some years, with great approbation, by several gentlemen of distinguished character in Philadelphia" (e). The work was well received both here and abroad, for so late as 1828 Dr. Thatcher writes: "Dr. Rush used to quote it constantly in his lectures with praise. In some of the British journals this practice is mentioned as the most successful in England and in those countries where the disease still prevails" (f). Six years later he joined the Drs. Bond in founding the first hospital in America, and was one of its medical staff during his life, and the same year, because of the general interest in electricity awakened by Franklin during the preceding five years, was the first American physician to use that agent in disease, the case being that of Governor Belcher of New Jersey, who was afflicted with paralysis (g). He was an active trustee and clinical lecturer in the first medical school and a founder of the first medical society in 1765, as well as of the first medical library two years before. Indeed, as a friend and kindred spirit of Franklin, who was only a year older, he was partaker in almost every new foundation in this fruitful period of beginnings, and was even chosen first acting-president (as vice-president) of the new American Philosophical Association during Franklin's absence, in 1769, an organization always largely influenced by physicians. When, in 1775, four years before his death, there appeared for use of surgeons in the coming struggle, the first American surgical work, already quoted, by his nephew and special pupil, Dr. John Jones, the eminent New York

---

(e) In the copy referred to the first preface precedes the title page.
(f) Thatcher's Medical Biography.
(g) From an account in manuscript by Dr. Charles E. Cadwalader, the physician's great-grandson.

surgeon and the physician of Washington, his influence was acknowledged in its dedication, which says: "To you, whose whole life has been one continuous scene of benevolence and humanity, the most feeble efforts to soften human misery and smooth the bed of death, will, I know, be an acceptable present, however short the well-meant zeal of the author may fail of his purpose" (h). Eight years after his death, which occurred in November, 1779, in the midst of the contention about the commission of medical examiners that occupied him even at the advanced age of seventy-two, Dr. John Redman, in his inaugural as first president of the College of Physicians, paid the following fine tribute to "one, whose person, age, character and medical ability and respectable deportment to and among us, as well as his generous, just and benevolent temper of mind and great acquaintance with books and men and things, and proper attention to time and seasons, would, I am persuaded, have pointed him out as our first object." He owns there is no need to mention his name, "but I naturally recollect with pleasure the name of our worthy and well-respected brother and much-esteemed friend Thomas Cadwalader," whom "it would have been the highest gratification to me, as I believe it would to all who knew him, to have given our suffrages unanimously to place him at the head of such an institution."

Great contributor as he was to the progress of medicine, he was still greater as a man. It would be interesting, were this the place, to consider the eminent family to which he belongs, one of the first in national history, and to recount his own activities, as prominent as they were far-reaching, suggesting Rush in his wide interests, Franklin in his secret management of events, and Washington in his judicial poise as a leader. "Kadwaladyr" means "arranger of battles," a name peculiarly applicable to him, since he was chairman of the provincial board of war almost continuously from the French war of 1755 to near the close of his life (i).

(h) Dr. Jones, 1729 to '91, spent his early years and eleven at the close of his life in Philadelphia, but became famous in New York.

(i) It is interesting to note that a young student of Dr. Redman spent four years in the war as a surgeon and bore the title of Lieutenant John Morgan, his commission dated April 1, 1758.

Twelve years after Dr. Cadwalader began practice, and while the young native American physicians, Zachary, Shippen and the Bonds, were showing their power, the increased immigration from various regions and the consequent introduction of such "distempers," as smallpox, yellow fever and the like, alarmed the merchants and prompted the Assembly to take some measures of quarantine to prevent their introduction. An act of February 3, 1743, secured Province Island, a part of the west bank of the mouth of the Schuylkill, on which lazaretto buildings were erected and ships ordered to stop there. Various temporary measures were taken for the care of the sick who landed before and after this time. Almshouses were established by the Friends and by the city, and as a matter of course, some provisions for the sick were required in them, but there was one of these young physicians who, in his considerable visitation among the needy, for which he was especially known, conceived the idea of bringing them together in one place as a permanently instituted hospital. Heretofore medicine had been dependent on individuals and rose and fell with them, but to Dr. Thomas Bond belongs the honor of first (j) introducing the permanency of institutions into the medical history of this city and the founding of the oldest independent hospital in the United States (k).

Dr. Bond was born in Calvert County, Maryland, in 1712, and studied medicine under a Scotch physician there, Dr. Hamilton, but afterwards supplemented this instruction by attendance upon lectures in Europe, especially at the Hotel Dieu in Paris. In 1734 (l), at the age of twenty-two, he returned to Philadelphia and soon became active in his profession and in various enterprises of a

---

(j) In 1709, on the "25th of the ninth month," a meeting of Friends voted money toward negotiating with the proprietary "for an Hospital," but it seems not to have succeeded, and in 1712 the city began arrangements for an almshouse. Before they completed them the Friends' Almshouse was started, but had no real hospital department. The city's almshouse, now the Philadelphia Almshouse, had its first structure completed about 1731, and had a hospital department, the oldest in the colonies.

(k) Some authorities speak of Catholic hospitals in Canada and possibly in Mexico as slightly older.

(l) Dr. G. W. Norris, Morton and Woodbury give it two years earlier.

public character which were founded in that period. It was about the end of his sixteenth year of practice, 1750, that he decided to take measures toward securing the foundation of a hospital. Enlisting the aid of Dr. Zachary and Dr. Phineas Bond, his younger brother, men of a character not unlike his own, efforts were made to launch the project. "He was zealous and active in endeavoring to procure subscriptions for it," writes Franklin in his autobiography, "but the proposal being a novelty in America, and at first not well understood, he met with but little success. At length he came to me with the compliment, that he found there was no such thing as carrying a public-spirited project through without my being concerned in it. 'For,' he said, 'I am often asked by those to whom I propose subscribing, "Have you consulted Franklin on this business? And what does he think of it?" And when I tell them I have not (supposing it rather out of your line), they do not subscribe, but say they will consider it.'" Franklin headed the subscription and when he saw it needed provincial aid prompted a petition to the Assembly on January 29, 1751, asking for a place for the insane and those "whose Poverty is made more miserable by the additional Weight of a grevious disease, from which they might easily be relieved, if they were not situated at too great a Distance from regular Advice and Assistance, whereby many languish out their lives, tortured perhaps with the Stone, devour'd by the Cancer, deprived of sight by Cataracts, or gradually decaying by loathsome distempers; who, if the expense in the present manner of Nursing and Attending them separately when they come to town were not so discouraging, might again, by the judicious Assistance of Physic and Surgery, be enabled to taste the Blessings of Health, and be made in a few Weeks useful Members of the Community, able to provide for themselves and Families." A bill was prepared, but objections were offered, the chief being expense for surgeon's fees, which was met by these three physicians offering three years' service free, thereby also establishing a precedent, and the bill was approved on the 11th of May. In October the old Judge John Kinsey mansion, on the south side of Market below

Seventh (m) was secured temporarily, under the direction of Israel Pemberton and Dr. Thomas Bond, and on February 10, 1752, the managers of the medical staff invited those who had been appointed consultants, Drs. Graeme, Cadwalader, Moore (n) and Redman, to act on the first applications to the Pennsylvania Hospital. The first patient and first cured was Margaret Sherlock. The present site at Spruce, Pine, Eighth and Ninth streets was secured two years later.

From circumstances and ability as well, Dr. Bond continued to be the most prominent figure at the hospital for many years. In 1753 he reported a peculiar case of a worm in the liver to "Medical Observations and Inquiries," a London journal, and sent the specimen to Dr. William Hunter of that city. He was distinguished for his skill in surgery, and his operation of lithotomy in 1756 on the first case of stone at the hospital is the first record of this operation in America, antedating that in New York by four years. His subsequent cases of lithotomy were numerous. Three years later he published a paper in London on the use of Peruvian bark in scrofula, and ten years later, when the new medical school was begun, its founder requested him to give the first regular clinical lectures in America at the hospital he had established. Fortunately his words inaugurating them have been preserved.

"When I consider the skillful hands the practice of Physic and Surgery has of necessity been committed to in many parts of America," said Dr. Thomas Bond on the 26th of November, at his home (o), in his introductory lecture to his clinical course which began at Pennsylvania Hospital on December 3, 1766, "it gives me pleasure to behold so many worthy young men, training up in those professions, which, from the nature of their objects, are the most interesting in the community, and yet a greater pleasure in foreseeing, that the unparalleled public spirit of the good people of this prov-

---

(m) Old number, 172 High (Market) Street.

(n) Samuel Preston Moore, 1710-1785, was consultant until 1759, and served as Provincial Treasurer for fourteen years.

(o) Drs. Redman, Cadwalader, Shippen and the Managers were present with thirty students.

ince, will shortly make Philadelphia the Athens of America and render the sons of Pennsylvania reputable amongst the most celebrated Europeans in all the liberal Arts and Sciences. This, I am at present certain of, that the institutions of literature and charity already founded, and the School of Physic lately opened in this city, afford sufficient foundation for the students of Physic to acquire all the knowledge necessary for their practicing every branch of their profession reputably and judiciously. The great expense in going from America to England, and thence from country to country, and college to college, in quest of medical qualifications, is often a bar to the cultivation of the brightest geniuses amongst us, who otherwise might be moving stars in their professions, and most useful members of society." He farther on points out where "the clinical professor comes in to the aid of speculation and demonstrates the truth of theory by facts," and promises "to show you all the operations of Surgery and endeavor, from the experiences of thirty years, to introduce you to a familiar acquaintance with the acute diseases of our own country," notwithstanding "the season of my life points out relaxation and retirement." The hospital afforded an average of one hundred and thirty patients at that time, and had averaged over one hundred for two years. It was now fifteen years since Dr. Bond had proposed the institution to Franklin, and it was eminently fitting that he should begin the list of its great clinical teachers.

Six years later a contemporary writer (p) describes him at an operation: "I had the curiosity last week to be present at the hospital, at Dr. Bond's cutting for stone, and was agreeably disappointed, for instead of seeing an operation said to be perplexed with difficulty and uncertainty, and attended with violence and cruelty, it was performed with such ease, regularity and success, that it scarcely gave a shock to the most sympathizing bystander, the whole being completed and a stone two inches in length and one in diameter extracted in less than two minutes." The enthusiastic visitor was ready to rank such surgery with the fine arts.

(p) Letter quoted by Dr. G. W. Norris and written in 1772.

His medical skill was no less remarked upon. He introduced hot and cold bathing in treatment far more than anyone else, and was the first to secure the general use of mercury among the profession of the city. Even so early as December 4, 1776, at the age of sixty-two, he offered his own and his son's (q) services for hospital duty to the Committee of Safety, and both did excellent work. It will be recalled that he was one of the original founders of the American Philosophical Society and its first vice-president in 1743, and in 1782 delivered before it an address on "The Rank of Man in the Scale of Being, and the Conveniences and Advantages He Derives from the Arts and Sciences." He was also one of the founders of the college out of which came the University, and yet when, at the age of seventy-two, he passed away, March 26, 1784, his greatest honor lay in being the founder of the oldest hospital (r) and the first clinical instruction in the republic.

So intimately was his brother, Dr. Phineas Bond, associated with him in all these enterprises of medical and general progress, that it may fairly be said that where the one was there was the other also. He was five years younger than Thomas and only lived fifty-six years, dying in 1773, after a life so refined and scholarly that, writes Dr. Caspar Wistar, no member of the profession in the state "ever left behind him a higher character for professional sagacity, or for the amiable qualities of the heart." His education had been received in their Maryland home and in Europe, where he spent even more time than did Thomas, and visited Leyden, Paris, London and Edinburgh. His practice was extensive and purely medical. His service at the hospital covered twenty-two years. He was one of the original members of the first American Philosophical Society, and is happily remembered as one of the three or four organizers of the College of Philadelphia, now the University, in which was soon to appear still greater medical progress.

(q) Dr. Thomas Bond, Jr.
(r) Only four years later an eminent French traveler, M. de Warville, wrote so highly of it that he said there was but one in France to compare with it.

Another member of the hospital staff passed away the same year (1773), at almost exactly the same age (s) as Phineas Bond, one to whom, according to the statement of Franklin, is due the honor of having proposed the first medical library. This was Cadwalader Evans, who, after his studies under Thomas Bond, had his Atlantic voyage interrupted by a vessel of one of the three warring powers, Spain, France and England, and was persuaded to live in Hayti awhile and to spend two years of practice in Jamaica before finishing his studies in Edinburgh and London. He began a life service on the hospital staff in 1759, and three years later was no doubt impressed, as others were, by a present received by the institution from a famous physician of London, Dr. John Fothergill. This was a book recently published there, "An Experimental History of the Materia Medica, by William Lewis, F. R. S." It was presented for the use of students of the hospital and was prompted by the doctor's Franklinian purposes for medicine in general and also, no doubt, by his friendship for the brilliant son of Dr. William Shippen, Sr., who was at that time one of the managers and a member of the hospital medical staff. This was in July, 1762, and in May of the following year Dr. Evans' proposal bore fruit in an offer of the medical staff to use student fees for the founding of a library. It was signed, in order, by Drs. Thomas Bond, Thomas Cadwalader, Phineas Bond and Cadwalader Evans, and, being accepted, the library of the Pennsylvania Hospital was soon, and for long years, the best in the land.

This little incident of the book, with its connection with Dr. Fothergill and the Shippens in 1762 binds together three most interesting characters in the inception of medical education in America, and most happily associates them with the noble monument of Dr. Bond, the Pennsylvania Hospital. It may also serve to usher into the medical field a new generation, some of whose members are destined to outshine all their predecessors in the history of the profession on this continent.

It will be recalled that one of the managers of the hospital at

---

(s) Fifty-seven years.

this date, Dr. William Shippen, Sr., was, about thirty years before, one of the first native American students who was unable to finish his studies abroad, and that it was his keen realization of his loss that led him to urge his fellow student, Dr. Thomas Cadwalader, to give the first public medical lectures in America. He was five years younger than Cadwalader, born in Philadelphia in 1712, where he received both his liberal and professional education. He seems to have served his apprenticeship in the office of the Kearsleys, though most accounts of his life contain no reference to the fact (t), and, according to excellent authority (u), under Dr. Cadwalader's direction, "he took lessons in Anatomy and became, by study, a proficient in Chemistry and Natural Philosophy." At the age of forty-one he became one of the staff of the hospital and served until his resignation a quarter of a century later, when he had already retired from an extensive practice of the highest reputation. Though he lived to the ripe age of eighty-nine years, dying in 1801, a distinguished member of the Continental Congress, a vice-president of the American Philosophical Society, a founder of the College of New Jersey, now Princeton University, a trustee of the College of Philadelphia, and with even more honors, there was nothing that so characterized him as the love for higher education in medicine, born of his own regrets, and his purpose to train up his son, William Shippen, Jr., to the same profession and with the highest advantages that Europe could afford. Indeed, some eminent authorities (v) have intimated the probability that he trained his son with the definite hope of his becoming a public lecturer on medicine, which would be wholly in keeping with the oratorical powers already displayed by the young man while in Princeton.

In view of these facts it is interesting to notice the proceedings of a meeting of the hospital managers in the Warden's room of the Court House, the 8th of "the 11th month, 1762," with the

---

(t) Morton and Woodbury say he studied with Dr. John Kearsley, Jr.
(u) Dr. Caspar Wistar's Eulogium, 1809.
(v) Dr. Caspar Wistar and Dr. Joseph Carson; "but," says the former, "I have heard nothing in support of this opinion."

medical staff present, the Drs. Bond, Dr. Shippen, Sr., Dr. Redman and Dr. Evans, a meeting called "at the request of Doc'r William Shippen, Jun'r, lately arrived (w) from London" (x). He informed them that there had arrived seven cases containing anatomical drawings and models for the hospital from his friend Dr. John Fothergill of London, who had given him some verbal directions concerning them, and that he wished permission to use them in connection with a private school of anatomy he should open during the season. A letter from Dr. Fothergill to James Pemberton, dated the 7th of the 4th month preceding, was read, a part of which says: "I propose to send by Dr. Shippen a present to it (the hospital), of some intrinsic value (y), though not probably of immediate benefit. I need not tell thee that the knowledge of Anatomy is of exceeding great use to Practitioners in Physic and Surgery, and that the means of procuring subjects with you are not easy. Some pretty accurate anatomical drawings about half as big as life have fallen into my hands, and which I purpose to send to your hospital, to be made the care of the physicians and to be by some of them explained to the students or pupils who may attend the hospital. In the want of real subjects these will have their use, and I recommend it to Dr. Shippen to give a course of anatomical lectures to such as may attend. He is well qualified for the subject and will soon be followed by an able assistant, Dr. Morgan, both of whom, I apprehend, will not only be useful to the province in their employment, but, if suitably countenanced by the Legislature, will be able to erect a school for Physic amongst you that may draw many students from various parts of America and the West Indies, and at least furnish them with a better idea of the rudiments of their profession than they have at present the means of acquiring on your side of the water" (z). The cases were opened the next day and found to contain eighteen crayon drawings, three cases of anatomical models, a skeleton and a fœtus model, of which Dr. Caspar

(w) He arrived in May of that year (Wistar).
(x) The spelling of these minutes is not used farther.
(y) The drawings were estimated at £350 value in the hospital stock.
(z) History of Pennsylvania Hospital, Morton and Woodbury, 1895.

Wistar writes: "Dr. Fothergill "employed Rimsdyck, one of the first artists of Great Britain, to execute the crayon paintings now at our hospital, which exhibit the whole structure of the body at two-thirds the natural size; and the gravid uterus, with many of the varied circumstances of natural and preternatural parturition, of the full size. Jenty, an anatomist of London, is said to have made the dissections from which these paintings were taken." These were not the first signs of interest in a teaching museum at the hospital, however, for so early as April, 1757, Deborah Morris gave a skeleton for that purpose, the first gift of this kind recorded, and the real beginning of the first medical museum.

Dr. John Fothergill had been a substantial friend of the hospital long before this letter. The influence of such a friend at this stage of medical progress is of no indifferent interest. A Yorkshire Quaker of the same age as the elder Shippen, he was educated by those able founders of the Edinburgh medical school, headed by Monro, whose attention he attracted from the first. He graduated in 1738 and began practice in London in 1740. By 1748 his publications had given him European fame, and his mind touched so many sides of progress that probably no man of his time could be said more truly to be a medical Franklin. When he died in 1780, at the age of sixty-eight, he was president of the Medical Society of London, and medical education in Philadelphia and New York, with both of whose colleges' foundations he was associated, lost a valuable friend. His instinct to discover talent in young men was not less than his power to inspire them with the fructifying suggestiveness that characterized his own mind. It is of the greatest significance and importance that the first of the new generation of Philadelphia physicians should have had the good fortune to enjoy the friendship of such a man and to partake of his spirit.

William Shippen, Jr., was twenty-six years old as he stood before the hospital board, proposing the first foundation of systematic public lectures on Anatomy in the province (a), and prob-

(a) Dr. William Hunter gave anatomical lectures at Newport, Rhode Island, in the years 1754-5-6; he was a relative of the Hunters of London (Carson).

ably the first on the continent in Obstetrics, and he was undoubtedly the first who had the purpose of inaugurating medical school education in the Colonies, as distinguished from the apprentice system. Born in Philadelphia on October 21, 1736, he had been carefully educated under Mr. Finley, afterward president of the College of New Jersey, now Princeton University, and also at the latter institution under the presidency of Burr in 1754, where he graduated with high honor as valedictorian. His oratorical qualities were so remarkable on this occasion that the great evangelist, Whitefield, who was attending the commencement there, desired to win him for the ministry. Instead, however, he returned to Philadelphia and at once began the study of his chosen profession under his father. After three years thorough work he went to London in the autumn of 1757 and at once had the good fortune to be established in the home of the Hunters, under the direction of his younger brother, John, who then assisted Dr. William Hunter in anatomy. He also had the friendship and instruction of William Hewson, who assisted the Hunters for a time, and there began his intimate relations with Dr. Fothergill. Here, too, he attended the lectures of the accomplished accoucheur, Dr. McKenzie, and became so interested in obstetrics that he resided in the poor quarter in order to have greater advantages in that practice, and it was undoubtedly at this time that his preferences for that branch were determined. From London he went to Edinburgh and there became much attached to Cullen and the younger Monro, graduating under their instruction in 1761, with the very characteristic thesis: *De Placentae cum Utero Nexu*. Desiring to go to Paris, but encountering obstacles due to the existing war, his friend, Sir John Pringle, secured his services as medical attendant for a wealthy lady who was about to travel in Southern France. By this means he gained an intimate acquaintance with a number of Parisian physicians, among whom was the well-known Senac. On his return to America in May, 1762, he began practice with his father and opened the way for a private school of anatomy and midwifery in the fall, as soon as the season should warrant. The time was ripe for it; indeed, to use the words of Dr. Wistar, "we must conclude that Shippen could not have fixed upon any part of the new world, which, at that time, was more promising than Philadelphia. He was not disposed to neglect any of these advantages." He was equal to the situation, too: "Nature," says the same writer, "had been uncommonly bountiful in his form and aspect; his manners were extremely elegant; his pronunciation was fine; he belonged to a family proverbial for good temper; his father, during his long life of ninety years, had scarcely ever been out of humor, and he had a strong resemblance to his father. In his intercourse with men he was perfectly at his ease with the most stately—he could converse with the most ignorant so as to make them easy, but without affecting ignorance himself; he could mix with the lowest orders of society without imposing a painful restraint on them, while he preserved the manners of a well-bred gentleman. He was also particularly agreeable to young people. At this period he was known to almost every citizen of Philadelphia, and yet it is probable that there was no one who did not wish him well. This portrait is strongly colored, but there are yet (b) many amongst us who remember the original, and to them appeal for its truth."

Dr. Shippen undoubtedly believed that Philadelphia was ready to at least look forward to a fully equipped medical school, but there is no evidence that he had any fully developed plans of his own for it other than the establishment of a private school of Anatomy and Midwifery. This it was his mission to create, and, as a pioneer, to familiarize the public with the subject of medical teaching. In the only expression (c) he has left on the subject, there is the statement that in his introductory lecture he suggested the expediency of provision for medical teaching, but that he was waiting for another fellow-student's return to carry it into effect. It is by no means definite, and rather suggests that he fully appreciated the organizing powers of his friend, who was in Europe at the time he

---

(b) Wistar's Eulogium, 1809.
(c) Letter to the trustees of the College of Philadelphia.

was finishing preparations for his course of lectures in the autumn of 1762, which were an important preliminary to more systematized instruction. Early in November he announced (d) the course as follows: "Please inform the public that a course of anatomical lectures will be opened this winter in Philadelphia for the advantage of young Gentlemen now engaged in the study of Physic, in this and the neighboring Provinces, whose circumstances and connections will not admit of their going abroad for Improvement to the Anatomical Schools in Europe, and also for the entertainment of any Gentlemen who may have the curiosity to understand the Anatomy of the Human Frame. In these Lectures the situation, Figure and Structure of all the parts of the human body will be demonstrated and their respective Uses explained, and, as far as a Course of Anatomy will permit, their Diseases, with the Indications and method of Cure briefly treated of; all the necessary operations in Surgery will be performed, a Course of Bandages exhibited, and the whole conclude with an explanation of some of the curious Phenomena that arise from an examination of the Gravid Uterus, and a few plain general Directions in the Study and Practice of Midwifery. The Necessity and Public Utility of such a course in this growing Country, and the Method to be pursued therein, will be more particularly explained in an Introductory Lecture to be delivered the 16th Instant, at six o'clock in the Evening, at the State House by William Shippen, Jun. M. D. N. B.—The Managers and Physicians of the Pennsylvania Hospital, at a special meeting, have generously consented to countenance and encourage this Undertaking; and to make it more entertaining and profitable have granted him the use of some curious Anatomical Casts and Drawings (just arrived on the *Carolina*, Capt. Friend), presented by the judicious and benevolent Doctor Fothergill, who has improved every Opportunity of promoting the Interest and Usefulness

---

(d) The Pennsylvania Gazette of November 11, 1762. The building for his lectures was erected for the purpose in the rear of his father's residence, which was on Fourth street, north of Market. An alley-way led to it from Market street. This he used until Anatomical Hall was erected many years later on Fifth street, north of Walnut.

of that noble and flourishing Institution." The introductory lecture was well received and attended, but no record of it seems to have been preserved. Two weeks later it is announcd (e) that "Dr. Shippen's Anatomical Lectures will begin to-morrow evening at six o'clock, at his father's house in Fourth Street. Tickets for the course to be had of the Doctor, at five Pistoles each, and any gentlemen who incline to see the subject prepared for the lectures and learn the art of Dissecting, Injections, etc., are to pay five Pistoles more." Twelve students were in attendance, and thus was founded the first private school of anatomy in the province, the forerunner of the first medical college on the continent. This was not unattended with difficulties of various sorts, but they were subdued in the end. In December following the body of a negro, who had committed suicide, was turned over to Shippen for dissection, and those of all suicides and criminals thereafter for some time. Indeed, according to Watson, there was a most uncanny feeling abroad regarding the young medical school, so that not only was it necessary for Dr. Shippen to publicly announce that his subjects were entirely suicides, criminals and a few specially diseased subjects from the Potter's Field, but a mob of sailors was with difficulty restrained from demolishing his house and did succeed in breaking the windows. His innovations in midwifery, too, had to make their way slowly against public feeling adverse to men entering that field and against the opposition of the midwives, but his skill and persistence finally won, so that he gave lectures to both men and women and established a lying-in hospital in 1762 (f). In the field of obstet-

---

(e) The Pennsylvania Gazette, 25th of November, 1762.

(f) George W. Norris. As the first announcement of the first lectures of this kind on the continent, the following is of interest. This was in March, 1762:

"*Doctor Shippen, Junior*, proposes to begin his first course on midwifery as soon as a number of pupils sufficient to defray the necessary expense shall apply. A course will consist of about twenty lectures, in which he will treat of that part of anatomy which is necessary to understand that branch, explain all cases in midwifery—natural, difficult and preternatural—and give directions how to treat them with safety to the mother and child; describe the diseases incident to women and children in the month, and direct to proper remedies; will take occasion during the course to explain and apply those curious anatomical plates and casts of the gravid uterus at the Hospital, and conclude the whole with necessary cautions against the dangerous and cruel use of instruments. In order to make the course

rics Dr. Shippen must be accorded the honor of being the most powerful pioneer in America. The course of 1762-3 was so successful that in the spring he offered his services to the managers of the hospital, and on May 17 they announced that on the 21st instant Dr. Shippen would give lectures once a fortnight at the hospital also, and that students would be expected to pay "a proper gratuity" for the benefit of that institution. His regular course was repeated in the winter of 1763-4 and that of 1764-5, when the time had come for new developments, the first signs of which began to appear in May of the latter year.

The appearance together in so small a medical field as Philadelphia then was, of two such royal, highly organized natures as Drs. Morgan and Shippen, both conscious of the magnitude of the events they were enacting, and both fired by an ambition so splendid and intense that it was destined to mar their closing years with pathetic disappointment, was an event almost certain to be attended by abrasions in their relations, although they were intimate friends at times and fellows in most of the events of their lives. This last infirmity of noble minds profoundly influences both their lives and yet binds them, forever inseparable, in some of the most picturesque and pregnant events of American medical history. Both were cultured gentlemen of the highest type the age afforded; the one, Dr. Shippen, was calm, self-possessed, far-seeing, cautious, a pioneer of rare powers as a leader; the other, Dr. Morgan, fervent, impulsive, positive, and with the highest qualities of a statesmanlike organizer; of nearly the same age, the one was senior in practice by three years, the other senior in age by one year; engaged in the same events, the one was destined to precede at this time and

---

more perfect a convenient lodging is provided for the accommodation of a few poor women, who otherwise might suffer for want of the common necessaries on these occasions, to be under the care of a sober, honest matron, well acquainted with lying-in women, employed by the Doctor for that purpose. Each pupil to attend two courses at least, for which he is to pay five guineas. Perpetual pupils to pay ten guineas. The female pupils to be taught privately and assisted at any of their labors when necessary. The Doctor may be spoke with at his house, in Front Street, very morning between the hours of six and nine, or at his office in Letitia Court every evening."

the other at another. Thus in the story of events they are so independent, yet so united, that the life of the one cannot be understood without an acquaintance with that of his friend and rival. Thus, the pioneer of education became professor of Anatomy and Surgery (g) in the school the other had founded and in the first year of its organization, and so continued until his resignation, forty-one years later, at the age of seventy years. Ten years later, in 1776, with a record of having taught nearly three hundred and forty students, he enters the army as medical director of "the flying camp," while Morgan was Director-General of the Medical Department, and a year later Shippen succeeded him and remained at the head of the Department until his resignation in 1781. In practice Dr. Shippen was probably the ablest accoucheur in the colonies, and as a teacher of anatomy had no superior. Disappointment prematurely closed the career of Dr. Morgan in 1789, and scarcely a decade later, 1798, to Dr. Shippen came a sorrow that, says Dr. Wistar, "cut the sinews of his exertions and left him gradually to wither—the amiable victim of paternal affection." "His son," he says further, "had every advantage in education that good sense and knowledge of human nature, that respectable connections, and, finally, that money could procure for him; and, such were his talents and application that his proficiency was equal to his opportunities. He had often been caressed by Washington—he went abroad and visited France under the auspices of Jefferson—whilst in England he enjoyed the countenance of the late President Adams, and was on intimate terms with Lord Shelburne. His letters from those countries were so replete with information and good sense that they gave great pleasure to many persons to whom his delighted father used to read them. After four years of absence he returned and proved to be exactly what his father wished. He was not only a man of talents and information, but of great virtue and strong filial affection. Shippen would have loved him as a friend had there been no other connection between them. The regard excited by these qualities, added to the strong, natural

---

(g) Midwifery was added later.

affection of Shippen, produced an attachment to his son which has seldom been equaled. He seemed, like James Boswell, in the case of Samuel Johnson, to lose sight of himself, and forget that he also had a part to act, so fully was his attention absorbed by this endeared object. His strongest wish was, to pass the remainder of his life as his son's guest. He therefore gave him the fairest portion of his estate; and, to obtain leisure and exemption from care, procured the establishment of an adjunct professorship of Anatomy. But, alas! instead of realizing these fond hopes, Shippen had to endure a disappointment, the most painful which suffering humanity can experience. In 1792 his son began to complain of ill-health; the father devoted to him almost all his time, and consulted, occasionally, all his medical friends; but in vain. After a great variety of efforts for his relief, and much suffering on his part, he died in 1798. And the object, upon which Shippen founded hopes of comfort for the remainder of his life, and which he had contemplated with increasing tenderness for thirty years, was, forever,—done away. This overwhelming stroke did not prostrate him, for he appeared able to endure it; but it did him a greater injury, by destroying the interest he felt in every remaining object." But when ten years later his own death occurred on July 11, 1808, nothing stood out so prominently in his long career as his pioneer work in preparing Philadelphia for her career at the head of the medical education in the republic, and posterity will ever regard as the most important period of his life the three years preceding 1765, during which he presided over the young school of anatomy.

It was during the winter course of 1764-5 that Dr. Morgan, in London, wrote (h) to his friend, the celebrated Dr. William Cullen, of Edinburgh, in cordial intimacy: "I am now preparing for America, to see whether, after fourteen years' devotion to medicine I can get my living without turning apothecary or practicing surgery (i). My scheme for instituting lectures you will hereafter

---

(h) Dated "London, November 10, 1764."
(i) This is ten years before Dr. Jones' expression on this subject, quoted at the beginning of this chapter. Dr. Morgan introduced limitations of a specialist character.

know more of. It is not prudent to broach designs prematurely, and mine are not yet fully ripe for execution." This independent tone assumed on the eve of his departure, but ill accords with Dr. Fothergill's description of Morgan as Shippen's "assistant." Dr. Morgan was born in 1735, and was a year older than his fellow-student; if he did not begin practice sooner it was only because he spent far longer time in preparation. "It is now more than fifteen years," said he, in his announcement of methods of practice, "since I began the study of medicine in this city, which I have prosecuted ever since without interruption. During the first years I served an apprenticeship with Dr. Redman, who then did, and still continues to enjoy a most justly acquired reputation in this city for superior knowledge and extensive practice in physic. At the same time I had an opportunity of being acquainted with the practice of other eminent physicians in this place, particularly of all the physicians to the hospital, whose prescriptions I put up there for above the space of one year. The term of my apprenticeship being expired, I devoted myself for four years to a military life, principally with a view to become more skillful in my profession, being engaged the whole of that time in a very extensive practice in the army amongst diseases of every kind. The last five years I have spent in Europe, under the most celebrated masters in every branch of medicine, and spared no labor or expense to store my mind with an extensive acquaintance in every science that related in any way to the duty of a physician, having in that time expended in this pursuit a sum of money of which the very interest would prove no contemptible income. With what success this has been done, others are to judge, and not myself." Others had already judged, and this man of thirty years, rarely prepared to found the first medical college in America and rare exemplar for its students, was already a Fellow of the Royal Society of London, Correspondent of the Royal Academy of Surgery at Paris, Member of the Arcadian Belles Lettres Society of Rome, Licentiate of the Royal Colleges of Physicians in both London and Edinburgh, as well as Professor of the Theory of

Practice of Medicine in the newly-organized medical department of the College of Philadelphia, afterward the great University, the first professorship in the medical history of America.

It is interesting to observe that Dr. Morgan was of Welsh blood, born in Philadelphia, son of Evan Morgan, an old resident of the province in whose founding his countrymen had been so prominent. Like Dr. Shippen, he also had taken his preparatory studies at the Rev. Samuel Finley's academy at Nottingham, in Chester County, but instead of going to the college of New Jersey, returned to his native place and entered that other new institution of learning, the College of Philadelphia, founded in 1749 as an academy, and graduated in its first class, with the bachelor's degree, on May 17, 1757, at the age of twenty-two. He had begun his medical studies very early, under the youngest of the first group of native American physicians in Philadelphia, Dr. John Redman, whose long life of eighty-two years caused him to survive all his early contemporaries and most of his later, to become the Nestor of a third generation. During his six years' apprenticeship he served thirteen months as the second occupant of the office of apothecary to the hospital, resigning the 1st of May, 1756. Undoubtedly he carried on his medical and literary studies at the same time, and must have been connected in some manner with the hospital service of the French war even at this date. So little exact record is left of his early years that, considering his unusual ability, it seems reasonable to infer that he had been carried so far by the Rev. Mr. Finley, who was a college in himself, as to be admitted as an advanced student in college, and even that he did much non-resident work for his degree, received in 1757. At any rate, since he served four years in the French war, he must have enlisted in some part of its hospital service in 1756, and is known to have been on the Forbes' expedition (k), holding a lieutenant's commission, dated April 1, 1758, though acting chiefly as surgeon, in which capacity his superior officer chose to mention that he "did his duty very well." This is one of the earliest records of a Phila-

---

(k) Dr. Ruschenburger's History of the College of Physicians. Transactions of 1887.

delphia physician in military hospital service, this being in the last war waged by Britain and this province against a common enemy. On retiring from military service he began preparations for going abroad in 1760. He first went to London, where he studied under Hewson and the two Hunters, and became an adept in the art of making anatomical preparations by corrosion, which he was later to introduce on the continent of Europe. The following year he prepared for Edinburgh, bearing to Dr. William Cullen a letter from Franlin (l), who was then in London, stating that "the bearer, Mr. Morgan, who proposes to reside some time in Edinburgh for the completion of his studies in Physic, is a young gentleman of Philadelphia whom I have long known and greatly esteem; and as I interest myself in what relates to him, I cannot but wish him the advantages of your conversation and instruction." A biographer of Dr. Cullen (m), quoting this letter, says: "Mr. Morgan, who is mentioned in the foregoing letter, appears to have fully realized the expectations of his friend Dr. Franklin. He distinguished himself while in Edinburgh by a diligent application to his studies; published, on receiving the degree of Doctor of Medicine, an excellent inaugural dissertation on the subject of Suppuration (n); visited the principal hospitals of France and Italy before returning to his native country. After his return to America he took an active share in the institution of lectures on different branches of medicine in the College of Philadelphia, and in the establishment of a dispensary and of a medical society in that city. The progress of these institutions is minutely described in his letter to Dr. Cullen, toward whom he always appears to have felt and expressed a very grateful attachment." It was at Edinburgh that he gained his ideas of the constitution of a medical college and thus stamped

---

(l) Dated October 21, 1761.
(m) Dr. John Thompson, 1832.
(n) A copy of his thesis, dated July 18, 1763, may be seen in the Library at the University of Pennsylvania (and in that of the College of Physicians), "De Puopoiesi," etc. Dr. James Curry, of Guy's Hospital, in 1817, says that in this thesis Dr. Morgan anticipated Dr. Hunter in the theory that pus is a secretion from the vessels. His diploma hangs in the library of the College of Physicians.

upon the whole medical educational system of America the essential features of that school.

On the 29th of June, 1763, a friend writes from London: "Morgan is still in Edinburgh and will leave Edinburgh in about a fortnight," and again on September 1st: "Morgan has graduated at Edinburgh with an eclat almost unknown before. The Professors give him the highest character you can imagine (o)." It would seem from this that sometime late in 1763 he went to Paris, where, under the direction of M. Sue, he made farther studies in anatomy. While there he prepared the vessels of a kidney according to his system of corrosion, so finely, that, on account of his presentation of it before the Royal Academy of Surgery, he was afterward made a corresponding member of that body on July 5, 1764. But one member had seen the method before and Dr. Morgan claimed the honor of having introduced it in both Paris and Southern France. In the latter region and in Switzerland and Italy, he traveled during the spring and summer of 1764, visiting medical schools, hospitals and other public institutions, most interesting details of which have been preserved in his journal, and from which is taken the following account of his visit to the famous Paduan, Morgagni. He had left Rome on July 6, and the description is dated at Padua, July 24, 1764, and reads:

"I went to pay my respects to the celebrated Morgagni, Professor of Anatomy at Padua, to whom I had letters from Dr. Sevati, of Bologna. He received me with the greatest politeness imaginable, and showed me abundant civilities, with a very good grace. He is now eighty-two years of age, yet reads without spectacles, and is alert as a man of fifty. I found that he was unacquainted with anatomical preparations made by corrosion. I showed him a piece of kidney which I had injected at Paris, and which was finely corroded. Broken as it was, he was highly pleased, and saw at once the utility of such preparations. I apologized for the state it was in, from having brought it so far. He was pleased to answer, *ex ungue leonem*—that he saw enough from that small specimen

---

(o) Powel-Roberts' Corespondence, 1761-65, in the Pennsylvania Magazine.

to convince him of the excellency of such preparations. He acknowledged that he had never seen any preparations before in which the vessels were so minutely filled. Ruysch, he says, had sent him some of his preparations, in which the vessels appeared more like a confused mass than distinct, in the manner of this. I asked him what method he took to trace the vessels. He told me, he did (p) always in subjects where the inflammation was great, which made the vessels appear distinct and plain, but these were not durable as preparations made by injection. He then conveyed me into a small cabinet, where he showed me a great number of skeletons of the human fœtus, in a series, from a few weeks old, to nine months, and from that upward to an adult. Among others, a fœtus of six or seven months old, in which the form was complete, except near half of the spine— i. e., the back of it was wanting all the way up; nor had it ever either brain or spinal marrow. He showed me also a calculus, formed on a needle, in the bladder of a man, which had stopped up the urethra without forming any ulceration, or the least sign of a cicatrix of a wound. This, and the following which he showed me, are spoken of in his treatise, *De Sedibus et Causis Morborum*, viz., the second was a calculus formed on the point of a corking pin, which a female had introduced a little way into her bladder, which, being irritated thereby, contracted, and drew the pin into the bladder, so as to lay the foundation of a calculus, of which she died.

"He showed me, likewise, many curious preparations of the bones of the ear, and pointed out the spur-like process of the malleus which his master in anatomy, Valsalva, could never find till he showed it to him; also the three semi-circular canals, separate from all the other bones, with the five holes opening so as to be seen at the same time; also all the organs of hearing, with the external ear, the hard and soft parts together, freed from all

---

(p) This sentence is faulty, either in the original, or else by error of the copyist. The manuscript in the Historical Society is a copy, the original being in the possession of the family.

the surrounding hard bone; and, lastly, the internal cavity of the ear, with all the parts *in situ*, which he had so prepared as to see the different bones in their place without touching them at all. This he had done partly with a file and partly with a hard tempered knife, like adamant, and—a great deal of patience. He had sawed the cranium in two, as usually done in dissecting the brain, but acknowledged that if he had taken the temporal bone out, he could work much easier, as the surrounding bones would not have impeded the motion of his hand in dissecting.

"In this cabinet he had a series of portraits of old anatomists, his famous predecessors at Bologna, in which he pointed out a particularity with regard to dress; the necks of the first being covered with a kind of caul, like a modern monk's hook; this gradually lessened, and a fur lining took the place, but the neck less covered up, till at length they came to wear bands, which at first were small, and gradually enlarged to the greatest size. In this cabinet were the portraits—i. e., the heads—of two beautiful girls, done by Rosalba, in crayons. I asked, Who were these, and he told me as follows: 'That he had fifteen children, of whom remain two sons and eight daughters; every one, as they grew up, requested to become nuns, which he esteemed very singular, and that they entered by pairs into four different convents. When their time of probation expired, they were, at their own choice, to live in the world or take the veil, which last they all preferred; the two youngest going into the strictest order of Franciscans, where they go barefooted and always veiled. Before these were shut up thus for life, the celebrated female paintress, Rosalba, as a friend of Morgagni, drew these portraits and made him a present of them, before he knew she had any intention to draw them. As the others are of orders less strict, and may be seen without veils, there was less occasion for their portraits.'

"I presented him, before coming away, with my thesis, and he was so good as to do me the honor of making me a present of his late publication, 2 vols. folio, '*De Sedibus et Causis Mor-*

borum,' (q), of which there have been three different editions within these three years, being in the highest estimation throughout Europe, and all the copies of the first edition already bought up."

His Padua visit over, he went to Switzerland, and while at Geneva presented letters to Voltaire in his home at Ferney, on Sunday, the 16th of September, and made as great an impression on the great Frenchman as elsewhere, the account of which in his journal is as vivid as that written at Padua. Passing on to London, he writes a chatty outline of his continental visit, to Dr. Cullen, full of suggestive references; it is dated November 10, 1764, at London:

"Can you forgive me if, upon my being just returned from my tour through France and Italy, I write you but a very short letter till I have been here a week or two longer, and got myself a little composed. At present what with a crowd of acquaintances every day, and with the kindest intentions, breaking in upon that time I proposed to devote to writing to my friends, and the chaos of ideas which disturb my regular thinking at present, I find I cannot execute the task as I ought. Everything I tell you now must be rather broken hints, than a connected relation. I have not been able to see M. Senac while last in Paris. I was at Fontainebleau once with that view, but he was then for a night or two with the King at Choisy, which I knew not of at the time; and I was too much hurried to repeat the visit, as I wanted to reach London in time enough to sail in the fall for Philadelphia; I think I cannot now sail till toward spring. The most agreeable incidents happened to Mr. Powel and myself in our tour, which lasted about eight months. It was crowded with a great variety of the most interesting circumstances, full

---

(q) These, by his will, have been in the library of the College of Physicians since February, 1790, and at the foot of the first and second title pages respectively, in fading Latin phrases are: "Gift of the author to the most skillful and accomplished Dr. John Morgan," and "Gift of the author to Dr. John Morgan, highly deserving in anatomy," "Viro experientissimo et humanissimo D. Di Joanni Morgan Auctor" and "Viro de Re anatomico bene merito Do. Joanni Morgan Auctor."

of pleasing scenes for the most part, and of a nature different from and more agreeable than what I have been commonly used to. The order of our travels through Italy was Genoa, Leghorn, Pisa, Florence, Rome, Naples and its environs. After our return to Rome, it was on the Adriatic side of Italy, through Loreto, Bologna, Ferrara, Padua, Venice; we took Padua in the way again on our return, and passed through Vicenza, Verona, Mantua, the states of Parma and Placentia, to Milan and Turin. We crossed the Alps to Geneva, returned to Paris through Lyons, and from thence came to London about a week ago. We were in the suite of the Duke of York at Leghorn, Florence and Rome, where we were particularly presented to him, and had access to all the grand entertainments made for His Royal Highness, which were indeed superb, sumptuous and magnificent.

"We had a private audience with the Pope, four English gentlemen of us being presented at that time. He was affable and courteous. At Turin we had the honor of being presented to his Sardinian Majesty and the royal family, and obtained express leave of the King to see the fortifications of Turin, and those which defend the pass into his dominions by the Alps. When at Geneva we paid a visit to Voltaire, to whom we had a letter, and were entertained by him with most singular politeness—for us, I mean—perhaps usual enough in regard to Voltaire. . . . . There is a pretty good physical—I mean medical—university at Bologna, and Morgagni has a very crowded class at his anatomical lectures at Padua. There are some other schools of medicine in Italy; but, upon the whole, to me they seem behindhand— medicine not being in high repute, or cultivated with that spirit it ought to be. As to the grandeur of the ancients, from what we can see of their remains, it is most extraordinary. Arts with them seem to have been in a perfection which I could not have imagined. Their palaces, temples, aqueducts, baths, theaters, amphitheaters, monuments, statues, sculptures, were most amazing. The soul is struck at the review, and the ideas expand; but I have not leisure to dwell on these topics. I must return to the world where I now am just going—this as different from the former, the rest of Europe I have seen, as that from Italy, and really to me it does not appear more so. At Paris I took my seat in the Royal Academy of Surgery, of which I have the honor to be admitted as a corresponding member (July 5, 1764)—a distinction from a resident fellow. I am now preparing for America, to see whether, after fourteen years' devotion to medicine, I can get my living without turning apothecary or practicing surgery. My scheme of instituting lectures you will hereafter know more of. It is not prudent to broach designs prematurely; and mine are not yet fully ripe for execution. My best compliments to all your family, not forgetting them particularly to my Mamma Cullen, and to your eldest son. Believe me to be, with the greatest esteem, dear sir, your affectionate friend, and much obliged humble servant, JOHN MORGAN."

That winter in London was full of activity in maturing his plans for a new medical school. He was so confident of its outcome that he had already prepared his inaugural in Paris. He sought the aid of two former members of the board of trustees of his alma mater, Mr. Hamilton and Mr. Richard Peters, then residing in England; he conferred with and secured the approval of Drs. Fothergill, Hunter, Watson and Cullen; on February 15, 1765, not long before his departure, he secured the following letter for presentation to the board from Thomas Penn, one of its chief patrons:

"Gentlemen: Dr. Morgan has laid before me a proposal for introducing new professorships into the Academy for the instruction of all such as shall incline to go into the study and practice of Physic and Surgery, as well as the several occupations attending upon these useful and necessary arts. He thinks his scheme, if patronized by the trustees, will at present give reputation and strength to the Institution, and, though it may for some time occasion a small expense, yet after a little while it will gradually support itself, and even make considerable additions to the Academy's funds. Dr. Morgan has employed his time in an assiduous search after knowledge in all the branches necessary for the practice of his profession, and has gained such an esteem and love from persons of the first rank in it, that, as they very much approve his system, they will from time to time, as he assures us, give him their countenance and assistance in the execution of it. We are made acquainted with what is proposed to be taught, and how the lectures may be adapted by you, and since the like systems have brought much advantage to every place where they have been received, and such learned and eminent men speak favorably of the doctor's plan, I could not but in the most kind manner recommend Dr. Morgan to you, and desire that he may be well received, and what he has to offer be taken with all becoming respect and expedition into your most serious consideration, and if it shall be thought necessary to go into it, and thereupon to open Professorships, that he may be taken into your service. When you have heard him and duly considered what he has to lay before you, you will be best able to judge in what manner you can serve the public, the Institution, and the particular design now recommended to you."

Not long after securing this letter Dr. Morgan sailed for Philadelphia, and on his arrival pushed his plans with all vigor from the first. The board of trustees consisted of twenty-four members, of whom were five of the six members of the hospital staff, namely, Drs. Thomas and Phineas Bond, Cadwalader, the elder Shippen, and Redman; so intimately were the hospital and college connected already. His presentation was successful, and on May 3, 1765, says the minutes of the board, "entertaining a high sense of Dr. Morgan's abilities and the high honors paid to him by different learned bodies and societies in Europe, they unanimously elected him Professor of the Theory and Practice of Physic," and one of the institution's first graduates was inducted into the first medical professorship and the first established medical school on the western continent. Looking at it through the eyes of to-day it seems almost too insignificant to deserve the present resonant title of medical department of a university, but it need hardly be suggested that there is scarcely a great medical school or university in existence that did not begin in days of small things. It must be remembered, too, that both the city and country were comparatively of no larger dimensions, the former containing about twenty-five thousand inhabitants, and the latter less than three millions. Its greatness lies in its being an institution, and Dr. Morgan had precisely this idea of it. "What led me to it," said he, in his inaugural, "was the obvious utility that would attend it, and the desire I had of presenting, as a tribute of gratitude to my alma mater, a full and enlarged plan for the Institution of Medicine, in all its branches, in this seminary, where I had part of my education, being amongst the first sons who shared in its public honors. I was further induced to it from a consideration, that private schemes of propagating knowledge are unstable in their nature, and that the cultivation of useful learning can only be effectually promoted under those who are patrons of science, and under the authority and direction of men incorporated for the improvement of literature" (r).

All his plans of practice were subordinated to this institutional work. He proposed to limit it to a form of specialization, using specializing features of other occupations to illustrate whenever he spoke of it. He proposed to have time for investigation and preparation of lectures, and in consequence, said he, "my usefulness as a professor makes it absolutely necessary for me to follow that method of practice which alone appears to be calculated to answer that end."

He adopted a most advanced standard from the first, and almost immediately assumed a large and lucrative practice. In

---

(r) An interesting reference to his election, less than three weeks later, is found in the Powel-Roberts letters, previously quoted; it is dated at Philadelphia, May 21, and says: "Morgan comes home flushed with honors, and is treated by his friends with all due respect to his merit. He appears to be the same social, friendly man, not assuming the solemn badge so accustomed to sons of Esculapius. * * * * He has commenced Professor of the Theory and Practice of Medicine in the College, and intends publicly to open his scheme at next commencement. I hope the Doctor may meet with success in his undertaking, tho' I fear the mode of giving fees on attendance to the sick will be too refined for this paper-monied country."

the first place, he should be wholly a physician, and do neither the work of an apothecary nor surgeon, and that, too, on the principle that there should be professional surgeons (s) and apothecaries of the same high character as he proposed there should be in medicine. Indeed, he provided for this by bringing with him Mr. David Leighton, "educated in Great Britain both in pharmacy and surgery," and it is in no small measure due to Dr. Morgan that this city so early took so advanced a position in pharmacy. This method required a readjustment of fees, also, and on his first arrival he made it known that on his first visit he desired a retaining fee from the rich, though not from the poor, the rate being a pistole for the first visit, and a dollar for succeeding visits. This after a time was so misconstrued in some quarters that he chose to publish a full explanation of his whole system of practice, and while some of his standards were not generally adopted by the profession, he held to most of them himself and undoubtedly had a large influence on future city practice.

Commencement at the College occurred the same month, occupying two days, May 30 and 31, on both of which he delivered his inaugural, entitled "A Discourse Upon the Institution of Medical Schools in America." In this he gave a masterly outline of the various departments of medical study as then existing, the state of it in America, arguments for the institution of medical schools and the favorable conditions for study afforded by Philadelphia and the profession in that city, the steps already taken in that direction, the further steps necessary, answered objections as to the infant state of the colonies, and the mixed practice of the different departments of medicine, recommended the regular mode of practice, and finally gave a strong presentation of the advantages this institution would afford to students, the college, the city and the colonies, with an appeal to students and trustees in favor

---

(s) "Surgery calls for different powers and qualifications rarely united in one man. Are these all then to be blended with the apothecary, the botanist and chymist, which ought to be and are each of them separate and distinct in their very nature?" he writes in the account of his method of practice, published in connection with his inaugural as "An Apology."

of the project. "Never yet," said he, "has there offered a coalition of able men, who would undertake to give complete and regular courses of lectures on the different branches of medicine; and such an extensive field it is, as requires the united efforts of several co-operating together, to cultivate with success. As well might a parent take upon himself the private tuition of his son, and to make him master of all the different languages, arts, and sciences, which are generally deemed requisite, previous to his entering upon the higher studies of Law, Physic and Divinity; as that a physician, engaged in an extensive practice, should undertake to deliver to his apprentices, in a regular manner, the precepts of his art in all its branches. This is as impracticable as it is unreasonable to expect." He instances Edinburgh and how in but little more than forty years there had gathered there such great names as "Drummond, Dick, Clerk, Rutherford, Sinclair, Alston, Plummer, Monro, Whytt, Cullen, Hope, Black, and some others . . . . . now known wherever the knowledge of Physic is cultivated." He said if men were not ready for these positions, they would arise; one, besides himself, was already there. "It is with the highest satisfaction," said he, "I am informed from Dr. Shippen, junior, that in an address to the public as introductory to his first anatomical course, he proposed some hints of a plan for giving medical lectures among us. But I do not learn that he recommended at all a collegiate undertaking of this kind." He suggests when a chair of Anatomy is founded, that Dr. Shippen be chosen, and announces his own courses for the coming autumn. In one of his closing paragraphs he happily and truly describes the future:

"Perhaps this medical institution, the first of its kind in America, though small in its beginning, may receive constant increase of strength, and annually exert new vigor. It may collect a number of young persons, of more than ordinary abilities; and so improve their knowledge as to spread its reputation to distant parts. By sending these abroad duly qualified, or by exciting an emulation amongst men of parts and literature, it may give birth to other useful institutions of a similar nature, or occasional rise, by its example, to numerous societies of different kinds, calculated to spread the light of knowledge through the whole American continent wherever inhabited" (t).

In the autumn following, on the 23rd of September, the board met and as "Dr. William Shippen, Jr., applied by letter," to use the words of the minutes, dated on the 17th, he was unanimously elected Professor of Anatomy and Surgery. The letter reads:

"The institution of Medical Schools in this country has been a favorite object of my attention for seven years past, and it is three years since I proposed the expediency and practicability of teaching medicine in all its branches in this city in a public oration read at the State House, introductory to my first course of Anatomy. I should long since have sought the patronage of the Trustees of the College, but waited to be joined by Dr. Morgan, to whom I first communicated my plan in England, and who promised to unite with me in every scheme we might think necessary for the execution of so important a point. I am pleased, however, to hear that you, gentlemen, on being applied to by Dr. Morgan, have appointed that gentleman Professor of Medicine. A Professorship of Anatomy and Surgery will be accepted by, gentlemen, your most obedient and very humble servant,

"WILLIAM SHIPPEN, Junior."

Three days later, the 26th, announcements of the opening of the departments, signed by both, and of courses, signed by each respectively, appeared in the *Gazette*, the former being as follows:

"As the necessity of cultivating medical knowledge in America is allowed by all, it is with pleasure we inform the public that a Course of Lectures on two of the most important branches of that useful science, viz., Anatomy and Materia Medica, will be delivered this winter in Philadelphia. We have great reason, therefore,

---

(t) Bradford published the discourse, together with the prefatory "Apology," during the year, some of the original copies of which may be seen at the College of Physicians. The Pennsylvania Gazette said: "The perspicuity with which it was written and spoke drew the close attention of the audience, particularly of the gentlemen of the Faculty of Physic," as the profession was called.

to hope that gentlemen of the Faculty will encourage the design by recommending it to their pupils, that pupils themselves will be glad of such an opportunity of improvement, and that the public will think it an object worthy of their attention and patronage. In order to render these courses the more extensively useful, we intend to introduce into them as much of the Theory and Practice of Physic, of Pharmacy, Chemistry and Surgery as can be conveniently admitted. From all this, together with an attendance on the practice of the physicians and surgeons of the Pennsylvania Hospital, the students will be able to prosecute their studies with such advantage as will qualify them to practice hereafter with more satisfaction to themselves and benefit to the community. The particular advertisements inserted below specify the time when these lectures are to commence, and contain the various subjects to be treated of in each course, and the terms on which pupils are to be admitted.

"WILLIAM SHIPPEN, JR., M. D.,
"Professor of Anatomy and Surgery in the College of Philadelphia.
"JOHN MORGAN, M. D., F. R. S., etc.,
"Professor of Medicine in the College of Philadelphia."

The course announcements say that Dr. Shippen begins on November 14th. He seems to have used his own anatomical rooms, while Dr. Morgan's lectures were to begin on the 18th at the College, and were the first course on the practice of medicine given in the colonies. The former embrace sixty lectures and the latter three lectures a week, Mondays, Wednesdays and Fridays, at three o'clock, for "between three or four months." In the first, "the situation, figure and structure of all the parts of the Human Body will be demonstrated on the fresh subject; their respective uses explained, and their Diseases, with the Indications and Methods of Cure, briefly treated of; all the necessary Operations in Surgery will be performed, a course of Bandages given, and the whole will conclude with a few plain and general directions in the Practice of Midwifery." The second were to be on Materia Medica, and "to render these lectures as instructive as possible to students of

Physic, the Doctor proposes, in the course of them, to give some useful Observations on Medicine in general, and the proper manner of conducting the study of Physic. The authors to be read in the Materia Medica will be pointed out. The various substances made use of in Medicine will be reduced under Classes suited to the principal Indications in the cure of Diseases. Similar virtues in different plants, and their comparative powers, will be treated of, and an Enquiry made into the different Methods which have been used in discovering the Qualities of Medicines; the virtues of the most efficacious will be particularly insisted upon; the Manner of preparing and combining them will be shown by some instructive Lessons upon Pharmaceutic Chemistry: This will open to students a general Idea both of Chemistry and Pharmacy. To prepare them more effectually for understanding the art of prescribing with Elegance and Propriety, if time allows, it is proposed to include in this course some critical Lectures upon the chief Preparatives contained in the Dispensatories of the Royal College of Physicians at London and Edinburgh. The whole will be illustrated with many useful Practical Observations on Diseases, Diet and Medicines."

The young school passed its first year with success, and one of its professors, Dr. Morgan, at the commencement, on May 20, 1766, was honored with the Sargent gold medal of London for an essay on the advantages of a perpetual union of Great Britain and her American colonies. The following year Dr. Bond's clinical lectures, already referred to, were added, and his interest in the school and his ability combined led him to continue them for eighteen years, closing only with his death. During the summer (u) of 1767 a more formal organization (v) with provision for degrees for the class that would graduate the next May (1768) was made. This provided for two degrees, Bachelor and Doctor: For the former, "it is required (1) that such students as have not taken a Degree in any College shall, before admission to a degree in Physic, satisfy

---

(u) July 27th.
(v) This was made by the Provost, Dr. Smith, the medical members of the board and the two medical professors.

the Trustees and Professors of the College concerning their knowledge in the Latin tongue, and in such branches of Mathematics, Natural and Experimental Philosophy as shall be judged requisite to a medical education. (2) Each student shall attend at least one course of lectures in Anatomy, Materia Medica, Chemistry, the Theory and Practice of Physic, and one course of Clinical Lectures, and shall attend the Practice of Pennsylvania Hospital for one year, and may then be admitted to a Public examination for a Bachelor's Degree," preceded by private examination, and (3) satisfactory apprenticeship with a practitioner. The Doctor's degree could only be obtained three years after that of Bachelor and by a man twenty-four years of age, who should also prepare a thesis, somewhat after the manner of a Master's degree in liberal education, and it was proposed to make the degree equal to those of Europe. In the following winter, Provost William Smith delivered a course of lectures on Natural and Experimental Philosophy, beginning December 28th, and in January, 1768, a professorship in Materia Medica and Botany was created for a young man of twenty-seven years, a native of Germantown, near this city, who had just returned from Europe fresh from the teaching of the great Linnæus, and with the Edinburgh degree. This was Dr. Adam Kuhn, and in May, three months later, he gave his first course in Botany (w). On November 20th, preceding, Dr. Morgan had written to a friend (x), "I have twenty pupils this year at about five guineas

---

(w) Dr. Kuhn was born Nov. 17, 1741 (old style), son of a physician, Dr. A. S. Kuhn, under whom he studied. In 1761 he went to the University of Upsal, Sweden, until about July, 1764. After a year in London he went to Edinburgh, where he graduated on June 12, 1767, with the thesis *De Lavatione Frigida*. He also visited France, Holland and Germany, and returned to Philadelphia in January, 1768. He soon had a large practice and was one of several forming a society for inoculation of the poor for smallpox. He became a member of the hospital staff in 1775, and served twenty-two years, and was also one of the staff of the Philadelphia Dispensary. In the Revolution he had a long and valuable service as director-general of a hospital and otherwise. He served as both curator and councillor of the American Philosophical Society, and was a founder of the College of Physicians. He resigned his chair in the medical school in 1797. He died July 5, 1817, at the age of seventy-two. "In sound judgment," wrote Dr. Lettsom of London, "he greatly excelled. His talent for observation was profound. He was through life a studious reader."

(x) William Hewson of London.

each. Next year (1768) we shall confer the degree of Bachelor of Physic on several of them, and that of Doctor in three years after. New York (y) has copied us, and has six Professors, three of whom you know, to wit, Bard, Professor of Physic; Tennant, of Midwifery; and Smith, in Chemistry; besides whom are Dr. Jones, Professor of Surgery; Middleton, of Physiology; and Clossy, of Anatomy. Time will show in what lighte we are to consider the rivalship; for my part, I do not seem to be under great apprehensions." The candidates here referred to were examined from the 9th to the 16th, and publicly examined on the 18th of May, and on June 21, 1768, the first medical degrees awarded in America were those of Bachelors of Medicine conferred upon John Archer of New Castle County, Benjamin Cowell (z) of Bucks, Samuel Duffield and Jonathan Potts of Philadelphia, Jonathan Elmer of New Jersey, Humphrey Fullerton of Lancaster County, David Jackson of Chester County, John Lawrence of East Jersey, James Tilton of Kent County, Delaware, and Nicholas Way of Wilmington. The trustees grew enthusiastic and recorded in their minutes: "This day may be considered as the *Birth-day of Medical Honors in America.*" The ceremony occurred in the College building on Fourth street between Market and Arch, a building which had been erected over a quarter of a century before for the great evangelist, Whitefield.

Dr. Morgan continued to be the element of organizing power behind the young medical school, as well as the inspirer of various other advances, such as the establishment of the first medical society in 1765, of which little seems to have been recorded aside

---

(y) The medical department of King's College, then so-called, was organized in 1768, though preliminary measures were taken in July, 1767. They gave the first Bachelor's degree in 1769, and Doctor's in 1770, antedating Philadelphia in the latter, but not in the Bachelor's degree. It was not a real antedating, however, for the differences between Bachelor in Philadelphia and Doctor in New York was only one of name. Philadelphia's Doctorate was a Master's degree in medicine.

(z) Messrs. Cowell and Fullerton publicly debated whether or no the seat of vision was the Retina or Tunica Choroides; Messrs. Duffield and Way on "Questio num detur Fluidum Nervosum?"; an Essay "On Respiration" was delivered by Mr. Tilton; and Mr. Potts delivered "an elegant valedictory oration" "On the Advantages derived in the Study of Physic, from a previous liberal education in other sciences." Messrs. Potts and Tilton soon became prominent in the medical department of the army.

from the statement of its existence. He became the intimate friend of a brilliant young man, ten years his junior, who was just finishing the last of his six years' apprenticeship under Dr. Redman when Dr. Morgan was founding the new school, and seems to have practically decided upon him as the next addition to the faculty at this time, for he maintained an intimate correspondence with him during the three years the young man was in Edinburgh and finally secured his election. This was Dr. Benjamin Rush, who, from his entrance on his duties in the year 1769, was destined to be not only the greatest figure in the history of this school, but also possibly in the annals of American medicine itself. When funds were required for the College, Dr. Morgan was selected by the Provost, Dr. William Smith, to make a tour of the West Indies for the purpose of raising them, and about three thousand pounds were the proof of his success. These aggressive and able organizing powers made him the first object of attention of the authorities when a medical director of the newly raised Continental armies was needed, and, in opposition to the judgment of his friends and at a loss of a lucrative practice, he accepted appointment, on October 17, 1775, as Director-General and Physician-in-Chief of the American Hospital under Washington. This event was to him the beginning of woes unnumbered, which form a large part of the medical history of the Revolution itself. It is enough here to state that he satisfied his superior officer, General Washington, who himself was later on to be harassed by secret cabals, but nobly as he brought order out of chaos, in the effort to create an army medical department while the army itself was being created, his enemies were too strong and the shock of his undeserved dismissal by Congress on January 9, 1777, acknowledged by that body afterward, was so severe as to be the beginning of the end to him. He never recovered from it. Whether he was right or not, need not be argued, and there is abundant evidence that his dismissal was due to far more enemies than one; he attributed this injustice to his successor, Dr. Shippen, who seems not to have secured the cordial good will of either Morgan or Rush. On the reorganization of the Medical school at the

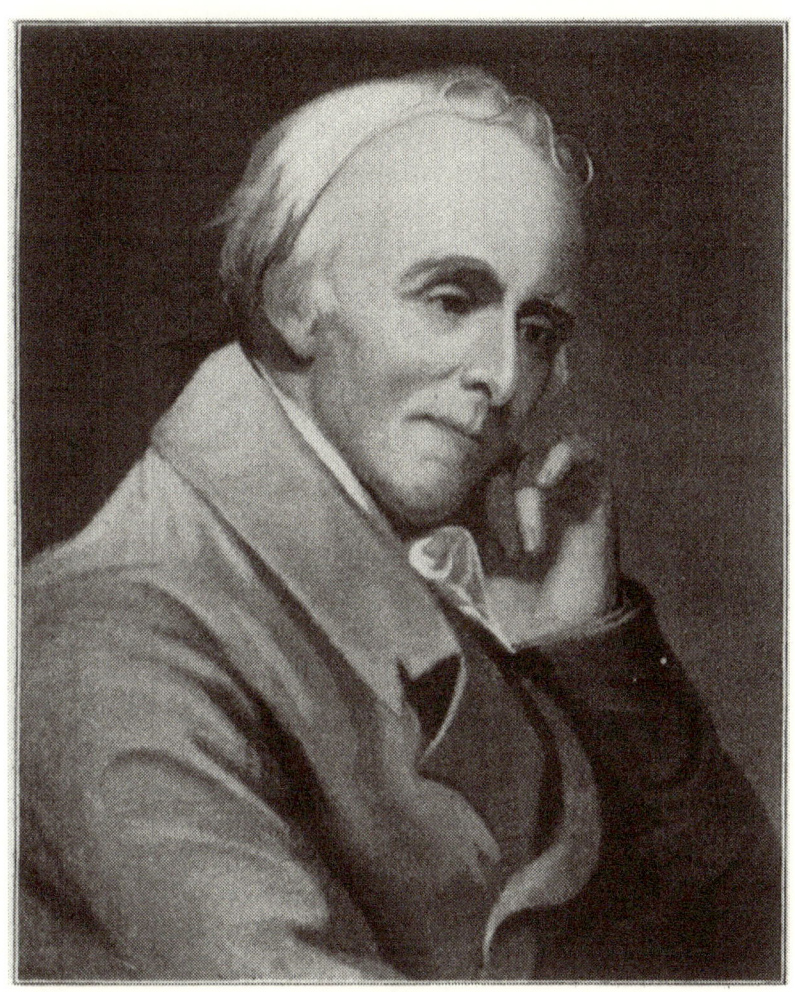

BENJAMIN RUSH.

close of the war, these two memorialized the Board on February 28, 1781, objecting to serve if Dr. Shippen were also to serve. The Board, however, strove for harmony and re-elected them all, though Dr. Morgan seems not to have performed the duties of the office (a). In 1785 his wife died, leaving no children, and, four years later, after Congress had endeavored to repair the wrong it had done, disappointment had finished its work and death occurred in October, 1789, at the early age of fifty-four years. He was buried on the 17th under the middle aisle of St. Peter's Church (b). His loss of interest in his professorship was gradual and it was held open to him until the last year of his life. He was one of the original founders of the College of Physicians, and one of its first board of censors, and had long been a leading member of the American Philosophical Society, before which, in the years immediately succeeding his return from Europe, he had read four papers, also serving as one of its curators. Dr. Morgan, however, seemed to be by nature an organizer, one whose powers were awakened to their highest operation only in the act of creation, and whatever else his life produced it is enough that he founded the first institution of medical education in America, and thus became the father of medical schools on this continent.

When, in 1775, Dr. Morgan was called to the head of the army medical department, the medical department of the college had been in existence ten years, and the faculty embraced five members, with an attendance of thirty or forty students. They were mentioned in the announcement as follows: Theory and Practice of Medicine, John Morgan, M. D.; Anatomy, Surgery and Midwifery, William Shippen, Jr., M. D.; Materia Medica and Botany, Adam Kuhn, M. D.; Chemistry, Benjamin Rush, M. D.; Clinical Medicine, Thomas Bond, M. D.; with lectures on Natural Philosophy by the

---

(a) Much of this, however, was due to the disorganized condition of the school itself in the reorganization of changing college to university.

(b) The picture of Dr. Morgan that is best known is from a painting, made by Angelica Kauffman in Rome in 1764, which is in the possession of relatives at the old family estate, Morganza, Pa. A good copy is owned by the College of Physicians.

Provost, Rev. Dr. William Smith. When this list was completed in 1769, says Dr. Carson, "like the School itself, the Professors would, in these days, be considered juvenile; but in the vigor of their youth, they were capable of accomplishing great things, and failed not in their endeavor. Rush was but twenty-four years old; Kuhn but twenty-eight; Shippen thirty-three; and Morgan thirty-four. Bond had only arrived at the age when experience is supposed to bring the greatest wisdom; he was over fifty years." This Faculty was the nucleus of that notable group of men which arose about the stalwart figure of Rush, after the struggles of the dark days of the Revolution, and made the medical department of the University of Pennsylvania a rival of Edinburgh herself. Indeed, the early days of the two schools were remarkably similar: Monteith and others had given anatomical lectures as early as 1694 in Edinburgh, as had Shippen and others before him; Alexander Monro had been appointed to the first professorship, that of the Institutes of Medicine, in 1720, as Morgan was to his chair in 1765; Other professors were added in 1724 and '26, as Shippen, Bond, Kuhn and Rush were in years succeeding Morgan. Monro and his confrères were educated in Leyden and adopted Leyden methods and the traditions of Boerhaave until they were modified by Cullen, as Morgan and his companions were educated in Edinburgh, adopted her traditions and the system of Cullen, until Rush arose to modify them; as Boerhaave was revered and followed at Edinburgh, so Cullen was revered and followed in Philadelphia, and Benjamin Rush became his greatest prophet.

The new medical department had already begun to dominate the medical profession of Philadelphia, and, like the city itself, was beginning to feel the approach of the great crisis several years before it announced itself at Lexington and Bunker Hill, and also before there was attached to the Declaration of Independence, as if in prophecy of his greatness, the signature of that one of her faculty whom the entire medical world still delights to honor. The colonial period may be said to have closed in the medical annals of Philadelphia when the founder of her medical school was called to be

Director-General of the Medical Department of the Continental Army in 1775.

Before that period closed, however, there arose to prominence in connection with the increased activity of the medical school, a new institution, of the greatest medical interest, destined to rival the Pennsylvania Hospital, not only in the coming war, but in subsequent medical history. This was the hospital ward of the Almshouse, or "Bettering House," as it was popularly called. The first buildings of this institution had been erected about 1731-2 on the "green meadows" surrounded by Third, Fourth, Spruce and Pine streets, and new quarters were opened in 1767 several blocks due westward between Tenth and Eleventh and the streets before mentioned, only the second block west of the Pennsylvania Hospital (c). The earliest record of physicians in attendance occurs in the following year, 1768, when Drs. Thomas Bond and Cadwalader Evans were appointed, although it is altogether probable that it had medical attendance, and possibly a sick ward, as early as its foundation in the "green meadows." It was not, however, until 1772, when a proposition was made to its managers to increase its usefulness by allowing students to be trained there, that official measures were taken to enlarge its staff. Drs. Bond and Cadwalader Evans had been allowed to instruct students in an obstetrical clinic as early as 1770 (d), "the first obstetrical clinic." On March 25, 1774, however, Drs. Adam Kuhn and Benjamin Rush, professors, Samuel Duffield (e), one of the first graduates, Gerardus

---

(c) It was removed to its present quarters on the west bank of the Schuylkill in 1834, where its common name, Blockley Hospital, grew famous, and where it soon, 1835, received its present name, Philadelphia Hospital.

(d) Philadelphia Hospital Reports, Vol. 1, History by Drs. D. Hayes Agnew, Charles K. Mills and others.

(e) Drs. Samuel Duffield, George Glentworth and Gerardus Clarkson, born respectively in 1732, '35 and '37, were the real contemporaries of Morgan, Shippen, Rush and Kuhn, being of almost the same age. Dr. Duffield, of whom there is little record, was born in 1732, and educated in Philadelphia, where he received his degree of Bachelor of Medicine of 1768. He served as curator and councillor in the American Philosophical Society, was surgeon in the navy and superintendent of the naval hospital of the province. In 1777 he was elected member of the Continental Congress, and was one of the founders of the College of Physicians. He was physician to the city poor, the Board of Health and the Yellow Fever

Clarkson (f) and Thomas Parke (g), having offered their services gratuitously, were chosen to the staff. The hospital department of the "Bettering House" was now of the first importance, both to the sick poor who had to be sent to the almshouse, and as an adjunct to medical education in the new medical school. It was to these wards on Eleventh street, that the Acadian Evangeline, grown old, sought her lover Gabriel, and found him dying.

"Then in the suburbs it stood, in the midst of meadows and woodlands;
"Now the city surrounds it; but still, with its gateway and wicket,
"Meek, in the midst of splendor, its humble walls seem to echo
"Softly the words of the Lord: 'The poor ye always have with you.'"

Orphan Asylum of 1793. He died in December, 1814. He and Benjamin Duffield were of different families.

(f) Dr. Gerardus Clarkson, a native of New York of 1737, became the stepson of the famous divine, Rev. Gilbert Tennent, under whom his education was begun. After studying under Dr. Thomas Bond he went to Europe in 1760, and after successful study returned to Philadelphia. He was one of the founders of the College of Physicians and its first treasurer. He was a member of the first medical society and of the American Philosophical Society, and served as a trustee of the University. He was "a pious, affectionate, modest, beloved physician," and died on September 19, 1790.

(g) Dr. Thomas Parke, the youngest of the staff, was only twenty-five, born in Chester County, Pa., in 1749 (old style). The classical teacher, Robert Proud, of this city, educated him and Dr. Cadwalader Evans was his preceptor for three years, after which, in 1770, the new college gave him the degree of Bachelor of Medicine. Then after two years, 1771-3, in London and Edinburgh, he returned to practice in partnership with his preceptor. In 1777 he became one of the staff of the Pennsylvania Hospital and served for forty-five years. He was the last of the founders of the College of Physicians to become its president, and he also served as a curator of the American Philosophical Society. He was one of those who did noble service in the pestilence of 1793, and was known among his medical brethren as "truly a peacemaker," a man of solid qualities rather than brilliance. He died January 9, 1835.

CHAPTER II.

THE REVOLUTIONARY PERIOD—1775 TO 1825.

IN APRIL, 1775, after arms had been gathered by Dr. Joseph Warren, president of the provincials, hostilities opened. The attack was begun by the English on the night of the 18th, and early the following morning Warren sent three messengers, Dr. Samuel Prescott, Paul Revere and William Dawes, to arouse the neighboring people. In this mission Dr. Prescott alone succeeded, Revere and Dawes being captured by a party of British soldiers. Dr. John Brooks led his militia against the British at North Bridge, and nine other physicians that day bore arms or gave medical aid. The sick and wounded were carried to private houses, which were used as hospitals. A provincial army was gathered about Boston, and on the 8th of May a committee was appointed to examine surgeons (a). On June 19th, Drs. Church, Taylor and Whiting were given charge of medical arrangements. On the 19th of July the Continental Congress at Philadelphia also appointed a committee of three to discuss the subject, and two days later Washington wrote from Camp Cambridge of the pressing necessity in that quarter for a medical director. On July 27th a temporary system was adopted, suitable for an army of 20,000 men, and Dr. Benjamin Church, who had been a confidential agent from that province to Congress, was elected director and physician of the hospital department. Beside him there were to be four surgeons,

---

(a) This was the first examining board of the Continental armies, and that they at once instituted a high standard is evinced by the fact that but eight out of the first fourteen recommended surgeons were accepted. Dr. Church was at the head of this committee. From that day, May 8, 1775, this high standard has been maintained.

one apothecary, twenty surgeon's mates, one clerk, and two storekeepers; and to every ten of the sick, one nurse. The duty of the director was "to furnish medicines, bedding, and all other necessaries, to pay for the same, superintend the whole, and make report to and receive orders from the commander-in-chief." Dr. Church was to appoint the surgeons, and they to choose their mates. Each regiment had its surgeon, who was to care for such sick as were not ill enough to be sent to the general hospital. These surgeons immediately began to complain of their supplies, their relative rank, and various other matters, and thus began within the department a conflict that grew fiercer and fiercer, until someone had to be sacrificed. It seemed that the policy of organization had to be almost fought out, and the rivalry of the regimental surgeons and their jealousy of the Director-General, combined with meager supplies, all resulted in an order for an investigation, September 7th. This order stated that, "Repeated complaints being made by the Regimental Surgeons, that they are not allowed proper necessaries for the use of the sick, before they became fit objects for the General Hospital, and the Director-General of the Hospital complains that, contrary to the rule of every established Army, these Regimental Hospitals are more expensive than can be conceived, which plainly indicates that there is either an unpardonable abuse on one side, or an inexcusable neglect on the other." During all of September the investigation lingered, when, to the amazement of all concerned, a new and disgraceful development closed further need for it, as far as the Director-General was concerned. On October 5th General Washington wrote to Congress that a court-martial trial had proved that Dr. Church had either unwisely or treasonably carried on a cipher correspondence with the enemy. Congress ordered his confinement, and later he embarked for the West Indies on a vessel which was never heard of again. Twelve days after Washington's letter was written, Congress at Philadelphia considered three names with the view of appointing a successor to the late Director-General. These were Dr. John Morgan, the founder of the new medical school at the continental capital,

Dr. Isaac Foster, surgeon of the hospital in Cambridge, and one of the army surgeons, Lieutenant-Colonel Hand, another Pennsylvanian. Dr. Morgan was chosen on the 17th of October, less than three months after the organization was effected. Of his appointment, Dr. J. M. Toner (b) says: "The success which had attended the medical department of the College of Philadelphia under his guidance was of itself a first-class endorsement. His ability as a surgeon, his character as a man, his patriotism, and his influence as a citizen were well known to the public. Therefore no more fitting appointment of chief medical officer could have been made." He had from the first, and never lost, the earnest sympathy, support and confidence of Washington, and on receiving his commission at once reported to headquarters at Cambridge. He found that of the army of 19,365 men in the neighborhood of Boston 2,817 were sick, and that smallpox, typhus and typhoid fevers, diarrhœa and dysentery were rife. "He set to work," says one account (c), "to introduce more systematic arrangements in the management of the hospitals; the wards were cleaned out, and men sent back to their regiments, the number of surgeon's mates in hospital reduced, and the surplus officers transferred to vacancies in the regiment, and he subjected the medical officers to another medical examination and caused those who were disqualified to be discharged." Congress referred all appointments to him and, notwithstanding the approaching winter and scanty supplies, together with the alarming increase in smallpox, the department was beginning to appear well ordered. The difficulty in obtaining supplies was so great that Dr. Morgan was compelled to appeal to the "Publick." This difficulty was experienced in every department of the army, but was more glaring in the presence of physical suffering. This, however, seems to have been more or less relieved. A more serious difficulty was the increasing jealousy of his powers of appointment and direction, which were so great that Congress was compelled to modify them and

---

(b) Medical Men of the Revolution.
(c) Brown's Medical Department of the United States Army.

give more authority to the regimental surgeons. The chief difficulty, however, arose in the army created under General Schuyler during the summer, to operate with the Canadians above Albany and with a fleet to be raised on the lakes. His sick were gathered in a hospital at Ticonderoga, and on August 5th he wrote that, as one-fifth of his 500 men were sick, he should be compelled to secure a surgeon in Albany to take charge of them. This he did on the 27th following, nearly two months before Dr. Morgan's appointment. This surgeon, a native of Maryland who had been educated at Philadelphia, was Dr. Samuel Stringer, and on the 14th of September, while the Church investigation was going on, he was commissioned by Congress, Director of the Hospital and Physician for the Northern Department, as General Schuyler's army was called, with power to appoint as many as four surgeon's mates, otherwise to be under the Director-General. Congress itself, however, seemed to be uncertain as to the powers necessary for the Northern Department to do its work, and finally increased them and also appointed a naval surgeon for the lakes. A conflict of authority now arose between Drs. Morgan and Stringer, neither of whom was the real cause of it. Stringer conceived his position to have the same relation to Schuyler's command that Morgan's had to Washington's, and as he had been in service before Morgan was appointed, and Congress was changeable in its directions, he insisted on an equality of position, although the law was plain as to Morgan's headship of the whole medical department. During the winter, while both the New England and New York armies were strengthening their forces, the friction seemed to be in abeyance, but when, in the middle of March (1776), the British began to withdraw from Boston beaten, and to advance upon New York, the removal of operations southward made the situation in the medical department more acute than ever, not only from this but from new rivalries. New armies had been raised to the southward, where the British had attacked and burned Norfolk, Virginia. The Southern Department was now organized with its general hospital at Williamsburg, Virginia.

Indeed, by this time there were five army departments, Eastern, Northern, Canadian, Middle and Southern, though there seems to have been but three general hospitals. Washington now began to move toward New York, and on April 3rd Dr. Morgan was directed to transfer the general hospital to that city. This was done successfully, and the hospitals were soon in excellent order. Meanwhile, Dr. Morgan had recommended changes in the organization to adapt it to any increase in the army. He advised the appointment of a surgeon and five mates to every five thousand men, with other provisions making the department to consist of a director-general, directors of each hospital, and other officers as before, with a complete system of reports and responsibilities. This plan was adopted by Congress on July 17th, but Dr. Stringer was so determined in his encroachments, that Congress was compelled to define his position, in an act of August 20th, to the effect that: "Dr. Morgan was appointed Director-General and Physician-in-Chief of the American Hospital (d). That Dr. Stringer was appointed Director and Physician of the Hospital in the Northern Department only." At the same time, a druggist was appointed at Philadelphia to act as purveyor of supplies for the whole medical department, Dr. William Smith, later on Arch street, between Front and Second streets, being the appointee.

Seven days after this law was passed, came the disastrous battle of Long Island, in which Washington lost nearly a thousand men and was compelled to leave New York. Dr. Morgan made special arrangements for hospitals in anticipation of the action, but all plans were now disorganized, and hospitals were scattered up the Hudson at Peekskill, which seemed to be Morgan's headquarters, at Fishkill and other places. Albany was full of the sick. The battles of Harlem Plains on September 16th, White Plains on the 26th, the loss of Fort Washington on November 16th and

(d) As Washington's was the largest and the main army, the Medical Department under him was of course the main one. This army was always spoken of as the Continental Army, although Washington had charge of all, so this manner of speaking of the "American Hospital" was used in the same way. Other hospitals were divisions of it.

of Fort Lee two days later, drove the disheartened army into winter quarters in New Jersey. These events raised up armies instantly all through the middle colonies, and the camps and hospitals became largely concentrated in this region. Meanwhile, as early as October 9th, the new army in New Jersey had needed a hospital, and Congress, so far as is known, without consulting either General Washington or Dr. Morgan, appointed Dr. William Shippen, Jr., to be director not only of the hospitals in that state, but also of the flying camp and Jersey militia. This act seemed plainly intended to reduce Dr. Morgan to some approach to an equality with the new appointee. It decreed, "That no regimental hospitals be for the future allowed in the neighborhood of the general hospital. That John Morgan, Esq., provide and superintend an hospital at a proper distance from the camp for the army posted on the east side of Hudson's River. That William Shippen, Jr., Esq., provide and superintend an hospital for an army in the State of New Jersey," and that they each make weekly returns to Congress and the commander-in-chief. The appointment "seems," says Dr. J. M. Toner, "to have been brought about by the general discontent of the people and the army, and by the friends of Dr. Shippen, who had influence with Congress, and possibly his own solicitation. The resolution of Congress in October, which enlarged his authority and power, would seem to give color to this hypothesis. His view of the duties assigned him by Congress was not promptly acquiesced in, or understood in the same way, by commanders generally, and led him to write complainingly on the subject to General Washington. The General's reply not being satisfactory, he then wrote on the same subject, and complains to Congress, and even reflects on the course of Dr. Morgan and General Washington. Dr. Shippen's letters are diplomatic, and show that he felt confident that he and Congress had come to an understanding on the subject of the future medical management of the hospital department."

The wavering attitude of Congress in not enforcing the medical system it had adopted, was in a large measure due to the pressure of the regimental surgeons who had the sympathy of their Colonels in resisting what they regarded as the policy of building up the general hospital system at the expense of the regimental service, and also to the rivalry of directors of hospitals, supported by their Generals, who desired their departments to be practically independent of all authority but that of Congress. A frank and manly letter from Dr. Morgan, even so early as August 12th, in regard to appointments he had made in the Northern Department, illustrates certain features of the situation: "After all I have said," he writes the President of Congress, "I cheerfully submit the propriety of my conduct in making the before-mentioned appointments in the general hospitals, and am desirous of conforming strictly to my instructions. If I have exceeded my commission, it has been for want of knowing the designs and resolves of Congress, or their being misunderstood. Should the Congress on that footing annul my appointments and make others, I must at least stand acquitted of intentionally going beyond the line of duty; and it will behoove Congress to be more explicit in respect to its intentions, for if the Congres does not suppose the appointment of any new surgeon rests with me, of what use is it to recommend one to me for my approbation? I must pay an implicit obedience to their simple recommendation. In that case, I do not imagine there will be the same security for harmony, or for having the business of the hospital so well executed, as where the choice of surgeons is left to the Director-General, which is an additional incentive to industry and an obliging behavior in the surgeon thus freely elected to approve himself worthy of the choice. Be that as it may, whenever the path of duty is plain, I shall endeavor to walk steadily in it, having no design or inclination to exceed those bounds which the good of the service or the wisdom of Congress may prescribe to me." On the 24th of September, Washington thus described the situation in a letter to Congress in unmistakable language. "No less attention should be paid," said he, "to the choice of surgeons than other officers of the army. They should undergo a regular examination, and if not appointed by the Director-General and surgeons of the hospital, they ought to be subordinate to, and governed by, his directions. The regimental surgeons I am speaking of, many of whom are very great rascals, countenancing the men in sham complaints to exempt them from duty, and often receiving bribes to certify indispositions with a view to procure discharges or furloughs. But independent of these practices, while they are considered as unconnected with the general hospital, there will be nothing but continual complaints of each other—the director of the hospital charging them with enormity in their drafts for the sick, and they him for denying such things as are necessary. In short, there is a constant bickering among them which tends greatly to the injury of the sick, and will always subsist until the regimental surgeons are made to look up to the Director-General of the hospital as a superior. Whether this is the case in regular armies or not, I cannot undertake to say; but certain I am, there is a necessity for it in this, or the sick will suffer. The regimental surgeons are aiming, I am persuaded, to break up the General Hospital, and have in numberless instances drawn from medicines, stores, etc., in the most profuse and extravagant manner for private purposes."

It will be seen from these extracts, that beside the purposes of Dr. Stringer in the Northern Department there was a new element of even more formidable dimensions entering into the situation when, on November 1st, Dr. Shippen reported to Congress concerning his sick at Perth Amboy, Elizabethtown, Fort Lee, Brunswick and Trenton, as follows: "I have not yet taken charge of near two thousand that are scattered up and down the country in cold barns, and who suffer exceedingly for want of comfortable apartments, because Dr. Morgan does not understand the meaning of the honorable Congress in their late resolve, and believes yet they are to be under his direction, although they are on this side Hudson's River. He is now gone over to take General Washington's opinion; as soon as I review the General's orders on this subject, I shall exert my best abilities to make the miserable soldiery comfortable and happy." On the 3rd, Washington had written to him, "it is my desire that they may remain under his (Dr. Morgan's) direction," and on the 9th Dr. Shippen wrote to Congress for further directions, saying he had not taken any of the Continental army's sick, "because Dr. Morgan differs in opinion with me concerning the meaning of Congress, and because General Washington desires they may remain under his care, as you will see from the enclosed letter from his Excellency, the General, who makes no distinction between my appointment in July and your resolves in October, and, in my opinion, has not seen the latter, which expressly says all the sick on this side of the North River shall be under my care and direction."

The repeated defeats of the Continental Army caused general dissatisfaction, as was but natural. Washington's policy was severely and openly criticised by Adams, and more secretly condemned by the noted Conway Cabal. Mismanagement was nowhere more apparent than in the Medical Department. But when, in November, Dr. Morgan was upheld by Washington, and Dr. Shippen by the members of Congress who were unfriendly to the General, it needed only the concentration of troops in the Continental capital, the mingling of officers and congressmen in Philadelphia society, and the large proportion of sick in the city, to bring about a better condition of affairs. Decided action was taken during December, when the first considerable movement of the sick toward the capital was directed by Dr. Thomas Bond, Jr. (e), who had immediate charge of the hospitals at Elizabethtown, and who had proposed the plan of establishing hospitals at Darby, Marcus Hook, Wilmington and New Castle, rather than at Bethlehem, Reading, Lancaster, Bristol and other inland towns. The former plan was preferable on account of the more convenient transportation by water which it involved. General Mifflin had directed Dr. Bond to load the sick on transports and go to Phila-

---

(e) Dr. Thomas Bond, Jr., of whom there seems to be little record, was surgeon of Gen. John Cadwalader's original battalion of the Revolution, rose to be an assistant director-general, and in 1781 was chosen medical purveyor of the entire army.

6

delphia, so that Dr. Bond., Jr., wrote to his father asking him to request the Council of Safety to prepare for them. He suggested the use of the Pennsylvania Hospital and other buildings, and on December 4th, the memorable founder of that hospital presented his son's letter to the Council, with a most touching offer of his own services, saying: "When I see so many of friends and valuable citizens exposing themselves to the horrors of war, I think it my duty to make them a tender of the best service in my power, upon the condition that I can have the joint assistance of my son in the great undertaking, who, I am certain, you will find on inquiry, has already distinguished himself in this department. As I am told many of the sick are near the city, the sooner the matter is concluded on the better." The next day these suggestions were acted upon favorably and the sick troops, who were already arriving daily, were provided for. This general movement brought out nearly all the medical talent in Philadelphia that was not already in service.

It was thoroughly evident, even in December, that Congress was taking the direction of the war more and more into its own hands, and became still more so while Cornwallis was forcing Washington over the Delaware into Pennsylvania. It was also plain that it was directing the medical department with a large degree of independence of former laws. The jealous spirit of independence of the provinces made it necessary to allow both provincial and Continental armies, and this also caused confusion in the medical departments. The inland towns were finally chosen as hospital sites in preference to those on the river, and on December 3rd, the Moravian Brethren at Bethlehem received word from Dr. John Warren, who signed himself "General Surgeon of the Continental Hosp.," that by General Washington's direction they were to prepare buildings for the "General Hospital," (f) and later, on the same day, Drs. Warren and Shippen came and secured the "Brethren's House," while on the day following, 250 sick were installed. Of these 110 died before the winter closed. It would seem from a

(f) Moravian Souvenir. Prof. W. C. Reichel.

journal already referred to (ff) that Dr. Morgan must have been at Bethlehem during the next few weeks in December. This appears from the following extract: "1777, January 8, Dr. Morgan and surgeons received orders to repair to the army in New England." The meaning of this becomes evident when it is known that on the day following, January 9, 1777, Congress "resumed the consideration of the medical committee, whereupon, *Resolved*, that Dr. John Morgan, Director-General, and Dr. Samuel Stringer, Director of the Hospital in the Northern department of the Army of the United States, be and they are hereby dismissed from any further service in said offices," and that a general invoice should be returned to Congress from the departments. The immediate occasion of this was the persistent refusal of Dr. Stringer, supported by General Schuyler, to be subordinate to the Director-General. This insubordination was carried so far that he refused to make returns or enroll or pay surgeons that were sent to him. The blow had fallen on Dr. Morgan, who had not failed to do his duty, and that, too, to the satisfaction of his superior, the head of the army. "His reputation," says the late Dr. Toner, a writer who has made the most careful study of the whole subject, "was sacrificed, and his eminent abilities lost to his country."

When it is recalled that republican government in this country was in the experimental stage, and that majority government, with its peculiar weaknesses, had been voluntarily chosen because of its freedom and safety, it will not be necessary to seriously impugn the motives of any one of those concerned in these events. In all majority governments there is always ground for honest difference of opinion as to policy, method and execution, and each opinion has perfect right to endeavor to secure a majority. Nor is the heated recrimination of such a period of special value for a true historical perspective. When, on December 17th, not long after his arrival at Bethlehem, Dr. Shippen wrote to Colonel Richard Henry Lee, of Congress, proposing a reorganization of the whole medical wing of the army on independent de-

---

(ff) Moravian Souvenir. Prof. W. C. Reichel.

partment lines responsible to Congress, he voiced for medicine only what others were demanding in other lines. He proposed three independent departments, corresponding to the Northern, Middle and Southern armies, and "to each of these the following officers:" One director and surgeon-general, three assistant directors, ten surgeons or physicians, twenty mates, one apothecary-general and four mates, one quartermaster-general and three deputies (to every hundred sick), and other subordinate officers in proportion. He adds: "The director-general and sub-directors to be chosen by Congress; the physicians, surgeons and apothecaries by the directors; the mates by the physicians and surgeons after a strict examination; all other officers by the directors. Not less than this, in my opinion, will induce men properly qualified to engage; and any other will be dear at any price." This plan was abandoned before the ensuing spring, when General Washington secured the admission into the service of Dr. John Cochran of New Jersey, who, in conjunction with Dr. Shippen, formulated a plan almost wholly patterned after the complicated system of the British army, in which the numerous distinctions of social rank had created a profusion of offices. It was probably a compromise between the independent spirit of the provinces and Washington's desire for a unified service. In accepting this plan, which provided for a director-general of the whole service, three, for each of the three departments, a deputy director-general, a physician-general, a surgeon-general, and an apothecary-general, an assistant director and commissary for each of the hospitals, senior physicians and surgeons, second surgeons, mates, stewards and nurses, and likewise a physician and surgeon-general for each army to have control over the regimental surgeons and their mates, General Washington, in qualified terms, said: "The number of officers mentioned in the enclosed plan, I presume are necessary for us, because they are found so in the British hospitals." The plan was adopted on April 11th, (1777) next. Dr. Shippen was chosen director-general of all the service; Dr. Benjamin Rush, who had left Congress, was chosen surgeon-general of the hospital of the middle department (g); and Dr. John Cochran, physician and surgeon-general of the army of that department; while other surgeons from various parts of the land were selected to fill the remaining offices.

From the above, it is manifest that the chief control of the Medical Department of the Revolutionary Army was in the hands of Philadelphia men, and that an account of their administration of its affairs is practically identical with the medical history of this period. Dr. Shippen was handicapped from the first by being the object of fierce resentment from the friends of Morgan, but a man who had coolly, but with iron will, faced hostile public sentiment when introducing men accoucheurs and dissections of the human body, was not to be easily diverted from his purpose. The attacks upon him were even more malignant than those upon Morgan, and scarcely any more outrageous are recorded in the annals of ward politics. The passions of war, however, should not divert attention from careful consideration of conditions that were far more fruitful of explanation of events than passions. Results must never be measured aside from conditions, and as the events of the fatal year of 1777 move on, one must be prepared for a condition of things that has never been paralleled in this country except in the South during the civil war. Strictures that have been passed upon the medical department of this period seem to have been based far more largely on the records of recrimination than upon general conditions of the whole army and the entire country as well. Revolutionists are not generally a people of luxuries and rarely of sufficient necessities to keep even the vigorous from hardships and suffering. When gentlewomen of the land are foregoing even what would be common necessities in ordinary times, a war hospital is not to be compared with one in a city in times of peace. The British were aiming at Philadelphia, and it was a wise foresight that sent the hospitals inland, although this measure was bound to increase suffering. The gen-

---

(g) Dr. Rush was transferred to be physician-general of the same hospital on July 1st following, to fill the place of a resignation.

eral hospital (h) at Bethlehem, under the immediate supervision of Director-General Shippen, whose headquarters for two considerable periods were in that town, may well serve as a type of the army hospitals of the Revolution. It is true that, because of its size and the dangers which were, in those days, inevitably associated with a large collection of sick and wounded, it is probably the severest type that could be selected. Whether it be due to the frequent removal of these military hospitals or to the fact that their reports were essentially defective, the fact remains that scarcely any records of their work have been preserved.

The Moravians at Bethlehem, accustomed to a community system, had spacious buildings suitable for hospital purposes and nowhere else could the sick and helpless have received more tender consideration. The building mostly used was the "Single Brethren's House," which was "eighty-three by fifty feet," says a recent writer (i); "in height three stories, and above, a broken roof, surmounted by a belvedere forty feet long—a fine specimen of the style of building to which the Moravians of the last century were partial. The interior was arranged so as to separate the youths from the single men, on the first floor, four rooms being assigned to each. On the second floor were the refectories and extra rooms. In the summer of 1762 an east wing, and in 1769 a west wing were added, in which some work-shops for the trades conducted by the inmates were fitted up." A part of this building and some others were what awaited Drs. Shippen and Warren on the 3rd of December, 1776. The Rev. John Ettwein, who had made the arrangements for the reception of the sick, became the hospital chaplain, and it is in his journal that we find the fullest information concerning them. The deaths during December amounted to sixty-two, many of these being doubtless due to exposure and fatigue on the trip overland. Many of the criticisms of these hospitals were unnecessarily severe. At a time when the

(h) The term "general hospital," as used in the Revolution generally, means the main one of Washington's army, although technically it included every other hospital in the service as a division of it.

(i) John W. Jordan, in the Pennsylvania Magazine. 1896.

soldiers in the field were exposed to the greatest hardships it was not to be expected that their condition could be improved by wounds or illness, or that the bed of a hospital could be one of luxury. Dr. Shippen reported on the 17th of December in a letter to Colonel Lee that all the sick had been removed to Bethlehem, Easton and Allentown. He suffered the loss of an infant son during the month, and on Christmas day was suddenly ordered to the front, where Washington's army was about to move on Trenton. By the close of March, one hundred and ten had died, and in obedience to orders received on the 27th, the thirty remaining convalescents started for the army. What few were unfit to be moved, remained, so that the last did not leave until July 7th.

As has been seen, there had been sick soldiers at Philadelphia, brought there by Dr. Bond, Jr., as early as December 6th previous, and the Pennsylvania Hospital, the "Bettering House," and other houses had been used for their accommodation. The number of sick was continually changing on account of convalescence or death, so that when Dr. Shippen removed the general hospital to Philadelphia on March 27, 1777, provision was already largely made for them. As early as September 5, 1776, the Council of Safety had applied to President Wharton of the Almshouse Hospital at Eleventh and Spruce streets, for quarters for some of the Continental army's sick who were suffering from dysentery. As they were not granted, Colonel Francis Gurney was ordered to take military possession of the hospital on October 23rd. The sick were put in the southeast wing, and the building was held until the capture of the city. The records of the Pennsylvania Hospital mention no use of that institution, although some individual cases were there treated, until the arrival of the sick of Dr. Thomas Bond's (Jr.) transports in December (1776), about two months later.

On the 8th of January (1777) following, a number of sick soldiers and sailors and Hessian prisoners were received, and many more from that time on until the British occupation. When Dr. Shippen arrived, not only the Spruce and Pine street institutions were full of sick, but other houses also, among them being Carpenter's mansion on Chestnut street, between Sixth and Seventh streets, and the residence on the southeast corner of Market and Sixth streets, recently deserted by Mr. Galloway, the Tory lawyer. The sick had to be classified and a convalescent hospital was opened at Peel Hall, now a part of the Girard College estate. Early in the year, smallpox appeared and carried off large numbers. A letter of John Adams in July states that (j) there had been two thousand interments in the Potter's field, now Washington Square. "The Potter's field of Philadelphia," says Dr. James Tilton (k), "bears melancholy testimony of the fatal effects of cold weather on the military hospitals in the fall of '76 and the succeeding winter. Instead of single graves, the dead were buried in square pits, in which the coffins were placed in ranges, cross and pile, until near full, and then covered over." The first of the two darkest years of the Revolution was half gone and supplies were becoming more and more uncertain as the enemy pressed closer upon the capital. Tories showed signs of encouragement, while patriots grew restive under what they conceived to be the meager results of Washington's management. The criticism of the medical department, already alluded to, grew fiercer, and Dr. Morgan's friends seized the opportunity to repair the injustice that had been inflicted on him. Morgan was in Boston, whence during August he had written an elaborate defense of his services. This was published and laid before a congressional committee on the 9th of the month, with a request for an investigation, which Congress promptly provided for on September 18. A result, however, was not reached until June 12th of the next year (1778), by which time the current experience of the hospital service convinced them that medical men could not perform impossibilities, and they "resolved that Congress are satisfied with the conduct of Dr. John Morgan while acting as director-general and

---

(j) Scharf and Wescott.

(k) On Military Hospitals, 1813. The strictures of Dr. Tilton, who became head of the department in the winter of 1812, are as severe as anyone's, but Dr. Tilton, successful as he was in 1812, had no Revolution to deal with, and besides had a fixed government behind him and the experience of the Revolution to guide him.

physician-in-chief of the general hospitals of the United States, and that this resolution be published." One of the principal critics of the management of the medical department was Dr. Rush, who, on October 1st (1777), wrote to a member of Congress (l) saying: "It is now universally said that the system was formed for the director-general and not for the benefit of the sick and wounded. Such unlimited powers and no checks would have suited an angel." In another letter of the same month he says: "There are nearly as many officers as men in our army. Every regiment has a surgeon with one or two mates." "We shall never do well till you adopt the system made use of in the British hospitals. The industry and humanity of the physicians and surgeons are lost for the want of it. While I am writing these few lines there are several brave fellows expiring within fifty yards of me from being confined in a hospital whose air has been rendered putrid by the sick and wounded being crowded together" (m). The prominence of Rush, both in medical and political circles, gave to his criticisms unusual weight. The system of crowding the sick into large general hospitals was one of the chief points criticised by medical men, some of whom were seeking to make a radical change in the whole service, as others, who were discontented with Washington's management, were endeavoring to accomplish in the army.

The discontent was increased by Washington's unsuccessful effort to resist the advance of the enemy at Brandywine and by the consequent orders to evacuate Philadelphia. The general hospital was, in September, again removed to Bethlehem, Easton, Northampton and other inland towns. Director-General Shippen, whose objections to the removal of the hospital had been overruled by Washington, wrote to the Rev. Mr. Ettwein to again prepare to receive the sick and wounded. "It gives me pain," said he, "to be obliged by order of Congress, to send my sick and wounded

---

(l) Letter to John Adams. Atlantic Monthly of May, 1895.
(m) Letter written from Reading after the hospitals had been again distributed to inland towns.

to your peaceful village, but so it is. Your large buildings must be appropriated to their use. We will want room for two thousand at Bethlehem, Easton, Northampton, etc., and you may expect them Saturday or Sunday......... These are dreadful times, consequences of unnatural wars. I am truly concerned for your Society and wish sincerely this stroke could be averted, but 'tis impossible." This was received on Tuesday, September 19th. On Sunday evening the first of the sick and wounded began to arrive, and by the 22nd of October, above four hundred and fifty were at Bethlehem alone. One hundred more, sent by Rush, arrived a week later, whereupon Dr. Shippen urged Congress to make greater provision of supplies, as many of the men were unable to return to the army simply for want of clothes. In December, another detachment from New Jersey arrived in the sleet and rain, and now there were above seven hundred crowded into the "Single Brethren's House." The consequence of this overcrowding was a "putrid fever" so fatal that, by the end of the month, the number of deaths, since the removal, amounted to over three hundred. This fearful mortality was due, said the director-general, to "the want of clothing and covering necessary to keep the soldiers clean and warm, articles at that time not procurable in the country; partly from an army being composed of raw men, unused to camp life and undisciplined, exposed to great hardships, and from the sick and wounded being removed great distances in open wagons." "Owing to the crowded wards," said Dr. William Smith, one of the hospital surgeons, "and the want of almost every necessary, it was impossible to prevent an increase of the infection, and the suffering of the sick could not be attributed to negligence or inattention of surgeons and physicians." Even such household utensils as brooms were only to be obtained by levying on the homes of the village. One surgeon states that, in his three months' attendance there, between eight and nine hundred were admitted. Late in December, it was announced that the hospitals were again to be removed to the west of the Schuylkill, but this was not accomplished until April 12th. On the 26th, the superintendent of removal reported to Washington, who had, on the first of the year, been given complete direction of the hospitals, that from January 1st to April 12th, "eighty-one soldiers died; twenty-five deserted; one hundred and twenty-two were discharged and sent to the army; eleven were at the shoe factory (in Allentown), two attending on sick and wounded officers, and all the rest removed from the hospital" (n). It is estimated that "upward of five hundred" deaths occurred at Bethlehem alone and the death rate at Reading, Lititz, Ephrata, and other places was in proportion. "It would be shocking to humanity," wrote Dr. James Tilton, the head of the medical department in the war of 1812, "to relate the history of our general hospital in the years 1777 and 1778, when it swallowed up at least one-half of our army, owing to a fatal tendency in the system to throw all the sick of the army into the general hospital, whence crowds, infection, and consequent mortality, too affecting to mention."

Meanwhile, on the 26th of September, 1777, the second day after the first detachment of the sick had reached Bethlehem, the British had entered Philadelphia. General Howe at once took possession of the Pennsylvania Hospital for his sick, and held it until the 17th of the following June. In November, he also took possession of the Almshouse Hospital, ejecting the paupers and replacing them with the sick and wounded. Philadelphia had her full share of sick during the rest of the war, but there was no such wholesale concentration as in the days when the British were closing in about her environs. The records of the Revolution in all departments are very meager, and those of the medical department for 1778 and on to the end of the struggle are no exception to the rule. Dr. Rush gave up his position as physician-general of the middle department early in 1778 and made such an attack on its management that Congress decreed certain reforms, among them one providing that the deputy-directors of each department

---

(n) Mr. John W. Jordan, in his article, previously referred to, states that this is the only report to be found, from this hospital, in the various departments at Washington, D. C.

should give their whole attention to purveying. Dr. Rush was joined by Dr. Morgan in an attack that had for its avowed purpose the bringing of the director-general to trial for maladministration. Congress, as already stated, had begun the investigation of Dr. Morgan in September, 1778, and acquitted him on June 12, 1779. Then a trial of Dr. Shippen was inaugurated, but the court and Congress exonerated him also. In 1780, Dr. Rush, who, four years previously, had signed the Declaration of Independence, became a member of the convention for the adoption of a federal constitution, and the same year witnessed the reorganization of the medical department upon a simpler plan, Dr. Shippen being retained at its head. In June, 1871, however, being anxious to resume his work in the medical school, he resigned his post, and was succeeded by Dr. John Cochran, and Philadelphia's control of the medical department of the army was at an end.

It is not possible to make a complete list of Philadelphia physicians who served in the Revolution or to define the exact nature of their services. An approximate one may be made by comparing the first directory of physicians extant, issued two years after the war, with the government lists, as recorded by Dr. J. M. Toner. Dr. Barnabas Binney was a hospital surgeon; Dr. Thomas Bond, Sr., served as examining surgeon, while his son, Dr. Thomas Bond, Jr., beginning as surgeon's mate, rose to the office of assistant director-general of the middle department; Dr. Thomas Cadwalader, who died in the midst of the war, was a surgeon; Dr. Gerardus Clarkson attended the sick under the direction of the Council of Safety; Dr. John Colhoun was a member of the Council of Safety; Dr. William Currie was a surgeon and "furnished medicines;" Dr. Benjamin Duffield attended the pest house; Dr. Samuel Duffield became a surgeon in the navy; Dr. George Glentworth was a surgeon; Dr. James Dunlap was a surgeon in the navy; Dr. Nathan Dorsey, who was in the city in 1783, was surgeon's mate on the ship Defense; Dr. Wilson, a partner of Dr. Bond in 1873, also served; Dr. Robert Harris was surgeon's mate; Dr. James Hutchinson served in the navy hospital; Dr. Michael Jennings was a surgeon; Dr. David Jackson was a surgeon; Dr. John Jones, surgeon and examiner; Dr. Adam Kuhn became a director-general of hospitals; Dr. Samuel Preston Moore was provincial treasurer; Dr. John Morgan; Dr. Jonathan Morris was one of the Council of Safety; Dr. Otto was director of the hospital at Valley Forge; Dr. Peter Peres was a surgeon; Dr. Thomas Parke "attended soldiers;" Dr. Rittenhouse, superintendent of construction work, was probably not a practitioner; Dr. Benjamin Rush; Dr. Shippen, Sr.; Dr. William Smith, Sr., "surgeon-general of hospital at Philadelphia," and William Smith, Jr., druggist of the Continental army; Dr. Joseph Redman, Jr., a surgeon; Dr. Caspar Wistar "assisted wounded soldiers," and Dr. B. Van Leer was a member of the Council of Safety. The list is necessarily only suggestive as to the duties performed by the individuals mentioned. The medical leaders of Philadelphia in the Revolution were too immediately concerned in the revolutionary struggle to find time to make scientific observations on the diseases of the war. Scarcely any records of their work have been preserved. About four years after the surrender at Yorktown, however, on July 22, 1785, Dr. Rush jotted down a few observations (o) that are of interest: "The principal diseases," he writes, "are putrid fevers. Men, who came into the hospitals with pleurisies, rheumatisms, etc., soon lost the types of their original diseases, and suffered or died with the putrid fever. This putrid fever was often artificial, produced by the want of sufficient room and cleanliness. It always prevailed most, and with the worst symptoms, in winter. A free air, which could only be obtained in summer, always prevented or checked it. Soldiers billeted in private houses escaped it, and generally recovered soonest from all their diseases. Convalescents and drunken soldiers were most exposed to putrid fevers. The remedies that appeared to do most service in this disease, were tartar emetic in the beginning, gentle doses of laxative salts, bark, wine, (two or three bot-

---

(o) They were written for a member of the Literary and Philosophical Society of Manchester, England, and were reprinted in the London Medical Journal of the following year.

tles a day in many cases), and sal volatile. In all these cases where the contagion was received, cold seldom failed to render it active. Whenever a hospital was removed in winter, one-half of the patients generally sickened on the way, or soon after their arrival, at the place to which they were sent. The army, when it lay in tents, was always more sickly than when it lay in the open air; it was always more healthy, when kept in motion, than when it lay in an encampment. Militia officers, and soldiers, who enjoyed health during a campaign, were often seized with fevers upon their return to the *Vita Mollis*, at their respective homes. There was one instance of a militia captain, who was seized with convulsions, the first night he lay on a feather bed, after lying several months on a mattress and on the ground. The fever was produced by the sudden change in the manner of sleeping, living, etc. It was prevented, in many cases, by the person lying, for a few nights after his return to his family, on a blanket before the fire. I met with several instances of bubos, and ulcers in the throat, as described by Dr. Don Monro; they were mistaken by some of the junior surgeons for venereal sores, but they yielded to the common remedies of putrid fevers. Those patients in putrid fevers, who had large ulcers, and even mortifications, on their backs or limbs, generally recovered. There were many instances of patients in putrid fevers who, without any apparent symptoms of dissolution, suddenly fell down dead, upon being moved; this was more especially the case, when they arose to go to stool. Those officers who wore flannel shirts, or waistcoats, next to their skins, in general, escaped fevers, and diseases of all kinds. Lads under twenty years of age were subjected to the greatest number of camp diseases. The southern troops were more sickly than the northern or eastern troops. The native Americans were more sickly than the Europeans. Men above thirty and thirty-five years of age were the hardiest soldiers in the army. Perhaps this was the reason why the Europeans were more healthy than the native Americans; they were more advanced in life. The troops from Maryland, Virginia and North Carolina sickened for the want of salt provisions. Their strength and spirits were only to be restored to them by means of salt bacon. I once saw a private in a Virginia regiment throw away his ration of choice fresh beef, and give seven shillings and sixpence apiece for a pound of salt meat. Most of the sufferings and mortality in our hospitals were occasioned not so much by actual want or scarcity of anything, as by the ignorance, negligence, etc., in providing necessaries for them. After the purveying and directing departments were separated (agreeably to the advice of Dr. Monro), in the year 1778, very few of the American army died in our hospitals." The last fact, however accurate it may be, is probably to be explained by mere coincidence. The experience of '76 and '77 surely had no small part in securing better service, and other general causes operated to the same result. The work of the director-general, Dr. Shippen, like that of any other leader in a terrible conflict, was not without its errors and weaknesses, but it is doubtful whether those who, while free from his responsibilities, advanced other theories of management, were able to regard it from an unbiased judicial standpoint.

In one sense, a war always closes gradually, and long before the surrender at Yorktown the physicians of Philadelphia had begun to resume the duties of peace. The medical school and hospitals were reopened, but not without the difficulties attendant upon reorganization. This was especially true of the College. A new generation was in control. Many of the first group of native American physicians were incapacitated or had died. Undoubtedly the faculty of the medical school was by far the most dominant element in Philadelphia medicine. It'will be of interest to observe who were the active practitioners, and where they were located, two years after the war; in other words, to "take stock" of the medical profession of that period. The earliest list of physicians which has been preserved is one made "soon after" 1783, and two years later, 1785, the first directory (p) was issued. The

(p) Francis White's Philadelphia Directory. A copy of this is in the Historical Society's library. John McPherson issued one the same year, but the society has found no copy of it. Neither of these lists is more than approximately complete and only includes those who were well known in active practice. Dr. Shippen, Sr., for instance, is not mentioned.

differences between the two are but slight, so accurate results may be reached by their combined study. The physicians, like the city itself, were located chiefly about the banks of the Delaware: Benjamin Rush, M. D. (q), of the firm of Rush and Hall (r), was on Second street, between Chestnut and Walnut; William Shippen, Jr., M. D., was not far away, on Second, between Walnut and Spruce; John Morgan, M. D., was near by, on Second street, at the corner of Spruce; Dr. Bond, of Bond and Wilson (s), was also on Second street, between Market and Arch streets; John Redman, M. D., was near also on Second street, between Market and Arch streets; John Jones, M. D., had left New York, and was around the corner on Market street, between Second and Third streets; Adam Kuhn, M. D., was on Second street, near Walnut; Gerardus Clarkson, M. D., was on Pine street, just above Front street, and his son, William Clarkson, B. M., was around the corner on Front, between Pine and Union streets; Samuel Duffield, B. M., was on Chestnut, just above Second street; and Benjamin Duffield, M. D., was on Front street, between South and Almond streets; Nathan Dorsey was on Front street, between Walnut and Spruce streets; John B. Foulke, B. M., was on Front street, between Market and Arch streets; George Glentworth, M. D., was on Arch street, between Front and Second streets; John Carson, M. D., was on Third street, between Chestnut and Walnut streets; Barnabas Binney, who had settled in Philadelphia during 1777, was on Arch street, between Fourth and Fifth streets; Abraham Chovet, M. D., the well-known Tory, was in the same neighborhood, on Race street, between Third and Fourth streets; William Currie was on Second street, corner of Pine street; Samuel Griffitts (t), B. M., was on Union street, above Second; John Morris, B. M., was on Chestnut street, below Second; William Smith, B. M., was on Arch street, below Second; Thomas Parke, B. M., was on Fourth street, between Chest-

---

(q) The degrees are given in White's Directory, 1785. This is the better list of the two, and more accurate, even for 1783 or '84.
(r) Dr. James Hall.
(s) Probably Thomas Bond, Jr., as his father died in 1784.
(t) "Samuel K. Griffith" in Watson's list, an error.

nut and Market streets; Benjamin Say, physician and surgeon, was on Second street, between Arch and Race streets; James Hutchinson was on Second stret, between Walnut and Spruce streets, near Dr. Shippen; Drs. Jackson and Smith were on Second street, between Market and Chestnut streets; Robert Harris was on Spruce street, between Second and Third; Peter Glentworth was on Front street, between Market and Arch; Joseph Redman was on Market street, between Fifth and Sixth; James Dunlap was also near by on Market street, between the same streets; Joseph Goss was on Fourth street, near Walnut, although he had been on Front street; Joseph Phiffer, a German, was on Second street, near Vine, and Peter Peres, a Frenchman, was on Second street, "near the Barracks," at the corner of Brown street; John Kehlme (u) was on Race street, near Second; Frederick Rapp was on Third street, near Vine; Samuel Shober was on Front street, near South; Thomas Shaw was at Front and Callowhill streets; Benjamin Van Leer was on Water street, near Race; George Lyle was on Front street, "near Pool's Bridge;" Michael Jennings was on Moravian alley, near Race street; Dr. Farbley was on Story street, near Third; and James Batchelor (v) was on Water street, near Catherine. It will be seen from the above that physicians were clustered in the neighborhood of Second street, and that none were west of Sixth; also that there were about fifty physicians in a population ranging within a thousand or so of forty thousand inhabitants. It will be seen, as events move forward, that the most influential among them was he, who, nearly ten years previously, had signed the Declaration of Independence, and had subsequently been one of the framers of the constitution of his native State. Dr. Benjamin Rush was the instigator and promoter of many a useful project which, but for his influence in medical and political circles, would probably have been postponed or abandoned.

In August, 1783, in the course of a correspondence with Dr.

(u) "Kelhmle," Dr. Rush spells it.
(v) Not in White's Directory. Watson's list contains it and also a name which is undoubtedly a misprint of Dr. Kuhn's name.

Samuel Powel Griffitts, who was then in London, he had suggested the founding in Philadelphia of a society similar to the College of Physicians in London This young man was of such a character as to attract the notice of thoughtful men, his seniors. He was only twenty-four years of age at the time of his correspondence with Rush. Born in 1759 in Philadelphia, a member of the Society of Friends, his liberal education was acquired in the College and his professional in the Medical School, under the preceptorship of Dr Kuhn. Like his friend Wistar, he had charge of the wounded in the late war. In 1781 he went to Europe, studied in Paris and Montpelier until June, 1783, and then proceeded to London. In the autumn of that year he went to Edinburgh, but returned in the spring of 1784 to London, and in the fall was at home in Philadelphia. During the following year, 1785, a visitor, Dr Henry Moyes, who was delivered a course of lectures in Philadelphia on natural philosophy, suggested to Dr. Griffitts, and to his uncle, Samuel Powel, the project of a free dispensary. It was well received, and after consultation with Drs. Rush, Hall and Morris, a meeting of managers and physicians was held on February 10, 1786, with the object of obtaining subscriptions for the charitable enterprise. Before the end of the month the necessary funds were pledged; temporary quarters were secured in Strawberry alley, and on April 12th, the Philadelphia Dispensary, the first institution of its kind in America, was formally instituted.

The original staff of the Dispensary was composed of Drs. Samuel P. Griffitts, James Hall (w), William Clarkson (x), John Morris (y), John Carson (z), and Caspar Wistar, attending physi-

(w) Dr. Hall died in 1801. He was Lazaretto physician and is buried in the grounds of the Lazaretto.

(x) Dr. Clarkson was born in 1763, was educated at Princeton, graduated Bachelor of Medicine at Philadelphia in 1785, but in 1793 became a Presbyterian minister. He died in 1812.

(y) Dr. Morris, 1759-93, graduated Doctor of Medicine in 1783 at Philadelphia and was one of the two medical victims of yellow fever in 1793.

(z) Dr. Carson, 1752-94, was also short lived. He was a graduate of Edinburgh Medical School, was surgeon of city cavalry, a trustee of the University, and held other offices.

cians, with Drs. Jones, Shippen, Kuhn and Rush as consultants. The Dispensary was afterward moved to 127 South Fifth street. It was the object of Dr. Griffitts' unwearied devotion, as proved by the fact that he visited it daily, with few exceptions, "for more than forty years." In 1789, Dr. Griffitts became professor of Materia Medica and Pharmacy in the medical school. He was one of the founders of the College of Physicians, and at the time of his death was its vice-president. He was also a member of the American Philosophical Society, and of various humane societies, while, in the annals of the various epidemics of yellow fever that devastated the city, his name is one of the brightest. He was the chief founder of the Friend's Asylum for the Insane at Frankford. He lived to the age of sixty-seven and died on May 12, 1826.

While the Dispensary was founding, Dr. Rush saw that his long-meditated project of founding a College of Physicians was ripe for execution. At this time there were, besides Rush, about sixteen physicians who were members of the American Philosophical Society, as well as of other scientific and social organizations. Rush himself was also a member of the society founded by Morgan, and was, probably, also a member of the American Medical Society of 1773 (a). The new organization was to be on a different basis from any of these societies. It was to be for medicine what the Philosophical Society was for general investigation and to partake largely of the character of the medical "colleges" (as European societies of a certain official character were called) of London and Edinburgh. He corresponded with Dr. Lettsom of Lon-

---

(a) The Society founded by Morgan was "The Philadelphia Medical Society," which included in its membership Drs. John Kearsley, Jr., Gerardus Clarkson, James A. Bayard, Robert Harris and George Glentworth. The American Medical Society lasted for many years, and then a new Philadelphia Medical Society was organized in 1789, and incorporated in 1792, which had a vigorous career down to 1846. This seemed to be the general society, while the College of Physicians had a different character, and the Academy of Medicine and its successor, the Medical Lyceum, both small and temporary, ceased by the latter being merged into the general society in 1816. Nearly all the members of these other three societies were also members of the general society, for Rush, Barton, Physick and Chapman were among its presidents.

don, who heartily approved of the undertaking, and suggested that the college should include foreign members. "Set your men of science," said he (b), "upon studying your own country, its native and improvable productions. Your resources would influence Europe, your reflections would instruct her." During 1786, there were many conversations on the subject, and it is probable that Dr. Rush drafted more than one "constitution" for the new society. There are, however, no records of the first two or three meetings, which were undoubtedly held late in that year. From the most careful scrutiny of all references to the first meeting for formal organization, it would seem that this occurred on the first Tuesday in October, although there may have been preliminary conferences in September (c).

In all probability, the constitution was adopted at the October meeting. The objects of the new organization are indicated in the opening words of that instrument: "The Physicians of Philadelphia, influenced by a conviction of many advantages that have arisen in every country from Literary institutions, have associated themselves under the name and title of the College of Physicians of Philadelphia. The objects of this college are, to advance the Science of Medicine, and thereby to lessen Human Misery by investigating the diseases and remedies which are peculiar to our country, by observing the effects of different seasons, climates, and situations upon the Human Body, by recording the changes that are produced in diseases by the progress of Agriculture, Arts, Population and manners, by searching for medicines in our Woods, Waters and the bowels of the Earth, by enlarging our avenues to knowledge; from the discoveries and publications of foreign countries, by appointing stated times for Literary intercourse and communications, and by cultivating order and uniformity in the practice of Physick." It provided that the membership should consist of twelve senior Fellows and an indefinite number of juniors, all to be local residents, and of associate members elsewhere. How

---

(b) 1785.
(c) History of the College of Physicians, by Dr. W. S. W. Ruschenberger, 1886.

many and who were present at that meeting can only be conjectured.

When it came to a choice for president, there was little or no hesitation. All eyes naturally turned to one of the first group of native American physicians, who had recently retired from pracice, at the age of sixty-four. This was Dr. John Redman, a companion of Cadwalader, who had died seven years before, and of Bond, whose death was but two years distant. Dr. Redman was learned and dignified, and his ideal of the nature of the physician's calling was a noble one. This is manifest from the following toast which he once proposed: "The dignity and success of the healing art: And long health, competent wealth, and exquisite happiness to the industrious practitioner, who makes the health and comfort and happiness of his fellow mortals one of the chief ends and delights of his life, and acts therein from motives that render him superior to all the difficulties he may have to encounter in the pursuit thereof." Drs. Rush and Morgan were old students of Redman and probably were active in promoting his election. Dr. Redman was a native Philadelphian, born February 27, 1722, and educated, like many of his contemporaries, at Tennent's Academy. He passed his apprenticeship under Dr. Kearsley, practiced for some years in the Bermudas, and finally spent a year or more in Edinburgh, Paris, Leyden and London, graduating at Leyden in 1748. He joined the Pennsylvania Hospital staff in 1751 and continued a member of it for nearly thirty years, and was both a trustee of the College of Philadelphia and a member of the Philosophical Society. He published "A Defense of Inoculation" in 1759, and, after a long and distinguished career as a practitioner, he had retired only two years before he was called to the first presidency of the College of Physicians. After a faithful service of more than eighteen years in this office, feeble health obliged him to resign, and about three years later, 1808, he died at the advanced age of eighty-six years.

For vice-president they chose the distinguished author of "Wounds and Fractures," who, for the previous six years had been a citizen of the city of his ancestors. Dr. John Jones, born in 1729, on Long Island, where his father, Dr. Evan Jones, had removed, after studying under his father and Dr. Cadwalader, went to Europe and continued his studies in Edinburgh, London, Paris, and the University of Rheims, from which latter he was graduated in 1757. Settling in New York, he became a surgeon in the Colonial army during the French war, and in 1768 was made Professor of Surgery in King's College. His work on surgery, published in 1775, has already been referred to. It was intended for the use of surgeons in the army and navy, and was certainly a most opportune publication. When Jones returned to Philadelphia, in 1780, he was fifty-one years of age and immediately assumed prominence as a surgeon of great dexterity. He was the physician of Washington, Franklin, and other prominent men, and was a man of the highest character in every phase of life. He would certainly have succeeded to the presidency of the College, as Dr. Redman wished, had the latter been permitted to resign. He died in 1791, at the age of sixty-three, Redman surviving him for about seventeen years. "Few persons," says an account of him, "possessed more of those engaging qualities which render a man estimable, both professionally and otherwise, than Dr. Jones. His conversation was most pleasing. His language flowed in an easy, spontaneous manner, and was animated by a vein of sprightly but always unoffending wit, which delighted while it secured attention. He was a belles-lettres scholar; was observant, and possessed a good memory; and was ever a most agreeable, entertaining and instructive companion."

The first treasurer of the College was Dr. Gerardus Clarkson, who has already been noticed, and for secretary was chosen Dr. James Hutchinson, who was destined to be the most distinguished medical victim of the yellow fever epidemic of 1793. The censors were very properly composed of the old faculty of the medical school, Drs. Shippen, Morgan, Rush and Kuhn. The first meetings, it is said, were held in the old College building at Fourth and Arch streets. At the second meeting, Dr. Redman was unable to be present, and it is believed that his inaugural address, which has been preserved, was delivered at the third meeting, in December, 1786. Of this supposed fact there is no other proof than that derived from the internal evidence of the address itself, and from a study of the earliest minutes of the College. The address was filled with excellent advice to the Fellows, some of whom, said he, "I have the honor to call my professional children," and he felt it, he said, both his "duty and inclination, as your oldest member, and especially as your president, and as very becoming to us at the commencement of this our Institution, in your name and on your behalf, to acknowledge the Supreme Being to be our Sovereign, Lord and Ruler." For some reason, the constitution was not signed until the first Tuesday in January (2), 1787, which was probably the date of the first full meeting, and has always been treated as the real birthday of the College. Those who signed it did so in the following order: The twelve seniors, Drs. John Morgan, John Redman, John Jones, William Shippen, Jr., Adam Kuhn, Benjamin Rush, Gerardus Clarkson, Samuel Duffield, Thomas Parke, James Hutchinson, George Glentworth (d), Abraham Chovet (e); and the following juniors: Drs. Andrew Ross, William

---

(d) Dr. Glentworth was the same age as Dr. Morgan, having been born in 1735, in Philadelphia. After his academic education he was apprenticed to a Dr. Peter Sonmans, of whom little is known, except that he had an extensive practice, was a member of the Philosophical Society, and died in 1776. Dr. Glentworth was a junior surgeon in the British army until 1755, when he went to Europe. After three years he graduated at Edinburgh, and, returning, became a partner of his preceptor. In 1777 he became a regimental surgeon, and later a senior surgeon in the military hospital. He died in 1792, a faithful and able physician, and a mild, friendly, intelligent patriot.

(e) Dr. Chovet, born in England in 1704, was nearly eighty-three when he signed the constitution. He was educated in London, is believed to have been a lecturer of the Barbers' and Surgeons' company, and is known to have come to Philadelphia some years before the Revolution from the West Indies because of a slave insurrection. He was an eminent anatomist and had an excellent wax collection of models made by himself, which he used in public lectures as early as 1775, and which is now in the Wistar and Horner Museum of the University. He was a Tory and experienced some annoyance on that account, but his mirthful and fun-loving temper carried him safely through what, to one less happily constituted, might have been serious dangers. His death occurred in 1790, at the advanced age of eighty-six, when he had only ceased visiting patients but a few weeks.

W. Smith, James Hall, William Clarkson, William Currie, Benjamin Say, Samuel P. Griffitts, John Morris, Nathan Dorsey (f), Benjamin Duffield, John Carson, John Foulke, Robert Harris, John R. B. Rodgers (f), Caspar Wistar, Jr. (f), and James Cunningham (f). The constitution was revised in November following (1787), and has been signed by every Fellow since elected. At the next meeting, February 6, 1787, Dr. Rush read the first paper, "On the Means of Promoting Medical Knowledge." This may be considered as the medical scientific constitution of the organization, in which its policy is first distinctly formulated. "I feel peculiar pleasure," said he, "in reflecting, that the late revolution, which has given such a spring to the mind in objects of philosophical and moral inquiry, has at last extended itself to medicine, and in less than five years after the peace, before the human faculties had contracted to their former dimensions, a college of physicians, formed upon principles accommodated to the present state of society and government in America, has been established in the capital of the United States." He proceeds to show its value as a semi-official "college," in the European sense, in virtue of which it can command attention from the public and government, influence legislation, and publish a Dispensatory (which "will be one of the first objects of our attention"); and also as a society holding the same relations to medical science as the Philosophical Society to science in general. He announces that a library, the germ of the present superb collection, has been already begun. In fact, the purposes of the College, as announced by Rush, are of the noblest character, and it is partly owing to his prestige that they have ever since been kept in view. One cannot read this address without imbibing the lofty spirit and pure scientific temper that stamped themselves upon the institutions that arose with the federal constitution. At the very next meeting, the College began its practical work by appointing a committee, almost prophetic of pes-

(f) These names were probably added later, for their election in full did not occur until April, and the published membership of February did not include them, and did include a John Lynn, whose name was dropped for some reason.

tilence to come, on Meteorology and Epidemics, a body that reported regularly for ninety-five years (g). A pharmacopœia (h) was proposed the next year for use of the College, and in 1789 a circular letter was issued to the profession of the land to secure co-operation in the establishment of a national pharmacopœia. This year witnessed the first governmental recognition of the College, also, and its incorporation. 1790 (i) was notable for a eulogy on Cullen by Dr. Rush, which brought the institution into world-wide notice, as it was probably the best extant estimate of the character and work of the great Edinburgh leader. The influence the College now began to have in the medical world was due not only to the fact that its leaders were distinguished medical men, but quite as much, if not more, to the fact that they were, necessarily, observers in a new medical field, toward which the eyes of the world had been turned by the course of public events.

The new institution was, in a sense, both complementary and supplementary to the medical school, which, in 1791, began its career as the medical department of the University of Pennsylvania, and which undoubtedly dominated the medical thought of the nation for more than a score of years thereafter. It is unnecessary, at this point, to go into the details by which the change from province to state, during the decade succeeding the war, led to the erection of two colleges and two medical schools out of the same material that had composed one, or to explain how, on September 30, 1791, they coalesced as the University of Pennsylvania. In an introductory lecture, Dr. Rush congratulated his hearers "upon the union of the two Medical Schools of Philadelphia under a charter founded upon the most liberal concessions by the gentle-

---

(g) Composed at that time of Drs. Carson, Griffitts, Morris, Hall, and William Clarkson.

(h) The committee included Drs. Redman, Jones, Kuhn, Shippen, Rush, Griffitts, Wistar and Hutchinson. Dr. Morgan proposed one for the province in May, 1787, the first, and Griffitts had been especially interested in this subject in a private way. The first effort of this kind was made for the army by Dr. William Brown at Valley Forge.

(i) 1791 witnessed the election of the first associate member in the person of Dr. James Tilton, of Dover, one of the first graduates of the medical school.

men who projected it, and upon the purest principles of patriotism in the Legislature of our State. By means of this event, the ancient harmony of the different professors of medicine will be restored, and their united efforts will be devoted, with accumulative force, toward the advancement of our science." This was a prophecy whose fulfillment was largely due to the brilliant talents and indefatigable zeal of him who uttered it. The new faculty of 1791-2 that inaugurated the new era were: For Anatomy, Surgery and Midwifery, William Shippen, and Caspar Wistar as adjunct; for Theory and Practice of Medicine, Adam Kuhn; for Institutes of Medicine and Clinical Medicine, Benjamin Rush; for Chemistry, James Hutchinson; for Materia Medica and Pharmacy, Samuel P. Griffitts, and for Botany and Natural History, Benjamin Smith Barton. Some of these chairs were soon vacated, but, for the next twenty years, the Professor of the Institutes and Clinical Medicine remained at his post, inculcating his doctrines, and impressing his methods upon the minds of hundreds of students.

Events were soon to try him, as few men have been tried, but amid the direst misfortunes, his constancy remained unbroken. There began in that calamitous year of 1793 events that were destined, ere long, to wrest from Philadelphia the proud position of metropolis, although without diminishing, in the slightest degree, her medical prestige. The city, by the end of the century, included a population of about 70,000, and undoubtedly contained about 50,000 when the yellow fever appeared. Instead of growing westward, it had spread up and down the Delaware frontage, so that even so late as 1798, says a current account (j), "the buildings do not at present extend over half the ground designated in the original plan; as the inhabitants, from obvious commercial advantages, have preferred the Delaware front rather than the Schuylkill; hence, at present, the houses extend nearly three miles north and south along the Delaware, and about three-quarters of a mile due

---

(j) History of the Pestilence Commonly Called Yellow Fever, etc. Condie and Folwell, 1798. This account makes a very conservative estimate of population, at 55,000 to 60,000 in 1798.

west toward the Schuylkill. They are chiefly built with bricks, from two to five stories high; the streets are regular, wide and airy, except Water street, which occupies the space between the bank upon which Front street is built, and the river, which was originally designed for stores. It is the narrowest, yet one of the most populous in the city," and was considered "a disagreeable street." "Where Dock street is now built," the account runs, "in former years was a swamp or canal, with a small stream of water running through it, extending from the river to Third street, which became a general nuisance, and a common reservoir for the filth of a large part of the city." This was then covered by an arched street running from beyond Sixth street in the Potter's field down to the river, but its apertures along the way were still offensive. Pegg's run in Spring Garden was another marshy nuisance, and the central cemeteries behind were regarded as a source of disease. Refugees and immigrants had greatly increased the population, while the number of physicians, in 1793, was about fifty-six (k).

Philadelphia had not been visited by yellow fever for more than thirty years, and this long period of immunity had given rise to a false sense of security with regard to its recurrence. There had been a fearful epidemic in 1699, when, according to a letter of Isaac Norris, there were two hundred and twenty deaths out of a population that could scarcely have exceeded 2,000. According to Dr. Rush: "The yellow fever, which I take to be exactly the same distemper as the plague of Athens, described by Thucydides, has been five different times in this city." Dr. Bond remarked in the course of a lecture in 1766: " 'Twas in the year forty-one, I first saw the horrid disease, which was then imported by a number of convicts from the Dublin gaol. The second time it prevailed, it was indigenous from evident causes, and was principally confined to one square of the city. The third time, it was generated on board of crowded ships in the Port, which brought in their passengers in health, but soon after became very sickly.

(k) There were fifty-six mentioned in the directory of 1791, together with nine barber-surgeons, cuppers and bleeders.

I here saw the appearance of contagion like a dim spark, which gradually increased to a blaze, and soon after burst out into a terrible flame, carrying devastation with it, and, after continuing two months, was extinguished by the profuse sweats of Tertian fevers." The years he refers to are 1741, '47 and '62, the two latter being the only years mentioned by Dr. Rush after '41. Bond's description is undoubtedly based upon the epidemic of 1762, the last, which Dr. Redman was now able to recall for the benefit of the profession (l). He said he believed that Dr. Bond had cases in 1762 as early as the second week of August, that the epidemic reached its height the week after the middle of September, and ceased early in November. It began in some tenements near the corner of Front and Pine streets, and was believed to have had its origin in a case brought from Havana. It spread from this point southwardly three or four squares and westwardly from the river to about Third or Fourth streets. At the height of the epidemic Dr. Redman had treated daily from eighteen to twenty cases of the disease. The city was now nearly four times as large as in 1762, and as the metropolis and the capital of the United States, was in a condition of great commercial prosperity. "Not to enter into a minute detail," writes Mathew Carey (m), "extravagance, in various forms, was gradually eradicating the plain and wholesome habits of the city." In July, 1793, the Cape François refugees arrived. On August 5th, (n), Dr. Rush visited the child of Dr. Hodge, which died two days later. This is the earliest case reported by him, although he admits that during the child's illness he was mistaken as to its nature. On the 18th, Dr. Say called Rush in consultation in the case of Peter Ashton, who died the same evening. On the next day, Drs. Foulke and Hodge called him in to consult in the case

---

(l) His manuscript is in the library of the College of Physicians.

(m) A short account of the "Malignant Fever," etc., by Mathew Cary, one of the public committee, January, 1794.

(n) Dr. Isaac Cathrall had a case as early as the 3rd, though it was not known to be yellow fever. Physicians "who had entered into practice since 1762," says Dr. Currie, "were entirely unacquainted with it at the time of its occurrence in Philadelphia, in the year 1793."

of the wife of Peter Le Maigre in Water street, between Race and Arch, and, on coming out, the three physicians noticed, on the wharf, a heap of putrid coffee, which had been discharged from the damaged cargo of a vessel. This putrid coffee was the nucleus of one of the fiercest medical controversies that have ever arisen in Philadelphia. Drs. Rush and Foulke regarded it as the origin of the fever, and this opinion was defended by Rush with the greatest ability and the utmost pertinacity. He now declared his belief that the above-mentioned cases and many others belonged to a malignant type of bilious remitting yellow fever. The Governor now asked the Secretary of the College of Physicians, Dr. Hutchinson, who was also consulting port-physician, to investigate the epidemic. On the 22nd, the Mayor gave orders for cleaning the streets. On the 25th, the College of Physicians met and proposed an address to the public, and Dr. Rush urged the people to clean the wharf. Dr. Hutchinson reported, on the 27th, that the epidemic had gained considerable headway and was chiefly raging in Water street, near Race and Arch, and also at Kensington, and was fast spreading. He also raised the question whether it had not originated in Kensington. The city register showed that about one hundred and fifty had already died from the disease. The public had already taken alarm. "The removal from Philadelphia," writes Carey, "began about the 25th, or 26th of this month (August); and so great was the general terror, that for some weeks, carts, wagons, coaches and chairs were almost constantly transporting families and furniture to the country in every direction. Many people shut up their homes wholly; others left servants to take care of them. Business then became extremely dull. Mechanics and artists were unemployed and the streets wore the appearance of gloom and melancholy." The increase in the number of cases was so great that the guardians of the poor were obliged to secure additional quarters for the sick. With this object, they rented a circus tent that had been lately in use, and this tent was the beginning of the Municipal Hospital. Nurses could not be secured; the patients were left to die alone or possibly to recover, and the people threatened to burn the tent. It was then decided to use the old mansion of William Hamilton, known as Bush Hill, and, as its owner was absent, the Governor took possession of it on the 31st, and it was turned into a hospital. By this time the guardians had abandoned the poor committed to their charge. "The consternation of the people of Philadelphia at this period," says Carey, "was carried beyond all bounds. Dismay and affright were visible in almost every person's countenance. Most of those who could by any means make it convenient, fled from the city. Of those who remained, many shut themselves up in their houses, and were afraid to walk the streets. The smoke of tobacco being regarded as a preventive, many persons, even women and small boys, had segars almost constantly in their mouths. Others, placing full confidence in garlic, chewed it almost the whole day; some kept it in their pockets and shoes. Many were afraid to allow the barbers or hairdressers to come near them, as instances had occurred of some of them having shaved the dead and many having engaged as bleeders. Some, who carried their caution pretty far, bought lancets for themselves, not daring to be bled with the lancets of the bleeders. Many houses were hardly a moment of the day free from the smell of gunpowder, burned tobacco, nitre, sprinkled vinegar, etc. Some of the churches were almost deserted, and others wholly closed. The coffee house was shut up, as was the city library, and most of the public offices—three out of the four daily papers were discontinued," the *Federal Gazette* being the exception. "Many," he continues, "were almost incessantly employed in purifying, scouring and whitewashing their rooms. Those who ventured abroad had handkerchiefs or sponges impregnated with vinegar, or smelling bottles full of the thieves' vinegar. Others carried pieces of tarred rope in their hands or pockets, or camphor bags tied around their necks. The corpses of the most respectable citizens, even of those who did not die of the epidemic, were carried to the grave on the shafts of a chair, the horse being driven by a negro, unattended by a friend or relative, and without any sort of ceremony. People hastily shifted their course at the sight of a hearse coming toward them. Many never walked on the footpath, but went in the middle of the streets, to avoid being infected in passing by houses wherein people had died. Acquaintances and friends avoided each other in the streets, and only signified their regard by a cold nod. The old custom of shaking hands fell into such general disuse, that many shrank back in affright at even the offer of the hand. A person with a crape or any appearance of mourning, was shunned like a viper. And many valued themselves highly on the skill and address with which they got to windward of every person whom they met. Indeed, it is not probable that London, at the last stage of the plague, exhibited stronger marks of terror than were to be seen in Philadelphia from the 25th or 26th of August, till pretty late in September."

Many of the leading people of the city had already gone to summer homes. President Washington was at Mount Vernon. On September 12th, a meeting was held, at which ten citizens volunteered to do what was necessary to help the guardians of the poor (o). The hospital at Bush Hill had become such a terror to the people, that they refused to enter it until almost ready to die; a fact which accounts for the frightful mortality in that institution. Besides, although it was attended by competent physicians, their efforts were not seconded by the nursing, which counts for so much in the treatment of yellow fever. On the 15th, Stephen Girard and Peter Helm voluntarily assumed the management of Bush Hill, the former having full charge of the interior work, containing 14 rooms, and this heroic action on the part of these philanthropists did much to restore public confidence. Drs. Deveze and Benjamin Duffield (p), the former one of the refugees from Cape François, and three resident physicians, did excellent

---

(o) Their number was afterward increased to twenty-six, four of whom died.

(p) Dr. Duffield was a native of Bucks county, Pennsylvania, born in 1753, the son of Edward Duffield, and an early member of the American Philosophic Society. He was educated at the College of Philadelphia and at the medical school, having had Dr. Redman as his preceptor, but the stormy period of his closing studies in 1774 allowed no commencement. He also studied in Edinburgh. He was in the military hospital at Reading, and was a public lecturer on midwifery. He died in 1799.

work in the hospital. Under the new management, about one thousand patients were admitted to Bush Hill, of whom nearly one-half died. This hospital, however, was only for the poor, and its inmates represented but a fraction of the sick. "Water street, between Market and Race streets, became a desert," writes Dr. Rush. "The poor were the first victims of the fever. From the sudden interruption of business, they suffered for a while from poverty as well as disease. A large and airy house at Bush Hill (q) about a mile from the city, was opened for their reception. This house, after it became the charge of a committee, appointed by the citizens on the 14th of September, was regulated and governed with the order and cleanliness of an old and established hospital. An American and French physician had the exclusive medical care of it after the 22nd of September. The contagion, after the second week in September, spared no rank of citizens. Whole families were confined by it. There was a deficiency of nurses for the sick, and many of those who were employed were unqualified for their business. There was likewise a great deficiency of physicians from the desertion of some, and the sickness and death of others. At one time there were only three physicians who were able to do business out of their houses, and at this time, there were probably not less than 6,000 persons ill with the fever. During the first three or four weeks of the prevalence of the disorder, I seldom went into a house the first time without meeting the parents or children of the sick in tears. Many wept aloud in my entry, or parlor, who came to ask for advice for their relations. Grief after a while descended below weeping, and I was much struck in observing that many persons submitted to the loss of relations and friends without shedding a tear, or manifesting any other of the common signs of grief. A cheerful countenance was scarcely to

---

(q) Bush Hill was the residence of Andrew Hamilton, the grounds of which occupied a tract about corresponding to the space between Twelfth and Nineteenth streets and Vine street and Fairmount avenue; except at one point between Sixteenth and Seventeenth streets, where it extended southward as far as Race street. The mansion and subsequent hospital buildings erected on this tract were all included by the public under the term "Bush Hill."

be seen in the city for six weeks. I recollect once, on entering the house of a poor man, to have met a child of two years old, that smiled in my face. I was strangely affected by this sight (so discordant to my feelings at the state of the city), before I recollected the age and ignorance of the child. I was confined the next day by an attack of the fever, and was sorry to hear, on my recovery, that the father and mother of this little creature died, a few days after my last visit to them. The streets everywhere discovered marks of the distress that pervaded the city. More than one-half the houses were shut up, although not more than one-third of the inhabitants had fled into the country. In walking for many hundred yards, few persons were met, except such as were in quest of a physician, a nurse, a bleeder, or the men who buried the dead. The hearse alone kept up the remembrance of the noise of carriages or carts in the streets. Funeral processions were laid aside. A black man, leading, or driving a horse, with a corpse on a pair of chair wheels, with now and then a half dozen relatives or friends following at a distance from it, met the eye in most of the streets of the city at every hour of the day, while the noise of the same wheels passing slowly over the pavements, kept alive anguish and fear in the sick and well, every hour of the night. But a more serious source of the distress of the city arose from the dissensions of the physicians about the nature and treatment of the fever. It was considered by some as a modification of the influenza, and by others as the jail fever. Its various grades and symptoms were considered as so many diseases, all originating from different causes. There was the same contrariety in the practice of the physicians that there was in their principles. The newspapers conveyed accounts of both to the public, every day. The minds of the citizens were distracted by them, and hundreds suffered and died from the delays which were produced by an erroneous opinion of a plurality of diseases in the city, or by indecision in the choice, or a want of confidence in the remedies of their physicians." He speaks of the religious feeling abroad, and of the spirit of self-sacrifice that prevailed, and adds, "but the virtues which were excited by our calamity, were not confined to the city of Philadelphia. The United States wept for the distress of their capital. In several of the states, and in many cities, and villages, days of humiliation and prayer were set apart to supplicate the Father of Mercies in behalf of our afflicted city." Provisions and supplies were sent to the afflicted city. It was, as Thacher says, "a memorable event in the history of the United States." The number of deaths remained below 20 a day until the 28th of August. By the middle of September it was ranging about 50, but rose to nearly 100 before the end of the month. On the 9th of October it went up to 102 and on the 11th it reached the highest point, 119, and for the next two days was but little below that figure. A refreshing rain fell on the 15th of October. By October the death rate had fallen to about 50 a day, and by the end of the month was about 20. The first week in November, the mortality was about twelve *per diem*, and it came down to 6 on the 9th, making the total mortality since August 1st, 4,044. The general estimate places it at 5,000, or about one-tenth of the entire population.

The most radical method of treatment, employed in this epidemic, and the one that attracted the most attention and the severest criticism, was that of Dr. Rush. Bleeding and purging were its chief features. "Never before," he writes, "did I experience such sublime joy as I now felt in contemplating the success of my remedies. It repaid me for all the toils and studies of my life. The conquest of this formidable disease was not the effect of accident, nor of the application of a single remedy; but it was the triumph of a principle in medicine. The reader will not wonder at this joyful state of my mind, when I add a short extract from my notebook, dated the 10th of September: 'Thank God! Out of one hundred patients, whom I have visited, or prescribed for, this day, I have lost none.'" The medication upon which he placed the strongest reliance is thus described: "It was," says Dr. Charles Caldwell (r), a pupil at the time, a "mixture of ten grains of calomel and ten of jalap—a dose which is now accounted mod-

(r) Autobiography of Charles Caldwell, M. D., 1855.

erate, at least, if not diminutive. But previously to that time calomel had never been so copiously administered in Philadelphia, nor, as far as I am informed, in any other part of the Middle or Eastern Atlantic States. From three to five or six grains of that article had been regarded until then as an ample dose." Many of his opposers called it "the dose of ten and ten;" Dr. Rush said: "Dr. Kuhn (s) called it a *murderous* dose! Dr. Hodge called it a *dose for a horse!* And Barton called it a *devil* of a dose!" Dr. Rush gave the prescription to the apothecaries, and, in fact, to anyone who would use it, and the former were taxed beyond their capacity to supply the demand for it. He does not hesitate to say that "not less than 6,000 of the inhabitants of Philadelphia probably owe their lives to purging and bleeding, during the late autumn." He employed five of his pupils to assist him, in compounding this prescription. Many physicians adopted the method, the first of them being Drs. Griffitts, Dr. Say (t), Dr. Pennington, and among the younger pupils, Drs. Leib (t), Porter, Annan, Woodhouse and Mease. It is not the province of the historian to discuss questions of therapeutics. Suffice it to say that the pertinacity with which Rush upheld his method as a specific in yellow fever, gave rise to fierce dissension, led to his resignation from the College of Physicians, and, in other ways, influenced his subsequent career.

The physicians did nobly, as a rule, and suffered greatly. "Rarely has it happened," writes Mathew Carey, one of the public committee, "that so large a proportion of the gentlemen of the faculty, have sunk beneath the labors of their dangerous profession, as on this occasion. In five or six weeks, exclusive of medical students, no less than ten physicians have been swept off, Doctors

---

(s) Dr. Kuhn, in a manuscript lecture in the College of Physicians, expresses himself thus: "Much the greater number, however, of those who died, as I am informed, were attended by gentlemen who were advocates of plentiful bleeding, and purging with calomel and jalap." He thinks the fact that the great mortality occurred after that treatment became prevalent is significant.

(t) Dr. Benjamin Say, 1756-1813, was a graduate of 1780, and active in humane societies. Dr. Michael Leib, 1759-1822, was a student of Dr. Rush. He became prominent in politics.

Hutchinson, Morris, Linn (u), Pennington, Dodds, Johnson, Glentworth, Phile, Graham and Green. Scarcely one of the practicing doctors that remained in the city, escaped sickness. Some were three, four and five times confined." Of these Dr. James Hutchinson, the most prominent, was port physician and secretary of the College of Physicians, a man whom Dr. Rush described as being "nearly as large as Goliath of Gath." He was a native of Bucks County, Pennsylvania, born in 1752, and received his education at well-known academies of the day, and at the College of Philadelphia, from which he was graduated with honors. After studying medicine under Dr. Evans, he went to London in 1774 and studied under Dr. Fothergill. On his return, in 1777, he bore dispatches from Minister Franklin at Paris, and when, in sight of the American coast, a British cruiser fired upon the ship, he braved the fire in an open boat and landed safely with his dispatches, leaving on the captured vessel his medical books and other personal effects. He soon entered the army as surgeon-general of his native province, served through the war, and also became a member of the Committee of Safety. He became a professor of Materia Medica and later of Chemistry, and was prominent in public affairs, having the friendship of Washington and other eminent leaders. Dr. Kuhn was called to see him on the last day of August, and continued to attend him until he himself became ill. Dr. Currie (v) visited him from this time until his death. Dr. Barton seems to have been called in consultation by Currie, and Dr. Rush also called and volunteered suggestions as to treatment. It is scarcely necessary to say that he recommended free purgation, not-

---

(u) Lynn is the proper spelling. The Glentworth above mentioned is not George Glentworth. The latter died in November, 1792. It may have been Peter Glentworth or another of that family, or Carey may have made a mistake. Dr. Rush speaks very highly of Pennington and Morris, whose deaths he witnessed.

(v) Dr. William Currie, a native of Chester county, Pennsylvania, was born in 1754, and, although educated for the Episcopal Church, became one of Dr. Kearsley's pupils and attended lectures at the medical school, although there is no record of his having received a degree. He was a surgeon of the Revolution, became a member of the Board of Health, and was senior physician of Magdalen Asylum. He was a prominent physician, an amiable man, although inclined to a love for satire. He died in 1828.

withstanding the fact that he had had "near thirty stools in three days." He died on the 7th of September. "Eminent as a practitioner, he fell a victim to his noble efforts in behalf of the humbler class of his fellow citizens."

When the epidemic came to an end, a warm controversy arose concerning the origin of the pestilence which had devastated the city. The results of the experience so painfully acquired were various. The best reports of autopsies were made, in the early part of the epidemic, at Bush Hill, by Dr. Philip Syng Physick, who had started in practice in the previous autumn, in association with Dr. Cathrall. The chief work of observation, that attended with the greatest public results, was performed by the College of Physicians, which body was clearly recognized by Governor Mifflin as the official organ of the profession. On October 30th, he addressed a letter to the College asking its advice concerning the means of preventing a recurrence of the epidemic. The questions of origin, contagiousness and treatment had divided the profession into two parties; Dr. Rush, whose opinions were widely accepted by the public, being the leader of a small minority, and Drs. Kuhn, Currie, Hutchinson, Barton and others, leading the majority. The contest became so bitter that, when a committee was chosen to answer the Governor, "the most rounded physician of Philadelphia" was omitted from the list, and a second committee finally reported in favor of origin by importation, contrary to the conviction of Dr. Rush. (w). Dr. Rush then felt obliged to resign from the College of Physicians, and in a letter of November 5th, 1793, accompanied by the presentation of an edition of Sydenham's works, he severed his relations with the institution he had been so active in founding. It was at this period that the influence of Rush, both with the medical profession and the public in general, was greatest, and he set out still more aggressively to promulgate his system of medical theory and practice.

(w) The publication of the opinion was not until the 26th; that, however, was merely incidental. Drs. Redman, Foulke and Leib dissented from it, although, as president, Dr. Redman signed it.

He published an exhaustive volume on the late epidemic, which remains to this day the authority on the fatal scourge of '93. In spite of their dissensions, however, the profession had done such valuable work that the Governor and Assembly, in March, 1794, asked the College for suggestions for a better health law. The result was the establishment of a law providing for a health office, with twenty-five inspectors, a health officer, a consulting physician, and a resident physician, at the lazaretto, or "marine hospital," as it was called. This body became known as the Board of Health and had especial charge of the "marine" and "city" hospitals, the latter referring to Bush Hill and its successors. It is the first legal ancestor of the present health board organization, although it did not assume the character of the modern board until some years later.

During the rest of the decade the yellow fever visited different cities in successive years. In 1793, Philadelphia was the only sufferer. In '94, she had but few cases, but havoc was wrought in Baltimore and New Haven; while in 1795, the fever visited New York, Norfolk and Charleston, and in '96 invaded Boston and some other places. Then, in '97, it returned with virulence to Philadelphia and carried off above 1,200. The epidemic of '97 began on a vessel at the Pine street wharf on July 23rd. Other vessels were attacked by the end of the month and the disease spread toward Southwark, with isolated cases throughout the city. Several physicians died, among whom were Drs. Annan (x), Pleasants and Thompson. One of the most important results of this epidemic, from an historical standpoint, had its origin in a letter of Governor Mifflin to Dr. Rush, dated November 6th, of which the following is an extract: "I have requested the opinion of the College of Physicians on the subject, but, as I understand that you and many other learned members of the Faculty do not attend the deliberations of that institution, the result of my inquiries cannot

---

(x) Dr. William Annan, who was one of the original Bush Hill attendants of '93 and a member of the College of Physicians, died October 4, 1797, a young man. Among those who were seriously ill, were Drs. Physick, Reynolds, Strong, Boys, B. Duffield, Hayworth, Church and Caldwell.

be perfectly satisfactory without your co-operation and assistance." Dr. Rush summoned his friends about him and prepared a report which emphasized the points at issue and especially that of the origin of the fever. It was signed by Drs. Benjamin Rush, Charles Caldwell, William Dewees, John Redman Coxe, Philip Syng Physick, James Reynolds, Francis Bowes Sayre, John C. Otto, William Boys, Samuel Cooper, James Stuart, Felix Pascalis and Joseph Strong. Most of these were young practitioners. Not long after, there appeared in The Weekly Magazine a notice that: "A Society for investigating the causes for the late mortality in this city is about to be instituted," and subscribers were directed to inquire at 41 Chestnut street. On the 8th of January, 1798, the above named and some other gentlemen formed "The Academy of Medicine of Philadelphia." Dr. Physick was president; Drs. Caldwell and Reynolds vice-presidents, and Dr. Sayre secretary. Other names mentioned in the scanty records of the Society are Drs. Budd, Heylin, Gallaher, Mease and La Roche. From the first official report of the Academy, dated March 20th, it is evident that its principal object was to promulgate what its members considered correct views of the nature and origin of yellow fever. The Society seems not to have lasted much more than a year or two, and some of its founders, six years later, organized the Medical Lyceum. The latter continued in existence for more than a decade. The American Medical Society still existed, and the Philadelphia Medical Society had been resurrected and included members of all societies in its weekly meetings. It does not anywhere appear that Dr. Rush, in founding the Academy of Medicine, had any intention of impairing the prestige of the College of Physicians; or that, in resigning from the latter, he had any other design than that of promoting harmony. In his brief letter of resignation he subscribed himself the "College's well wisher," and further testified his kindly feeling by presenting to the library of the institution a copy of Wallis' edition of the works of Sydenham (y).

The epidemic of 1798 was, in some respects, more severe than

(y) This copy is no longer in the library of the college.

that of '93. In April, an efficient Board of Health was constituted. Cases of yellow fever appeared as early as June 2d, and immediately stringent sanitary laws and rigorous regulations were enforced. Vessels arriving on the 5th of July from the West Indies were supposed, by some, to harbor the fever. It first prevailed extensively in Water Street, between Spruce and Walnut, and during the first week in August, there were fifty-three deaths. By this time, the city was being deserted more rapidly than in '93, and, probably, before the middle of September, three times as many persons as in the last-named epiemic, had fled. Some who had previously remained, now abandoned their homes. "The number who fled from the city," says one account (z), "has been estimated at three-fourths to five-sixths of the whole inhabitants; the total number of inhabitants has been estimated at fifty to seventy thousand." Drs. Physick and Cooper had charge of the City Hospital; Drs. Sayre, Mease and Kinlaid, were inspectors of the northern part of the city; Drs. Church and B. Duffield of the southern, and Dr. S. Duffield had charge of the poor. The malignancy and fatality were at first greater than in '93. The physicians who remained at their posts in the city were Drs. Rush, Griffitts, Mease, Wistar, Gallaher, Caldwell, Harris, Conover, Proudfit, Leib, Church, Boys, S. Duffield, B. Duffield, Parke, Stuart, Strong, Biglow, Kinlaid, Pfiefer, Yeatman, Trexo, Monges, Pascallis, La Roche and Devivier (a). Dr. Cooper was the first victim among the physicians. The City Hospital on Sassafras Street, on the east bank of the Schuylkill River, was in a bad place, and tents were substituted near Spruce and Chestnut streets, which were ready by the 24th of August. These accommodated nearly 2,000, and proved so advantageous that another camp was established at Master's Place, two miles north, on the Germantown road. The rate of mortality per day, beginning in the neighborhood of 20 as early as the 11th of August, crept up to near 50 by the 26th; it exceeded 100 on September 28th, when it reached 106, the highest

---

(z)) An excellent history by Thomas Condie and Richard Folwell, 1798.
(a) Drs. Currie, Sayre and Dewees are also said to have remained.

rate of the season. It dropped to near 50 about October 3d, and by November 5th, a total of over 3,645 interments was recorded. The estimate of 4,000 was believed to cover all the deaths in and near the city. The next year (1799) the disease first appeared in Penn street, and, according to the Board of Health, the mortality was 1,276. In 1802-'3-'5-'19 and '20, the disease prevailed more or less extensively, the mortality ranging from a minimum of 20 to a maximum of 400. These frequently recurring epidemics had a most disastrous effect upon the trade of Philadelphia, and "forever ruined its mere commercial supremacy" (b).

The most eminent physician in America was also the chief of the many heroes who battled with the pestilence. It was chiefly his writings on yellow fever that won for him from Europe the title of the "Sydenham of America." "When this grand production," said Dr. Lettsom of London, "uniting in an almost unprecedented degree, sagacity and judgment, first appeared, Europe was astonished. Even at this moment I cannot recall to mind the phenomena connected with the rise, progress and effect of that dreadful malady without admiration, and the conduct of the physicians without veneration. Contemplate this illustrious Professor, emerging from the prostration of strength induced by this fever; his aged mother dying; his sister a corpse; his pupils dead around him; flying from house to house, wherever infection is raging; at home, his apartments filled with supplicants diseased and dying; Death almost everywhere stalking over the victims from the raging pestilence; he, nevertheless, braves the uplifted and poisoned dart, emulating the Father of the Apollonean art at the plague of Athens and the descendants of Æsculapius at the siege of Troy. If there is an example of heroic fortitude—of disinterested exposure to peril for the public welfare anywhere recorded in medical history, superior to those which dignified this unappalled and luminous

(b) Address of Dr. S. Wier Mitchell, 1887. New York became first in population in 1810, when Philadelphia numbered 95,000. The first American novelist, Charles Brockden Brown, of Philadelphia, found material for one of his novels, Arthur Mervyn, in the worst of these years, '93.

Philanthropist, let that character be venerated as one of the first benefactors of mankind."

"La conduite du Dr. Rush," wrote the celebrated Zimmerman in 1794, "a mérité, que non seulement, la ville de Philadelphie, mais l'humanité entière lui élève une statue," and a century later an eminent member (c) of the profession in America said, in the calmer pose of educating them. Locating on Market street, just below and grown, and it seems not unlikely that he will remain forever with us, not it may be, as the greatest of our physicians, but as the first of our great physicians."

This estimate by a most competent critic, is correct in so far as it applies to Rush, the physician. He was, however, not only a great physician, but a great deal more. When, to his life work as a physician, are added his labors in the fields of politics, social science and philosophy, the sum total is such as to excite the highest admiration. Still an essential element of true greatness would have been lacking had not Rush been a man of the greatest firmness of purpose, united with stainless integrity. Taking him "for all in all," he stands out prominently amid a crowd of distinguished contemporaries and successors, as the *greatest man* in the medical profession of America.

It was unfortunate for his happiness in life, and perhaps also for his posthumous reputation, that he possessed so facile a pen and so eloquent a tongue. A man who is sluggish in repartee and who finds writing an insuperable task, may acquire a reputation for toleration and meek endurance of injury, which is properly to be ascribed to dullness and stupidity. Rush was ever aggressive in attack and resolute in defence, and, as is well known, he made many enemies; for it is one thing to convict and quite another to convince an antagonist.

Descended from Friends, although not a member of their Society, Rush, at the most impressible period of his life, had breathed the atmosphere of Princeton, which, as is well known, is

---

(c) Address before the American Medical Association, in 1889, by William Pepper, M. D., LL. D.

largely compounded of Scotch philosophy. Later, he became imbued with the scientific spirit of the day, of which his friend, Franklin, was the ablest living exponent. Nevertheless, Princeton's yearning for a constructive system, as the highest product of truth, dominated Benjamin Rush, from his school days with Finley down to the latest period of his life. This was the basis of his mental and moral character, and this it was which led to his differences with Washington and with the leaders of the medical profession. Washington was preëminently practical, and well knew that a republic, especially in its beginnings, must of necessity partake of the imperfections of its constituents. On the other hand, Rush longed for an ideal system of government, without sufficiently appreciating the fact that it would require ideal men to conduct it. The republic, as it was, was a sore disappointment to him. So with his conflict with the medical profession. Given a mind like that of Rush, dominated by the love of a constructive philosophical system, placed in a community dominated by the scientific spirit of Franklin, and misunderstanding and conflict were inevitable.

When the country closed with that awful decade of pestilence, Dr. Rush was fifty-five years of age and in his prime. Many of his contemporaries were dead; some had given up active life and from some he was estranged by his uncompromising adherence to his convictions of duty. The younger men of the profession, some of whom were to be the leaders of medical science in the future, were his most devoted adherents. The history of his life is as follows: He was born on his father's farm in Byberry Township (about fourteen miles northeast of Philadelphia) on the day preceding Christmas of 1745. It was in 1745 that Dr. Cadwalader published the first medical book in the province. John Rush, the great-grandfather of Dr. Rush, a favorite captain of horse in Cromwell's army, came to Pennsylvania after the death of the great Protector. James, the Captain's son, had a child, John, who was Benjamin's father. Both the grandfather and father of the doctor were gunsmiths, as well as farmers. John Rush, the father, and the Rev. Samuel Finley married sisters, who were earnest Presbyterians and women of great strength of character. Mr. Rush died when Benjamin was but six years old, leaving his widow, Susanna Morris Rush, and two children, Benjamin and a younger child, Jacob. They were so fortunate as to have for their guardian such a man as the excellent preacher and principal of Nottingham Academy. Mrs. Rush had great ambitions for her sons, and, upon her husband's death, at once removed to Philadelphia to earn money for the purpose of educating them. Locating on Market street, just below Second, she opened a grocery and provision store, with the sign of "The Blazing Star," and hallowed the place with her lofty aims. When Benjamin was about eight or nine years old he went to live with his uncle Finley in Nottingham, Maryland, about sixty miles southwest of Philadelphia, where the latter was the pastor of a church in the neighborhood, and head of Nottingham Academy. Rev. Samuel Finley, D. D., was famous both as a preacher and a teacher. He was subsequently called to the presidency of the College of New Jersey. Nottingham was an ideal location for an academy in those days. "The inhabitants of this retired spot," says Dr. David Ramsay, in 1813, "were plain country farmers, who cultivated so indifferent a soil that they could not derive a living from it without strict economy and the daily labor of their own hands. Their whole time was occupied in providing the necessary supplies for their support in passing through the world, and in preparing them for a better. To assist them in the latter, they enjoyed the blessings of public preaching and the faithful evangelical labors of one of the wisest and best of men. In their comparatively distressed situation, as to worldly matters, their morals were a virtual reproach to the inhabitants of many districts who enjoyed a much greater proportion of the good things of this life. Almost every dwelling house was so far a church that the reading of the word of God, and the offering up of family prayers, generally recurred every day; there were few, or rather no examples of, or temptations to, immorality of any kind." There was plain living and high thinking. "Among these people," he continues, "remarkable for their simplicity, industry, morality and religion, young Rush spent five years of his early youth in acquiring a knowledge of the Greek and Latin languages. Here also he learned much of human nature, and began to class mankind according to their state of society, a distinction of which he profited very much in his future speculations in political philosophy. The transition from the variegated scenes of Philadelphia to this sequestered seat of learning, industry and religious habits, could not fail of making a strong impression on his observing mind. He there acquired a reverence for religion—its consistent professors and teachers; a prepossession in favor of regular, orderly conduct, of diligence, industry, punctual attention to business, and in general of such steady habits as stamped a value of his character through life. In laying a solid foundation for correct principles and conduct he was essentially aided by the faultless example, judicious advice and fatherly care of the learned and pious Dr. Finley. This accomplished instructor of youth was not only diligent and successful in communicating useful knowledge, but extended his views far beyond the ordinary routine of a common education. He trained his pupils for both worlds, and in his intercourse with them had respect to their future as well as present state of existence. To young Rush he was devoted by peculiar ties; for he was fatherless and the son of the sister of his beloved wife. A reciprocation of affection took place between the parties, much to the credit and advantage of both. Benjamin Rush found a father in his Uncle Finley, and when adult, repaid the obligation in kind by acting the part of father to his son, James E. B. Finley, left an orphan when very young by the death of his father in 1766. This new obligation was gratefully acknowledged by the subject of it, particularly by giving the name of Benjamin Rush to his first-born son." These pleasant associations did much to influence young Rush, and his progress was so rapid that he entered Princeton in his fourteenth year under President Davies, and received his degree of Bachelor of Arts before the end of his fifteenth year, in 1760. He was educated in the profoundest sense of the term education, for he had a mind that naturally sought high levels and was led by instinct into the best channels in its search for knowledge. As he himself afterward said of another, he "possessed a great and original genius. By genius, in the present instance, I mean a power in the human mind of discovering the relation of distant truths by the shortest train of intermediate propositions. This precious gift of heaven is composed of a vigorous imagination, quick sensibility, a talent for extensive and accurate observation, a faithful memory and a sound judgment." The mind of Benjamin Rush was independent in its modes of thinking. He sought for the foundation principles that underlie the whole structure of truth. This characteristic, which manifested itself quite early in his career, was very marked throughout his life. The gift which he possessed of giving ready and forcible expression to his thoughts supplied him with another source of power, and most diligently did he labor to cultivate it by the study of rhetoric.

The time now came for his choice of a special life work. No field in America, among the professions, called more loudly for an investigating mind than that of medicine. Dr. Finley must have realized this, for he is said to have encouraged Benjamin Rush to enter it. The young man therefore began a six years' apprenticeship with Dr. Redman, according to the methods then adopted in professional training. Hippocrates was one of the first authors to whom he was introduced, whose works he translated into English; Sydenham and Boerhaave were also translated by him. The spirit of science now began to be awakened. His observations and experiments were as original and extensive as Franklin's were at his age. He made much of writing—"saved the thoughts other men throw away," and by his methods made of his mind a sort of mental laboratory and storeroom, which was of the greatest value in later years. At the same time, he thus improved his literary style. In his seventeenth year, 1762, he helped Dr. Redman in the yellow fever epidemic, writing his own observations of the disease. These, with Dr. Redman's own account, furnish the only records we possess of that plague. He was among Dr. Shippen's pupils that year also, and engaged with the greatest industry and enthusiasm in laying broad foundations in both medicine and general culture during the years of his apprenticeship up to the time of the founding of a medical school by Morgan. So close was his application that he only lost two days in those six years. He began his first public writing when nineteen years of age, and his pen was busy, ever after, on themes so varied, original and catholic that his medical writings form but one section of his work. His mind was as universal as Franklin's. So many-sided is he that no other figure in the medical history of Philadelphia is so difficult to portray, not because of the insufficiency of material for a biography of him, but because of his intense and profound personality (d). His description of Cullen is suggestive of himself. Alluding to his definition of genius already referred to, he says: "His imagination surveyed all nature at a glance, and, like a camera obscura, seemed to produce in his mind a picture of the whole visible creation. His sensibility was so exquisite that the smallest portion of truth acted upon it. By means of talent for observation he collected knowledge from everything he heard, saw or read, and from every person with whom he conversed. His memory was the faithful repository of all his ideas, and appeared to be alike accurate upon all subjects. Over each of these faculties of his mind a sound judgment presided, by means of which he discovered the relation of ideas to each other, and thereby produced those new combinations which constitute principles in science. This process of the mind has been called invention and is totally different from a mere capacity of acquiring learning, or collecting knowledge from the discoveries of others. It elevates man to a

(d) It is a well-known fact that much of his manuscript journal, autobiography, and the like, are reserved from the public, for the appearance of a biographer who can give him the sympathetic, impartial and adequate treatment he deserves. Only two or three short addresses and articles fitly representing his versatility exist. Ramsay has shown his character as a physician with sympathy; Richardson has given a glimpse of his catholicity of mind; Pepper has emphasized his ability as an organizer and his constructive genius, and Jackson has been his defender. Others give narrative or eulogy for the most part, so that his works are, after all, his best biography.

distant resemblance of his maker, for the discovery of truth is the perception of things as they appear to the Divine Mind." Rush himself certainly possessed the capacity for invention. Again, he says: "The difference between error and truth is very small." He listened to authorities great and small only so far as they carried conviction to his mind. "To believe in great men," said he, "is often as great an obstacle to the progress of knowledge as to believe in witches and conjurers. It is the image worship of science; for error is as much an attribute of man as the desire of happiness; and I think I have observed that the errors of great men partake of the dimensions of their minds, and are often of a greater magnitude than the errors of men of inferior understanding." This independent love of truth, without regard to its source, was so natural to him that it seemed absurd to him that some men should resent it. He would base his practice as readily upon a principle discovered by a comparatively unknown physician in a neighboring province as he would upon one of which Cullen or Sydenham were the discoverers. This feature of his mind is well illustrated in his essay on "Common Sense." "I consider it," he says, after giving Reed's definition, "as the perception of things as they appear to the *greatest* part of mankind. It has no relation to their being *true* or *false*, *right* or *wrong*, *proper* or *improper*. For the sake of perspicuity, I shall define it to be *Opinions and Feelings in unison with the Opinions and Feelings of the bulk of Mankind*. From this definition it is evident that common sense must necessarily differ in different ages and countries, and, in both, must vary with the progress of taste, science and religion. In the uncultivated state of reason the opinions and feelings of a majority of mankind will be wrong, and, of course, their common or universal sense will partake of their errors. In the cultivated state of reason, just opinions and feelings will become general, and the common sense of the majority will be in unison with truth." The result of this attitude of mind, in himself, led to his ignoring the common or prevalent ideas of his time. He discovered and advocated new principles in connection with such subjects as agriculture, temperance, slavery, suffrage, education, morals and religion. These were far beyond the appreciation of his own age, although accepted as axioms in our day. In some of his views he may be said to have been in advance of our own time. It is needless to say that the faults in the character of this great man were as great as his virtues, for they partook of the "dimensions of his mind." They can easily be magnified, however, out of all proportion to their relative importance in forming an estimate of his character. His was the attitude of the fearless reformer, who, acting through the courage of his convictions, marches on with unswerving purpose to the accomplishment of his ends. He "speaks with authority" to both high and low, knowing no height but truth and no depth but ignorance. This gave the force of originality to his criticisms, making them often as caustic as the acid of the chemist. Such was Rush at the age of twenty-one. In 1766 he left Dr. Redman's tuition, when Dr. Morgan was planning the establishment of a medical school, and went to the great University of Edinburgh, which "a Cullen supported and dignified." During the two years he spent in the Scotch capital, there is no doubt that he owed much to the influence of Cullen. He says of Cullen that "he appeared to have overstepped the slow and tedious forms of the schools, and, by force of his understanding, to have seized upon the great ends of learning without the assistance of many of those means which were contrived for the use of less active minds." Cullen "was an accurate anatomist and an ingenious physiologist. He enlarged the boundaries and established the utility of Chemistry and thereby prepared the way for the discoveries and fame of his illustrious pupil, Dr. Black. He stripped materia medica of most of the errors that had been accumulating in it for two thousand years, and reduced it to a simple and practical science. He was intimately acquainted with all the branches of natural history and philosophy. He had studied every ancient and modern system of physic. He found the system of Dr. Boerhaave universally adopted when he accepted a chair in the University of Edinburgh. This system was founded chiefly on the supposed presence of certain acrid particles in the fluids, and in the departure of these, in point of consistency, from a natural state. Dr. Cullen's first object was to expose the errors of this pathology, and to teach his pupils to seek for the cause of diseases in the solids. Nature is always coy. Ever since she was driven from the heart, by the discovery of the circulation of the blood, she has concealed herself in the brain and nerves. Here she was pursued by Dr. Cullen; and if he has not dragged her to public view, he has left us a clew which must in time conduct us to her last recess in the human body. Many, however, of the operations of nature in the nervous system have been explained by him; and no candid man will ever explain the whole of them, without acknowledging that the foundation of his successful inquiries was laid by the discoveries of Dr. Cullen." It was thus most natural that Rush should have chosen to become a physician rather than a surgeon, and that Chemistry should have proven his special field. His thesis was on a chemical experiment designed to discover what part fermentation had in digestion, and to prove that in three hours after deglutition, the aliment in the stomach did undergo acetous fermentation. The manner in which he used his own stomach as a laboratory was characteristic of him. His paper was executed in an elegant Latin and was entitled: *De Coctione Ciborum in Ventriculo* (e), "a performance so accurate in experiment," says Dr. Lettsom, "and so ingenious and lucid in diction, as to have placed him in a prominent and honorable point of estimation in that celebrated school." He received his degree in 1768 at the age of twenty-three.

Two interesting incidents of his student life may be noted. One occurred while he was in Scotland, the other after he went to London in the early winter of the year 1768-9. As has been said, President Finley of Princeton died in 1766, and Rev. Dr. Witherspoon of Paisley was chosen to be his successor, but declined. A year later he was approached again, the trustees of Princeton

---

(e) A copy, published by the Edinburgh School in 1768, is in the British Museum of London and the College of Physicians of this city. It is dedicated to Franklin, Redman, Shippen, Morgan, and Smith, and to Jacob Rush, his brother. He closes with a grateful tribute to Cullen.

choosing their brilliant young alumnus, Rush, to undertake the delicate task both of persuading Dr. Witherspoon to realize the importance of the great work open to him, and that of convincing the presbytery with which he was connected, that it was their duty to let him go. Dr. Witherspoon was an able disciple of the philosophy of Reid, and the Presbyterians of America wanted Princeton to become their leading institution. No man was better fitted than Rush to bring Witherspoon and Princeton together. The successful issue of the attempt may be said to have determined the subsequent career of Princeton—his beloved *alma mater*. That Rush was no less able in political than in philosophical controversy, is illustrated by the following incident:

Soon after he went to London, he attended, on one occasion, a society for general discussion, when the question of the American colonial controversy came up. A member was speaking in eloquent denunciation of the spirit of rebellion manifested by the colonists, and incidentally asserted that even if America had cannon she had not ball to fire from them. Dr. Rush arose, and "in his reply," says Dr. Lettsom, "he observed that if the Americans possessed no cannon-balls they could supply the deficiency by digging up the skulls of those ancestors who had courted expatriation from the old hemisphere under the vivid hope of enjoying more ample freedom in the new one."

That winter in London, and a portion of the following summer spent in Paris, closed his European experience, and he returned to Philadelphia, to join the faculty of the new school of medicine, and to commence the career which led him subsequently to find his name echoed from one end of the old world to the other, kings and emperors applauding his work and showing their appreciation of his deeds by medals of honor. Such was the man who began his work in Philadelphia in 1769 as the first Professor of Chemistry in the new medical school, the brightest ornament of its talented faculty. His twenty-two years in the chair of Chemistry helped to establish the reputation of the institution. After the reorganization of the school in 1791, he was for six years professor of the Institutes of Medicine, and, following the resignation of Dr. Kuhn, he included among his lectures those upon the Theory and Practice of Medicine, continuing to fill both chairs for sixteen years. The twenty-two years following were, however, the years of his greatest influence upon the medical history of America and the world. Indeed, it has been said that during this latter period "the history of Rush's work is largely the history of American medicine" (f). It was here that not only his mental and moral equipment, but also his splendid powers of expression, both oral and written, molded probably two-thirds of all the medical students of his time (g), comprising two generations. It has been estimated that he publicly taught considerably over two thousand students, while his office at home was always a hive of apprentices. These were not confined to the western continent, but included many students from Europe. The famous Cullen himself wrote of Rush in 1768 (h): "It is very convenient for me to write by Rush, for if I was to do it by some other hands, I should think myself obliged to give you the medical history of Europe, but I know he can give it to you in a better manner." Sixteen years later he wrote to Rush himself: "I shall always hold it as my highest honor that the founders of the medical school of Philadelphia were all of them my pupils, and if it can be known, I think it will be the most certain means of transmitting my name to a distant posterity, for I believe that this school will one day or other be the greatest in the world." Four years after this, 1788, he writes: "We have had for a year or two past much fewer gentlemen coming to us from America than formerly, and whether it is owing to their becoming wiser in judging that they can be as well instructed at home, or to any other cause, I cannot well determine." Again he says: "The medical school of Philadelphia, as the chief of a great empire, must

---

(f) Dr. Pepper's address.

(g) "We find, therefore, only five medical schools in existence in the United States in 1810," said Dr. N. S. Davis at the Centennial Medical Congress, "with an aggregate number of medical students in attendance of about 650, of whom about 100 received in that year the degree of either Bachelor or Doctor of Medicine. Two-thirds of this whole number were in the University of Pennsylvania."

(h) Letter to Dr. Morgan. Rush manuscripts at Ridgeway Library.

flourish more and more, while I am afraid the University of Edinburgh may decline with the declining state of Great Britain." It was about this time that Rush began to modify the system of Cullen that he had advocated. "In the autumn of 1789," says Dr. Ramsay, "I visited Dr. Rush and was received by him in his study. He said he was preparing for his next course of lectures in self-defense; that the system of Cullen was tottering; that Dr. John Brown had brought forward some new and luminous principles of medicine, but they were mixed with others which were extravagant; that he saw a gleam of light before him, leading to a more simple and consistent system of medicine than the world had yet seen, and pointed out some of its leading features." This system, which he ever after sought to work out, was characteristic of his mind, and was based upon "the unity of disease." "This wonderful vision," says one biographer (i), "may be thus explained. Excitement or Life is a unit, and this can be accurately divided into healthy and morbid only; hence there can be but one disease, that is, morbid excitement." This principle he worked out in his practice to a very large degree, though there is no evidence that he ever conceived his efforts to establish a complete system as more than a stage of medical progress. It is evident, however, that Rush yielded more and more to the dominance of his love for a philosophical system, and consequently grew farther and farther away from the spirit of inductive science which was so strong in his earlier years. The inflexibility with which he held to his system as a conviction is indicated by what he says of consultations, as early as 1793: "I have passed over the slanders which were propagated against me by some of my brethren. I have mentioned them only for the sake of declaring in this public manner that I most heartily forgive them, and that if I discovered at any time an undue sense of the unkindness and cruelty of those slanders, it was not because I felt myself injured by them, but because I was sure they would irreparably injure my fellow citizens by lessening their confidence

---

(i) Dr. Samuel Jackson (of Northumberland) in Lives of Eminent American Physicians and Surgeons. 1861.

in the only remedies that I believed to be effectual in the reigning epidemic. One thing in my conduct toward these gentlemen may require justification, and that is, my refusing to consult with them. A Mahometan and a Jew might as well attempt to worship the Supreme Being in the same temple, and through the medium of the same ceremonies, as two physicians of opposite principles and practice attempt to confer about the life of the same patient. What is done in consequence of such negotiations (for they are not consultations) is the ineffectual result of neutralized opinions."

When advised to leave the city in the epidemic, he said: "I resolved to stick to my principles, my practice and my patients to the last extremity." So far as in him lay he was determined that the principles he held should be universally recognized as forming the basis of scientific medicine. Opposing views might be as thick as tiles upon the housetops; he ignored them. This fearlessness of consequences subjected him to what was probably the fiercest attacks ever made upon any physician in the history of medicine. The assaults of his enemies reached their climax after 1793, when they assumed their bitterest form in a series of articles which appeared in "Porcupine's Gazette," and which were written by a most drastic satirist, William Cobbett. Cobbett was an Englishman, of Tory tendencies, in Philadelphia, who aspired to be an American Le Sage, under the cognomen *Peter Porcupine*. He began his vituperations in September, 1797, which soon became so scandalous that a libel suit was brought against him. Two years later, being convicted of slander, he was required to pay a fine of $5,000, which Rush is said to have distributed among the poor. This so enraged Cobbett that he went to New York and continued his publication under the name, *The Rush Light*, and which he finally removed to London. He imitated Le Sage's attack on Botallus, calling Rush "the Sangrada of America." Dr. Rush was once even challenged to a duel, a not uncommon episode in those times. Although his friends were as strong and loyal as his enemies were implacable, he sometimes wearied of the strife. His teachings, his character and the force of his example, however, only became the more widely influential. He was an acknowledged authority in medicine; learned societies at home and abroad honored him; governments of both hemispheres sought his advice on epidemics; the King of Prussia granted him a medal, and the Emperor of Russia presented him with a diamond ring. Similar testimonials from many other sources were not lacking. Hundreds of young men went forth from his teachings, inspired by him to lofty conceptions of professional usefulness. His public addresses, his writings and his conversation, were regarded by Rush as the chosen instruments by which his own earnest convictions of truth and duty were to be impressed on other minds, and he was ever ready and forcible in their use.

In his works, we have the most splendid achievements of his career. In comparison with these, the details of his life sink into insignificance. It is not the purpose here to enter into them (j). We have the following description of him as he appeared during the last five years of his life to a student (k): "He was above the middle height, very erect, rather slender, with small bones and rather thin, his hands and wrists, feet and ankles, being small and finely formed. His face was thin, nose aquiline, eyes beautifully

---

(j) Lives such as that of Dr. Rush cannot be condensed. He was great as a philosopher, a physician, a sanitarian, a politician, a statesman and patriot, an investigator, a writer, an orator, a leader, a teacher, a philanthropist, a diplomat, a Christian and a polished gentleman of the world. He was a friend of Paine, a student of Rousseau, a patron of Witherspoon and Nisbett, and the friend of the slave—so original and catholic were his sympathy and insight. He was a member of nearly all the great organizations of the time; he received the degree of LL. D. from Yale; he was the chief founder of Dickinson College, of the Society for the Protection of Free Negroes, the first to suggest the African Episcopal Church; he drafted the constitution of the Philadelphia Bible Society, and was treasurer of the Mint. His works on "Medical Inquiries and Observations," his "Essays, Literary, Moral and Philosophical," his "Lectures," his studies on the Mind, his editions of Sydenham, Pringle, Cleghorn and Hillary, his lay "Sermons," his fugitive contributions to the periodicals, and those unpublished were so numerous, powerful, and influential that they deserve to be treated in a separate work. No character in the annals of medicine offers a more interesting subject for biography. He deserves a great "Life" and a national monument.

(k) Dr. Samuel Jackson of Northumberland. The portrait of Dr. Rush that is best known is from a painting by Thomas Sully in 1812, and is said, by those who knew him, to be excellent.

set, large, blue, mild and benevolent; forehead broad and high; head long in the transverse diameter, and nearly bald from the crown forward; his hair clubbed behind and powdered; his face was of a fair and healthy complexion, not handsome or what is called fine-looking, for his cheeks were fallen in, many of his front teeth lost, and age and care had left its wrinkles. His countenance, in conversation, was highly animated; when reading to himself, or going abroad, it evinced intense thought, entire abstraction and firmness of purpose. His unfrequent smile was peculiarly gracious, but he hardly ever laughed. When walking the street, which was seldom, he was very erect, step firm, elastic and rather military, never using a staff, his arms folded on his breast; he uncovered to everyone, poor or rich, who uncovered to him, and his passing words were, 'I hope you are very well, sir,' uttered with habitually strong but mild voice. His dress was very plain, generally, of dark-colored cloth; he rode in a plain vehicle with two wheels and one horse, the same little negro by his side who had lived with him more than thirty years—master and man now grown old together. In this open carriage we saw him facing the storm the last winter of his life." In March, 1813, *"pneumonia typhoides"* became prevalent, and on April 14th, he was attacked. His friends, Drs. Mease, Dorsey, Griffitts and Physick and his son, Dr. James Rush, were in attendance. Dr. Mease was with him all day of the 19th, when his life closed, at the age of sixty-eight years. He was buried in Christ Church. "From one end of the United States to the other," says one of his students (l), "the event was productive of emotions of sorrow; for, since the death of Washington, no man, perhaps, in America was better known, more sincerely beloved, or held in higher admiration and esteem." "Another of our friends of '76 is gone, another of the co-signers of our country's independence," wrote Jefferson to John Adams, "and a better man than Rush could not have left us, more benevolent, more learned, of finer genius, or more honest." Posterity, Rush himself had said, "is to the physician what the day of judgment is to the

---

(l) Life of Rush in Delaplaine's Repository, by Charles Caldwell, M. D.

Christian," and posterity calls the great apostle of "the unity of disease," the Sydenham of America (n).

During the closing decade of Rush's life, practically the first decade of the new century, he was an elderly man in the sixties, while, almost without exception, every other member of the faculty of the University was about twenty years his junior. Most of these men were born between 1761 and '68. Several of them survived him but for a short time. Woodhouse died four years before Rush; Barton followed him two years later; Wistar only five years later; James survived him twenty-two years, and Physick and Dewees, twenty-four and twenty-nine years respectively. It was a decade of great activity and power in the development of medical science in Philadelphia; nearly every branch of the science was represented by strong men, who would have appeared even abler had they not been so closely associated with the towering figure of Rush, to whom not a little of their own activity was directly or indirectly due. Dr. James Woodhouse (m), one of his students, did excellent work in the chair of Chemistry from 1795 to his death in 1809, when he was succeeded by another favorite student, a grandson of Dr. Redman, Dr. John Redman Coxe, who had become prominent as the founder of medical journalism in Philadelphia, five years before. Dr. Philip Syng Physick, a special protégé of the doctor, had shown such originality in the field of surgery that Dr. Rush encouraged him in his purpose to become an independent lecturer on that subject, in 1800. The students of the University flocked to these lectures in such numbers

---

(n) Barton succeeded Rush as president of the Philadelphia Medical Society. Dr. Wistar was the successor of Rush in the presidency of the Society for the Abolition of Slavery.

(m) Dr. Woodhouse was a native Philadelphian, born in 1770; he received his Arts degree at the University in 1787, studied medicine with Dr. Rush and graduated in the first medical class, 1792, after the reorganization. He had medical service in the Indian campaigns of Gen. St. Clair, and showed such great ability in Chemistry in his student life that he was chosen to that chair over the eminent scientist, Dr. Adam Seybert. His lectures and experiments were so brilliant as to win from Priestley the high praise of being equal to any in Europe. He is said to have been the last of the American chemical leaders to believe in Phlogiston.

that in 1805 a division of the chair which embraced the subjects of anatomy, surgery and obstetrics was called for.

Shippen, and his associate Wistar, had heretofore lectured on these subjects. A new chair of Surgery was created, to which Physick was appointed, winning for himself the title of "the Father of American Surgery." Shippen, who had for some time allowed more and more of his duties to devolve upon his adjunct, since the appointment of the latter in 1792, was replaced by Physick in 1809. Upon Physick's assumption of the chair, Dr. Caspar Wistar announced his desire that a still further division be effected by the establishment of a chair of Obstetrics. This he secured in part in 1810, but not until the year Rush died, was midwifery fully recognized as a distinct branch of medicine, when Dr. Thomas C. James was appointed as the first Professor of Obstetrics in the University. To Dr. James, therefore, accrues the honor of giving this most important science its proper place in American medicine. Associated with James was a young man, Dr. N. Chapman (o). Upon the death of Rush, the subjects upon which he had lectured were apportioned among several chairs. Dr. Benj. S. Barton, who had followed Griffitts in '96, in the chair of Materia Medica, became Professor of Theory and Practice and the Institutes of Medicine. Born in 1766 in Lancaster, Pennsylvania, Barton was the son of an Episcopalian clergyman, whose wife was a sister of Rittenhouse. Early in life he came under the care of Rev. Dr. Andrews, later Provost of the University, and in 1782 joined his brother in Philadelphia and began study in the college and under Dr. Shippen's direction. His artistic and botanical tastes had shown themselves in boyhood, and in 1786 he went to Edinburgh for additional study. Here he won the Harveian prize from the Royal Medical Society for a botanical thesis; and the next year, while in London, he published his "Observations on Some Parts of Natural History." He became the friend of Lettsom, Hunter and other prominent men. After two years spent in Edinburgh he decided to take his degree from the University of Göttingen. After securing it he re-

(o) Young Chapman succeeded Barton in Materia Medica.

turned to London, and his reputation led to his election to the American Philosophical Society before he returned to Philadelphia. He was not twenty-three, in 1789, when William Bartram's chair of Botany was merged into a new chair of Natural History and Botany, which was created for Barton. He at once inspired his students with enthusiasm for the science; gave new interest to Bartram's Garden, founded an American Linnean Society, of which he was president, and established measures for the coöperation of students of natural history and botany in various parts of the country. He erected the first greenhouse in the city, in the rear of his Chestnut street residence, below Eighth. In his thirtieth year, he became Professor of Materia Medica, which position he held until the death of Rush. It was while he occupied this chair that he became still more widely known as the founder of a semi-annual periodical, "The Philadelphia Medical and Physical Journal," (1804-1809), the second journal of the kind in the city, and devoted more largely to botany than to medicine. It was thus he acquired the title of "the first teacher of Natural Science in this Atlantic world." He indeed "created a taste for these pursuits," says Dr. Carson, "that has never been lost in this community, and which has ultimately developed itself in permanent establishments for the cultivation of the Natural Sciences." He was the most natural successor to Rush in much of his work and thus received his later appointments. These he was enabled to fill but for a short time, when ill-health defeated his plans and closed his life December 19, 1815, at the comparatively early age of forty-nine years.

Another of the distinguished pupils of Dr. Rush, who probably owed his inspiration to the same great teacher, was Dr. John Redman Coxe, a unique figure among the medical men of Philadelphia, and the founder of medical journalism. Almost twenty years younger than Barton, who was a student of Shippen, he came under the influence of the earlier systems taught, and was so influenced by them that, as he was long-lived like his grandfather, he became the most notable illustration of the conservative teachings of an older time, and was, therefore, regarded by the adherents of a more modern medicine as an anachronism. This, however, in no way affected the good he did as the inaugurator of medical journalism in the summer of 1804, when so much activity was in progress. Dr. Coxe was thirty-one years of age when he conceived the idea of a journal. He was a native of New Jersey, born in 1773, and was educated in Philadelphia under his Grandfather Redman's care. "At an early period of my life," he writes in 1835, "I went to England, and after several years passed in the public schools, proceeded to Edinburgh, in my sixteenth year, under the direction of a well-established classical teacher, and with the intention of pursuing, during the summer months, the lectures on Botany, then given by Dr. Rutherford, and those on Natural History, by the Rev. Dr. Walker. I boarded at this time in the house of a surgeon and apothecary, by whom I was induced, thus early, to attend the hospital, and having spent nearly fifteen months in Edinburgh, returned to London towards the close of the year 1789, and during the following winter I attended two courses of anatomy and one of chemistry at the London Hospital, by Mr. Blizzard and Dr. Hamilton. In 1790 I left England for the purpose of more directly studying medicine under the direction of Dr. Benjamin Rush, with whom I continued until I obtained my degree here, in the University of Pennsylvania, of Doctor in Medicine, in 1794. Having, during four years' apprenticeship, attended the various lectures then delivered by Drs. Shippen, Kuhn, Rush, Wistar, Hutchinson and Griffitts, and having their respective signatures to my diploma, with the exception of that of Dr. Hutchinson, who, it is well known, fell a sacrifice to his active exertions during the eventful period of 1793, when the yellow fever spread terror and desolation through our devoted city." Of this period he says that, for four months, "I was not once absent from my post, and from the immensity of applicants for Dr. Rush's aid, he was obliged to transfer a very large portion to his students. Seldom, I believe, had I less than thirty to fifty a day to visit and prescribe for, and when necessary, likewise to bleed. Of four other fellow-students, three fell victims to their unwearied philanthropy, and the other was within the verge of existence in two several attacks." "Here, then, I had an ample field of experience, not readily to be forgotten, exclusive of that which I might be presumed to acquire during these years attending the practice of the hospital physicians, and also of a number of pauper patients committed to my charge by Dr. Rush, as was his usual custom, at a period when the Dispensary was just starting into full existence, and had not yet obstructed the proportion of that class of patients which fell to the care of every practitioner." Dr. Rush presented him with a commentary on Boerhaave for "his skill, fortitude, patience, perseverance and humanity" in that plague. In '94, he again visited London, Edinburgh and Paris, and studied in those cities until '97, when he returned and began practice and also was on the staff of the hospitals and Dispensary. It was in 1801 that he introduced vaccination into Philadelphia, by the successful vaccination of himself and his son (p). He had opened a drug store also, and late in the summer of 1804, actuated by the success of the New York *Medical Repository*, then seven years old, ventured upon the project of publishing a quarterly entitled *"The Medical Museum,"* with a section called the *Medical and Philosophical Register*. The first contribution was Mitchell's letter on the yellow fever in Virginia in 1741-2, and the only known medical record of Dr. Kearsley, Sr., contrasting the epidemic in this region with that of Philadelphia of the same date. Dr. Rush contributed an extended account of this disease in Baltimore in 1794. Other writers for the journal were Drs. James Stuart, J. C. Otto, J. R. Coxe, John Rush, Philip S. Physick, W. Baldwin, T. C. James and Horsefield. In his second number, Coxe records the advent of Barton's journal. Unlike the literary enterprise of the latter, the Museum had a vigorous existence until the close of the year 1811, and paved the way for similar journals, such as the "Repository," and the journals founded by Chapman, Hays

---

(p) Edward Jenner Coxe, M. D., was born in 1801, and received his vaccination fourteen days after his birth. His father himself was the first successful case of vaccination, November 9, 1801, the virus having been sent him by President Jefferson.

and others. In 1808 Dr. Coxe published a Medical Directory; he also published a Dispensatory, an exposition of Hippocrates, and other works. In 1809, he became Professor of Chemistry, and in 1818, of Materia Medica and Pharmacy; the latter position he held until his sixty-second year. He died at the advanced age of ninety years, in 1864. Dr. Coxe must always be regarded as the pioneer of medical journalism in Philadelphia.

Dr. Thomas C. James, the "amiable, gentle and accomplished gentleman," who received honors as the first Professor of Obstetrics, or "Midwifery," as it was then called, was seven years older than Coxe, and of the same age as Barton, whom he survived twenty years. He was named for his grandfather, Thomas Chalkley, a Quaker, favorably known as an author. Of Quaker parentage, he was born in Philadelphia and educated under the historian, Proud. He studied medicine with Dr. Kuhn, and received his Doctor's degree from the University in 1787. He spent about a year on the ocean, in 1788, as surgeon of the ship Sampson, in order to be able to finish his education abroad. In 1790, he began his studies in Edinburgh, London and on the Continent. In 1793, the year of the pestilence, he returned to Philadelphia. He was a scholarly man, of poetic talent, was active in nearly all the philanthropic, scientific and literary societies, and was one of the founders of the Historical Society of Pennsylvania. He is said to have been one of the first to introduce the use of anthracite coal as a fuel. He had given private lectures on Midwifery, with Dr. John Church, as early as 1802, and with such success that, on the separation of that subject from Anatomy, in the reorganization of the work of the University, he was chosen to the new chair in 1810, continuing to occupy it for nearly a quarter of a century. His was the uneventful life of a scholarly, refined and sensitive nature. Dr. William P. Dewees, a young man of ability, acted as his assistant from 1824, on account of his increasing age and infirmity. Ten years later, James resigned, only a year before his death, which occurred in 1835. His name will always be associated with the elevation of Obstetrics to an equality with the other branches of medical science, and the opening of lying-in wards in both the Philadelphia and Pennsylvania Hospitals.

The most notable figure of the active group of workers associated with Rush, however, were Wistar and Physick, the former five years older than James, and the latter two years younger; the one Professor of Anatomy and the other of Surgery. These two men and James, were the real successors of Shippen. Wistar was fifty-two when Rush died, James forty-seven and Physick fifty-five. The strong personalities in the College faculty were now to be found in the Departments of Anatomy and Surgery, rather than in Medicine. Dr. Caspar Wistar, like James, was a Friend, descended from the strong old Palatine German stock of Hilsbach, near Heidelberg. His mother's family were of English descent and came to America in the time of Penn. He had the assertiveness of the English, the solidity of the German and the gentleness of the Friend. His greatness arose largely from his popularizing methods as a teacher, as well as from his investigations. His lectures were abundantly illustrated and thus probably rendered his teaching more effective than that of any of his predecessors. His models and original anatomical specimens were excellent and numerous. Some of them, as that of the ethnoid bone, were made for the first time by himself. These specimens, with successive additions, formed the basis of the well-known Wistar Museum of the University. It was his practice to hold social gatherings at his home on Saturday evenings, to which prominent members of the profession were invited, and the purpose of which was to stimulate scientific research. These meetings are still continued, being perpetuated in his honor, under the name "Wistar parties." As has been said, he was fifty-two years old when Rush died, for he was born in Philadelphia on September 13, 1761. Educated in the Friends' School, he became known as a classical student of especial merit. He afterward went to the old academy or college. When at the age of sixteen, being a Friend and opposed to war because of his religious convictions, he offered his services in the care of the wounded at the battle of Germantown. After this experience, he was so convinced of his adaptation to medicine that he chose forthwith to prepare for the profession. Entering Dr. Redman's office, he studied under the old tutor of Rush and Morgan, and also under the celebrated Dr. John Jones, who had settled in the city, and who became so interested in him as to help him to establish himself in practice afterwards. He had the good, or bad, fortune to have his medical collegiate career divided between the medical school of the College and that of the University, graduating in the latter as Bachelor of Medicine in 1782, at the age of twenty-one. His examination offered amusing proof that the faculty were divided between Boerhaave and Cullen, and that Wistar, having mastered both, could give the views of either one or the other as he instinctively felt them to be preferred by his examiners. In 1783, he spent a year in London and then went to Edinburgh, where he at once became a prominent member of that select body, the Royal Medical Society, and was honored with its highest office for two years. He held a similar position in a society for the study of Natural History. Graduating in '86, with the thesis *De Animo Demisso*, he returned to Philadelphia. He joined the Dispensary staff the next year, and, in 1789, was called to the chair of Chemistry in the reorganized College of Philadelphia. He accepted it only to aid in uniting the schools. In 1792, after the union, he became assistant to Dr. Shippen, and succeeded him seventeen years later. For thirteen years before his death, which occurred in 1818, he gave Anatomy his chief attention and did much to enlarge its boundaries. In 1811, following the examples of his confrères, he published a text-book on Anatomy. This was a period marked by the production of the first text-books. Dr. Wistar became so eminent in his scientific and classical work that he was made vice-president of the American Philosophical Society and succeeded Thomas Jefferson as its president in 1815, holding that position at the time of his death. Three years later Chief Justice Tilghman said of him: "Surely, never was life more earnestly desired, never death more sincerely regretted than that of this genial and generous physician-teacher."

The year 1818 was not to close a decade of such losses as those resulting from the death of Shippen, Woodhouse, Rush, Barton, Kuhn and Wistar, without another victim in the successor of Wistar, Dr. John Syng Dorsey, a nephew and favorite protégé of Dr. Physick. Dorsey was only thirty-five when he died (in November, 1818), and yet he was so brilliant that he became an assistant to Dr. Physick two years after the chair of Surgery was created. He succeeded Barton in Materia Medica eight years later, and Wistar, still later, in Anatomy. He was a Philadelphian, born in 1783, and educated in the Friends' School. He studied medicine under Physick, from 1798, his fifteenth year, and made such remarkable progress that his course in the medical school of the University closed in 1802, when he was two years under the age required for graduation. Because of his ability the trustees were induced to suspend their rules and give him his degree. His thesis was on "The Powers of the Gastric Juice as a Solvent for Urinary Calculi." He finished his preparation for Surgery by a term of study in Europe in 1803-4. His literary talent showed itself by the production of a work entitled "Elements of Surgery."

The most eminent figure at the close of this period, after the death of Rush, was "the father of American Surgery," Dr. Philip Syng Physick, a man almost the exact opposite of Wistar in most respects—always afflicted with bodily weakness held up by a powerful will; sensitive and retiring, and impatient of the systems so vigorously advocated by his great friend, Rush. An evidence of his sensitiveness and delicacy is afforded by the following incident in his history. At the age of seventeen, he was taken to the medical College on Fifth Street, opposite Independence Square, to see an amputation for the first time. He almost fainted, and plead with his father to permit him to give up the study of medicine. He was always opposed to the practice of vivisection, and expressed himself strongly against it. Yet the keen, penetrating intellect of this man almost created the science and art of Surgery in America, which had come to be overshadowed by medicine. As an operator he was so distinguished that, at the age of sixty-three, he performed a successful lithotomy on the aged Chief Justice of the United States, John Marshall. Dr. Physick's father, Edmund

Physick, was agent of the Penn estate and had his country seat about seven miles up the Schuylkill River. When Philip, who was born in 1768, came to Philadelphia to attend the Friends' Academy, presided over by Proud, the historian, he lived in the family of the lady who afterward became the wife of President Madison. He later entered the University and graduated in 1785, with no especial desire to study medicine other than his wish to please his father. Beginning his medical studies in 1785 with Dr. Kuhn, he spent three and a half years with him, attending at the same time the lectures of the medical faculty. He went to London in 1789 and lived with Dr. John Hunter. While there he showed a remarkable gift in original research and experiment, and became house surgeon to St. George's Hospital. Dr. Hunter desired him to settle in London. In 1791, he obtained his license to practice from the Royal College of Surgeons, but the same year he went to Edinburgh, and was so able as to obtain a degree at the University after but one year's residence—the first American student, it is said, to win this distinction. His thesis, in 1792, was entitled *De Apoplexia*. In September he returned to Philadelphia and began practice at the age of twenty-five. It has been already shown how he bore the trials of the fearful pestilence in 1793, when, with Leib, Annan and Cathrall, he helped to form the first staff of Bush Hill Hospital. His greatest work in connection with this hospital was accomplished in '98 when he was resident physician. He did royal service in all those years of epidemic, as has been testified by Bush and many others. There is no doubt that his infirmities were increased by his exposures to disease at this time. In '94 he became surgeon to the Pennsylvania Hospital, but it was not until the third year of his work that he began to acquire a practice of any magnitude. His real fame dates from 1800, when, at the age of thirty-two, he began his private lectures. After the delivery of the first lecture, Dr. Rush came up, offering his hand, and said: "Doctor, that will do; you need not be apprehensive as to the result of your lecturing. I am sure you will succeed." The secret of his power seemed to be merely his splendid mastery of his subject, for otherwise he was not remarkable either as a speaker or writer.

From 1805, when the chair of Surgery was created by him, he was the great Philadelphia surgeon for the next thirty years. The many changes necessitated by death in the faculty of the University during the last thirteen years of his professorship led Dr. Physick to accept the chair of Anatomy, at the time of Dorsey's death. The loss of three such active men as Wistar, Rush and Dorsey in so short a time, was a calamity of no slight order, and necessitated some sacrifice. The transferrence of Physick from the chair of Surgery to that of Anatomy was always regarded as a misfortune for the University, as Surgery was eminently his specialty. His ill-health caused him to resign in 1831, and in November, 1837, at the age of sixty-nine, his life closed. His career was at its zenith, no doubt, during the closing years of the life of Rush. "What a glorious privilege was that enjoyed for nearly a decennial period by the students who attended the medical lectures in the University of Pennsylvania!" writes Dr. John Bell. "To pass from the amphitheater of the great teacher of Anatomy, Dr. Wistar, to that of Physick, the Father of American Surgery, and thence go and hear the prelections of Rush, the American Hippocrates, and the father of American medicine, the medical philosopher, the philosophical philanthropist, patient, learned, yet ever learning, diligent in collecting facts, and ready when the opportune moment came to expand facts into principles; whose purity of life, from boyhood to advanced age, was the practical commentary on his elevated ethics, and whose pen and tongue were enlisted in the advocacy of every theme that could give value to the independence of his country, by improving the health, cultivating the minds and preserving the morals of its people." It was at this time, then, that Physick won his renown. The honors that came thereafter were rather rewards than additions to his fame. He was president of the Philadelphia Medical Society for thirteen years before his death; and also was connected with many other prominent societies in Europe and America. His best energies, however, were devoted to the practical work of his profession.

The war of 1812 did not affect medical science in Philadelphia to any great degree (q), but it is rather remarkable that the changes induced in the faculty of the University by the deaths of so many prominent men should be coincident with the national calamity. The years succeeding the death of Rush constituted a period of reorganization in the medical profession of Philadelphia, and the process was attended by a long continued struggle, which lasted many years and centered around the person of a young man who organized a private medical school in 1817, called the "Philadelphia Medical Institute." This school attracted a large number of young men. Dr. Nathaniel Chapman and his associates, who all became members of the University faculty, were its founders, and so large was the work that it must have suggested the possibility of more medical colleges. Certain it is that the movement seemed to stimulate a desire for the establishment of a greater number of institutions for medical training.

(q) Dr. William E. Horner, Dr. Jackson, and a few others, served in the war.

CHAPTER III.

THE ANTE CIVIL WAR PERIOD.—1825 TO 1861.

Despite her fatal experience, Philadelphia nearly doubled in population during the first two decades of the century, allowing New York but a small margin of advance. In 1820, the city, with her 113,000 inhabitants, still spread along the Delaware River, Tenth and Eleventh streets being the western borderland, beyond which a physician's sign was rarely to be seen. Although some 25,000 people were added by 1825, there were only about a dozen more doctors than thirty years before; but, besides the physicians, sixty-nine in all, it is noteworthy that there were twenty-five "Cuppers and Leechers" (a), the largest list of the latter given at the close of any decade before or since (b). Whatever may have been the reason, whether the heavy losses among physicians during the epidemics, the more recent losses of so many eminent leaders, or other causes operating to bring about this condition, it is certain that the profession in the few years before and after 1825 was less numerous in proportion to general population than at any other time in the history of the city. It was a period of reconstruction and disaffection of various sorts, not the least being an awakening resistance to the old systems. It was a period of transition to the extreme skepticism that foreshadowed the modern scientific spirit, and one of restlessness that sought to work out toward new conditions. It is interesting to note that the most prominent leaders were Southern men from Virginia and the Carolinas. A new generation was coming to the front, and it will also

(a) Wilson's Directory, 1825. There were also ten midwives, seventy-eight nurses and eighteen dentists.
(b) There were but sixteen "cuppers and leechers" in 1860 when the population was nearly five times larger.

be of interest to see how it had begun the modern movement from such streets as Second, Third and Fourth to lower Mulberry, Chestnut, Walnut and Spruce. Dr. Physick was on Fourth; Drs. Coxe, James and Chapman were in the "York Building;" Dr. Samuel P. Griffitts, just the year before his death, was on Front street; Jonas Preston, whose name is given to Preston Retreat, was on Mulberry; William P. Dewees, James Mease, Thomas T. Hewson, William E. Horner, J. Rhea Barton and James Rush were all on Chestnut; Thomas Parke, now grown old, was on Rittenhouse place; Isaac Hays, J. A. Monges and Samuel Colhoun on Sansom; W. P. C. Barton and Joseph G. Nancrede were on Tenth; Samuel Jackson, William Darrach and Edwin P. Atlee were on Seventh street; William Gibson and Benjamin S. Janney were on Third; Mulberry street was full of a notable class: Samuel Emlen, Henry Bond, George B. Wood, Joseph Hartshorne, Charles D. Meigs, Samuel G. Morton, Joseph Parrish and John C. Otto; Pine street had Franklin Bache; on Walnut was Hugh L. Hodge; on Fourth was George McClellan, John Bell and William Rush; on Spencer street were Jacob Randolph, H. Neill, William B. Duffield and Alfred Drake; John K. Mitchell was on Fifth, also Elijah Griffiths, David F. Condie and Gouverneur Emerson; Benjamin H. Coates was on Front street, also J. Cooper, and Benjamin Rush Rhees; Anthony Benezet was on Shippen street; William Aitken on Ninth; John Allen on Fourth; John Eberle on Eighth; Lewis C. Gebherd on Sassafras; Caspar C. Gwyer at the Almshouse; Thomas Harris on Shippen street (c); Charles Lukens on Mulberry; Robert Abbott on Walnut; George T. Alberti on Fifth; M. Anderson on Pine; E. P. Atlee, Jr., on Vine; A. Baines on Beach; John Banks on Vine; G. H. Burgin on Chestnut; F. S. Beattie on Mulberry; D. Blenou at "Hamilton Village;" David Berton on Front street; J. R. Burden on Third; W. D. Brincklé on Vine; W. Burns on High (Market); J. F. Brooke on Fourth; W. C. Brewster on Fifth; J. Bullock on Mulberry; T. Coxe on Eighth; H. V. Carter on Fifth; T. Connell on Mulberry; W. Cheeks on Locust; J. Y. Clarke on Mulberry; J. Cornwell on Church alley; G. Colhoun on Front; Thomas Dunn on Vine; Ben-

---

(c) Samuel Harris lived in Camden.

jamin Ellis on Ninth; S. M. Fox on Sansom; S. Freedly on Second; D. Gallaher on Fifth; John Garrison on Beach; W. H. Geyer, G. Gillaspey on Eighth; John Goodman on Tenth; J. Green on Walnut; A. L. Gregory at Frankford; S. J. Griffiths on Callowhill street; R. E. Griffiths on Front, Thomas Hall on Eleventh; Richard Harlan on Third; J. C. Heberton on Fifth; W. S. Helmuth on Seventh; I. Heylin on Vine; John Hopkinson on Chestnut; Abraham Howell on Eighth; S. L. Howell on Fifth; Gideon Humphrey on Fifth; H. Huquenelle on Filbert; Robert Huston on Vine; John Jones on Third; J. Jeanes on Front; J. H. Karsten on Eleventh; James Kitchen, Jr., on Spruce; John Hehlme on Fourth; Harvey and Joseph Klapp on second; Alex. Knight on Front; J. F. D. Lobstein on Spruce; J. McCulley in Emlen's Court; Joseph Matthieu on Walnut street; J. Maurcu on Lawrence; Peter Miller on Mulberry; Robert Milnor on High (Market); William Milnor on Second; James Mitchell on Prune; John Moore on Seventh; Wilson Moore on Spruce; Nicholas Nancrede on Powell; Philip Pylz, Jr., on Cedar; John Perkins on Fifth; Manuel Phillips on Fourth; W. C. Poole on Ninth; John Porter on Sixth; R. Povall on Ninth; H. M. Read on Chestnut; T. Redman on Chestnut; I. Remington on Sixth; T. Ritchie on Front; C. Rohr on Third; J. Rose on Callowhill; John Rousseau on Pine; J. Ruan on Walnut; W. Rumsey on Third; H. Sansbury on Front; Thomas Sargent on Sassafras; George Schott on Seventh; J. S. Sharpless on Fourth; W. Shaw on Mulberry; T. Shrivers on Ninth; Nathan Shoemaker on Chestnut; D. C. Skerret on Tenth; James and F. Snow on Sassafras; I. C. Snowden on Walnut; R. Stevenson on Eleventh; J. Stewart on Eighth; J. Swan on Front; J. C. Thomas on Sassafras; J. L. Thomas on Second; Erasmus Thomas on Sixth; Gerard Trool on Fourth; A. B. Tucker on Fourth; H. M. and Samuel Tucker on Mulberry; J. A. Thackara on Spruce; J. Thomson in Thomson's Court; George and John Uhler on Front; A. Vantroy on Spruce; J. Van Zyle on Plum; J. F. Ward on Eighth; G. Watson on High (Market); and J. Webster on Eighth street. This embraced the entire list of Philadelphia physicians in active practice, with probably few exceptions, and is the last list small enough to be given in full. The general tendency of location is apparent, as also the tendency to groups among the older and younger leaders of the profession. Scarcely more than a half dozen of these men were above fifty-five years of age; these were Griffitts, Physick, Preston, James, Dewees, Parke and Monges, and Physick and Dewees were only fifty-seven. Many of the names better and more widely known to history, like Bache, Horner, McClellan, Wood, Mitchell and others, were those of men scarcely thirty years old, and the men who ranged near fifty were Mease, Caldwell, Hewson, Hartshorne, Parrish, Chapman, Coxe, Otto and Hare. Gibson, Jackson, W. P. C. Barton, Bond and Meigs were a medium between the two latter classes. The University faculty embraced Chapman, in the chair of Practice, with, two years later, Samuel Jackson as his assistant for the Institutes; Gibson in the chair of Surgery; Physick, who was in ill health, and his adjunct, Horner, in that of Anatomy; James and his adjunct, Dewees, both men of uncertain health, in the chair of Midwifery; Hare, the inventor of the oxy-hydrogen blowpipe, in the chair of Chemistry; Coxe in the chair of Materia Medica, and W. P. C. Barton in that of Botany. The repeated changes had excited a spirit of disaffection in spite of the fact that the University had strong men in some of its chairs, and that it had over twice as many students as any other school in the land. During the year it had 480 enrolled, out of 1,970 (d) medical students in the entire fifteen medical colleges of the United States. The only ones that approached it were Transylvania University with 235, the University of Maryland with 215, and the College of Physicians and Surgeons of New York with 196 students. It is probable, indeed, that this very aggregation of medical students in one school in a growing city was itself an impetus to larger facilities. The causes were numerous; it only required some slight events to set them in motion, and these were brought about as follows:

Every eminent practitioner had had his private pupils since the time of Griffith Owen, and many had given private and public lectures even after the University Medical School was founded, but

---

(d) These statistics were collected from professors in the various institutions and used by Thomas Sewall at his opening address at Columbian College, D. C., March 30, 1825.

it was reserved for Dr. Nathaniel Chapman, the popular and magnetic young Virginian, who entered the faculty, to conceive the plan of giving his private pupils more rounded and proportional advantages than he, alone, could give, by associating with him fellow preceptors as semi-specialists in other departments. He began this with Dr. Horner, as anatomist, in 1817, in the rear of his house, which was on the south side of Walnut street, the second door below Eighth street. The room used was the second floor of his stable, but from these small beginnings there soon arose an organization known as "The Medical Institute," of which, ten years later, it could be said it had "reached to the condition of a systematic and popular course of instruction," extending practically over the whole year, and registering over a hundred students for several years past. The third year Dr. Dewees joined it, as obstetrician, and soon after, Drs. Hodge, Bell, Samuel Jackson, J. K. Mitchell, and, for a time, T. P. Harris. It grew so rapidly that finally a charter was secured and a building erected on Second street, below Twelfth, with three spacious lecture rooms, that became the home of a new college twenty years later (e). The first of the two terms of the Institute was devoted chiefly to lectures, the second to examination, out of which the famous "Quiz" probably had its development. This extra-mural course prompted many others, and there is no doubt that, supplementary as it was intended to be, it served as training ground for both students and professors with a degree of freedom that would not be advisable in a university.

Here Dr. Chapman's peculiar power was manifested probably even more than in the University, for he was a man of great personal fascination, famous for his wit and humor, as well as ability. He was the Nestor of almost the entire period down to the civil war, and, after Physick, the acknowledged head of the American profession. The leader of that considerable body of Southern men such as Horner, Mitchell, Hartshorne, Caldwell, Meigs, Mütter and others, his ancestors were relatives of Sir Walter Raleigh, through whom a captain of British cavalry, the first founder of the family, received the ancestral estate about twenty miles above Richmond.

(e) Franklin Medical College.

Although the branch to which Dr. Chapman belonged is in Maryland, opposite Mt. Vernon, his father's estate was in Fairfax County on the Potomac, where Nathaniel was born May 28, 1780; so that he was thirty-seven years old when the germ of the Medical Institution came into existence. In due time he was placed at the classical school, founded by General Washington at Alexandria, where he met another Virginian, Joseph Hartshorne. Six years there, and some time in two other colleges, completed his literary course, but he had been at work in medicine under Drs. Weems of Georgetown and Dick of Alexandria so successfully that, in 1797, at the age of seventeen, he started for the University of Pennsylvania, and the private tutelage of Dr. Rush, who perceived his great powers at an early period, and undoubtedly favored his aspirations to a position in the faculty. Graduating in 1800 with a thesis on *Hydrophobia*, suggested by Rush, although he had previously prepared one on the sympathetic connection of the stomach with the rest of the body, which was characteristic and afterwards read before the Philadelphia Medical Society, Dr. Chapman then went to Europe and remained three years. He spent a year under Abernethy of London, who insisted so strongly upon the stomach and bowels as the seats of disease, that Chapman never after departed much from that line of medical theory. In 1801 he went to Edinburgh, where for two years he breathed the atmosphere of Cullen and his confrères, so that, to quote another, he was ever after "a most uncompromising vitalist and solidist" (f). Here, too, his personality won for him such friends as Brougham, Dugald Stewart and Lord Buchan, the last mentioned of whom gave him a public breakfast on his departure for Philadelphia in 1804; for he had already become something of a man of letters, and had even been a favorite contributor to *The Portfolio* under Dennie. His practice was remarkably successful from the first and his personality was equally forceful in this field. He soon gave a private course of Lectures on Obstetrics, which were so successful that in 1807 Dr. James sought his aid in the same field, in which he continued until the death of Rush six years later. He

---

(f) Dr. Samuel Jackson.

then took the chair of Materia Medica, and, in 1816, three years later, at the age of thirty-six, succeeded to the chief department of the chair of Rush himself, that of Practice (g). It was the next year that he began the original of the Institute, in which he lectured for about twenty years. While in the University his career was much extended by his founding a new medical perodical in November, 1820, four years after his election to the chair of Practice. This, the first permanent periodical, entitled *The Philadelphia Journal of the Medical and Physical Sciences*, still exists under the name, *The American Journal of Medical Sciences*. Years later it absorbed two other journals, and developed into one of the greatest medical periodicals of the land, as it is the oldest. His book on Therapeutics was a great work in its day, and his best known, although his other writings were numerous. He was long president of the Philadelphia Medical Society, and was, by acclamation, chosen first president of the American Philosophical Society, in 1853. The basis of his medical theory was *sympathy*, and he turned away from Rush's unity of disease and restored the older classification, modified by the prevailing spirit of the times; but his power was most characeristic as a lecturer, where he is described by Dr. Samuel Jackson, his adjunct, "as self-possessed, deliberate and emphatic. Whenever warmed with his subject, his animation became oratorical. Often the tedium of dry matter would be enlivened by some stroke of wit, a happy pun, an anecdote or quotation. He was furnished with stores of facts and cases, drawn from his own large experience and observation, illustrating principles, disease, or treatment under discussion. His bearing was dignified, his manner was easy, and his gestures were graceful. He had a thorough command over the attention of his class, with whom he always possessed an

---

(g) His rival to this chair was Dr. Charles Caldwell, a North Carolinian, born in 1772, of North of Ireland parentage. He was of an intense and ambitious nature, educated himself through great difficulties, began the study of medicine in 1791, and in 1795 finished his course in the University medical school. He was among the greatest controversialists of the day. He delivered clinical lectures at the Almshouse Hospital as early as 1807 and lectures on medical jurisprudence in 1810; said to be among the first on that subject. In 1815 he became professor of Geology in the University, and in 1819 left Philadelphia for the Chair of Medicine in Transylvania University at Lexington, Ky. He died in 1853.

unbounded popularity. His voice had a peculiar intonation, depending on some defect in the conformation of the palate, that rendered the articulation of certain sounds an effort. The first time he was heard, the ear experienced difficulty in distinguishing his words. This was of short duration; for, once accustomed to the tone, his enunciation was remarkable for its distinctness. Students would often take notes of his lectures verbatim." Such were some of the characteristics of the successor of Rush, who founded the Medical Institute in 1817.

The next year, 1818, another private lecturer, Dr. Joseph Parrish, after several years of successful teaching, found himself with thirty or more students, an increase which rendered it necessary to engage the young practitioner, Dr. George B. Wood, to assist him. Thus, writes that assistant over thirty years later, he "may be looked upon as one of the founders of that combined and more thorough scheme of private medical tuition, which constitutes a distinguishing professional feature of our city and our times." Dr. Joseph Parrish, born in 1779, was of an Anglicized Dutch lineage, his great-grandfather having the estate which a part of Baltimore now covers. His father, Dr. Isaac Parrish, settling in Philadelphia as a boy, became one of those gentle Quaker physicians, like his friend and his son's friend, Dr. Griffitts. Dr. Joseph Parrish followed the advice of Dr. Griffitts in seeking Dr. Wistar as his preceptor, and he graduated from the University in 1805. He was a favorite member of the staffs of the Dispensary, the City Hospital, the Almshouse Hospital, and the Pennsylvania, succeeding Dr. Physick in the last. His success in the typhus epidemic that took off Dr. Rush was notable. He succeeded Rush, Wistar and Franklin in the presidency of the Abolition Society. Dr. Wistar once said he "had the ambition of a Bonaparte and the benevolence of a Howard." He could have had a professorship for the asking, but he made to such overtures the significant reply: "My bark was made for quiet waters." He died in 1840 at the age of sixty-one. Meanwhile, his private school had risen and almost died with him. For the first twelve years it developed by adding two more assistants, Drs. Richard Harlan and Nathan Shoemaker, but in

1830 (h) it was further developed into the "Philadelphia Association for Medical Instruction," with a faculty composed of Drs. Parrish, Wood, S. G. Morton, J. R. Barton and Bache, to whom were afterward added Jacob Randolph, W. W. Gerhard, Joseph Pancoast and William Rush; this flourished for about six years and then gradually declined, though in 1818, when Dr. Parrish began his instruction near the rear of Christ Church, the school was about as large as that of Dr. Chapman, near Walnut and Eighth streets.

Two years later, in 1820, Dr. Jason V. O. Lawrance began the most permanent of these private institutions. It was situated at the upper end of Chant street (then called College avenue), on the North Side, and occupied the eastern of the two apartments which, under the name of *The Philadelphia Anatomical Rooms*, were destined to become to this city what the famous Windmill Street School of Hunter was to London (i). Lawrance was an original, scholarly lecturer, of striking qualities, that soon (in 1822) led to his becoming assistant to both the chairs of Anatomy and Surgery in the University; indeed, his lecture rooms were really intended as a summer school to cover the University's long vacation from April to November. He was a Southern man, native of New Orleans, born in 1791, and graduated from the University in 1815, so that he was twenty-nine years old when he opened his school in 1820. He lived only three years longer, however, as his career was cut short by the typhus epidemic of 1823. Before he died, his keen spirit of investigation led to his becoming one of a committee —Drs. Harlan and Coates being the others—of the Academy of Medicine (j), suggested by Dr. Chapman to determine whether the newly discovered absorbent vessels were the exclusive absorbents or not. He was investigating absorption by the brain when his

(h) About the same time Dr. William Gibson headed another association called the "School of Medicine," which included among its lecturers Drs. Jacob Randolph, Benjamin H. Coates, René La Roche, John Hopkinson, and Charles D. Meigs. It was of the same character and had a career similar to the "Association."

(i) History of the Philadelphia School of Anatomy, by Dr. W. W. Keen, 1875. This school lasted fifty-five years, while the London institution lived sixty-three. Dr. Parrish gave the first account of this work in an introductory lecture in 1857.

(j) The Academy of Medicine was not the old society of Rush's foundation. It was founded in 1821 with a view to discussion of the great changes then taking place and "for the improvement of the science of medicine."

death occurred, and his school went into the hands of another Southern man, Dr. John D. Goodman (k), who retired from practice and devoted himself to teaching with such ability that, in the following winter, 1823-24, he had seventy students. He soon added a library and reading room, and was joined by Drs. R. E. Griffiths and Isaac Hays; but on his departure in 1826 to New York the school was transferred to Dr. James Webster, who retained it four years until he, too, was called to a professor's chair (l). In 1841 the institution took the name Philadelphia School of Anatomy, and continued a famous training ground for professional chairs down to 1875.

In 1822, two years after Lawrance began, another private anatomical room was opened by Dr. Hewson over his stable on

---

(k) Dr. Goodman was born in 1794 in Annapolis, and was graduated in the University of Maryland in 1821. He was called to the chair of Anatomy in Rutgers Medical College, New York, in 1826. He did much to improve the professional feeling between New York and Philadelphia. He died in 1830.

(l) Dr. Joseph Pancoast reopened the rooms in 1831, and on his going to a chair in Jefferson eight years later, he was succeeded by Drs. J. Dunott and J. M. Allen as associate. In 1839 the west room was secured by Dr. James McClintock for his "Philadelphia School of Anatomy," which had been founded the year before at the southeast corner of Walnut and Eighth streets, but was compelled to move. In 1841 he was called to a professor's chair, and the whole building was united under the name of his school. Among other instructors since have been Drs. William R. Grant, D. Hayes Agnew, James A. Garretson, James P. Andrews, R. S. Sutton, W. W. Keen (who lectured the longest period of all), Dr. Richardson, Dr. H. Lenox Hodge, and a few others. Across the street from this school was one conducted by Dr. William S. Forbes, opened in 1856. "The Summer Association," which succeeded to the Parrish Association in 1842, began in the eastern building of the School of Anatomy with F. J. Meigs, J. M. Wallace, Robert Bridges, Francis Gurney Smith, and Joshua M. Allen. This school lasted until 1860, and also gave a new training ground for professors' chairs. Here lectured Drs. D. H. Tucker, W. V. Keating, J. H. B. McClellan, A. Hewson, John H. Brinton, Ellerslie Wallace, S. Weir Mitchell, Alfred Stillé, J. M. Da Costa, Francis West, James Darrach, Edward Hartshorne and others. In 1855 another association was formed called "The Pennsylvania Academy of Medicine," whose lecturers were Drs. W. W. Gerhard, Henry H. Smith, D. Hayes Agnew, Bernard Henry, R. A. F. Penrose, Mr. Edward Parrish and Dr. Edward Shippen. Two years later, Gerhard, Agnew, Penrose and Parrish began a quiz association. This was also good training ground for professors. Among others who experimented, lectured or quizzed in these various associations may be mentioned Drs. S. W. Gross, J. B. Brinton, Isaac Ott, H. C. Wood, Jr., Harrison Allen. F. H. Getchell, W. F. Jenks. James Tyson, J. E. Mears, J. S. Parry, O. P. Rex. O. H. Allis. Stanley Smith, H. Osgood, W. G. Porter, G. C. Harlan, George Strawbridge, W. W. McClure, J. Solis Cohen, E. G. Davis, Witmer, Duer, Dunglison. Maury, Warder, McArthur, Leaman, Hutchins, Leffman, Laughlin, Wilson. West, Greene. Willard. Curtin, Cheston, and Githens.

Library street, next the Custom House, and seven years later in Blackberry alley, in the rear of his residence, on Walnut street, above Ninth. He was a son of the celebrated London anatomist, William Hewson, whose widow came to America through the friendship of Franklin in 1786, and educated her son, Thomas T. Hewson, in his father's profession. Dr. T. T. Hewson studied under Dr. John Foulke, and enjoyed advantages of the highest character in Philadelphia and abroad. He settled in practice in 1806, and became especially known for his successful work as physician to the Walnut Street Prison, the Blockley Hospital, the Pennsylvania Hospital and other institutions. He was also the chief representative of the College of Physicians in the formation of the National Pharmacopoeia and the success of its final publication was largely due to him. He was president of the College of Physicians for twelve years, until his death in 1848. He was elected to the chair of Comparative Anatomy in 1816, and it was six years later that he opened his anatomical rooms with Drs. Harris, Meigs and Bache as associates (m).

About the same time, though a little earlier, in 1821, another lecture course was opened, which was destined to produce more momentous results than any of the others. This was begun, in a lecture room fitted up in connection with his office at the corner of Walnut and Swanwick streets, for the benefit of his private students, by a young physician of twenty-four years, full of the inspiration of his preceptors, Dorsey and Physick, and of a sufficiently original genius to stand out in striking relief against the dominant Southern element of the University. This was Dr. George McClellan, of whom, says his biographer (n), "Physick and Dorsey both predicted the future eminence." McClellan came of a Highland-Scotch and English ancestry, his great-grandfather being one of those who emigrated to Massachusetts after the battle of Culloden, while his grandfather was Gen. Samuel McClellan, of the Revolution. The mar-

---

(m) There was still another on Eighth above Jayne street, but by whom conducted is not known.

(n) Dr. W. Darrach, 1847.

tial spirit was reproduced in the Doctor's son, the late General George B. McClellan of the civil war. The Doctor himself had something of "the heart of a lion, and the eye of an eagle," and early evinced qualities that betokened success. Born in Woodstock, Connecticut, on December 22, 1796, he was educated at Woodstock Academy and was prepared to enter Yale College at the age of sixteen. This was in the days of Dwight and Silliman, and to the latter he became greatly attached, for his enthusiasm for chemistry, mineralogy and geology was characteristic of his academic course. Receiving at the age of eighteen his degree as Bachelor of Arts, he began study under Dr. Thomas Hubbard, afterward of the chair of Surgery in the New Haven Medical College. In 1817, he came to Philadelphia, to enter the University Medical School under the direct preceptorship of Dr. Dorsey. He soon became a resident student of "Blockley," the Philadelphia Hospital, where "he was the spirit and delight of the house," says his eulogist, and "he sometimes made trouble, easily quieted, though, for the people even then seemed intuitively to know that McClellan was appointed to be their head doctor, in spite of all the great doctors; and they let McClellan do anything." Graduating in 1819 (o), he at once entered upon a surgical practice of a bold and brilliant order, and two years later, in 1821, had so many private pupils that the Walnut street lecture room, already referred to, was opened (p). His classes became so large that he was soon compelled to rent a part of Rembrant Peale's Apollodorian Gallery, in the rear of his residence on George street, and to call to his assistance Dr. John Eberle (q), editor of the "American Medical

(o) His thesis was on "The Tying of Arteries."

(p) It is a notable fact that Dr. McClellan's ideas of the practical led to Jefferson Medical College instituting dispensary clinical instruction on May 9th before its opening session, the first school of the city to do so. Out of this grew the hospital of the College.

(q) Dr. Eberle came of German parentage. He was born in 1788 and graduated from the medical school of the University in 1809 at the age of twenty-one. Having ability as a writer he became editor of a political paper, until in 1818 he launched the *Recorder*. He soon issued also his well-known work on "Therapeutics," and it was about this time he joined Dr. McClellan. He taught Materia Medica and Theory and Practice in the first faculty of Jefferson and issued a work on the latter subject that is also well known. In 1831 he was persuaded to join a new Ohio school, projected by Dr. Drake at Cincinnati, as a rival to the

Recorder," a journal Dr. Eberle had started successfully in 1818, after the first two periodicals had passed away. McClellan's school was becoming more and more popular, and there is evidence at a very early period that he had in mind its development into a medical college. Even during his last session at the University, some projects for a new medical college were discussed and acted upon (r). Dr. W. P. C. Barton, professor of Botany in the University (appointed in 1816), drew up plans for a second school, and applied to the Legislature during the session of 1818-19, which effort, according to one account (s), came so near being successful that a meeting of the University students was called to gain an expression of their views. The committee appointed by them included Messrs. J. K. Mitchell as chairman, William Darrach, J. P. Harrison, S. H. Dickson and E. R. Craven, who reported a strong resolution against a second school. It was believed this would pass, but a student of Dr. James Rush, Benjamin Rush Rhees, arose to lead the opposition, and at the next meeting the report was defeated. The discussions of the next year waxed warm and lasted long in the Philadelphia Medical Society and in the press. In the spring of 1820 an incident occurred that involved the situation. A student, John G. Whildin, who was about to graduate at the University, was allowed to do so on condition that he should expunge certain passages from his thesis. This circumstance widened the breach between the friends of the University and those who were disaffected or in favor of a new school. It was during this period that Dr. McClellan undoubtedly started influences that tended to make his lecture room a rallying point for the new school party, for, says one writer: "Often had I conversed freely with Eberle and McClellan, in the city, in respect to the contemplated school," and, he continues: "Unexpectedly both paid me a visit, at my residence in Frankford, avowedly to

---

Medical College of Ohio, but they were subsequently united. He afterward occupied the chair of Theory and Practice in Transylvania, the year before his death, which occurred in 1838. He was a man of learning, but not of decision of character. He was eight years older than Dr. McClellan.

(r) Early history of Jefferson Medical College, by James F. Gayley, M. D., 1858.
(s) Dr. Thomas D. Mitchell in his life of Dr. John Eberle (Gross).

press me more closely to the advocacy of the cause. The daily papers had already opened a pretty fierce discussion of the merits of the case; and it was desired by both the individuals named that my pen should come to their aid. This service was rendered with all the energy I was able to carry into the contest, and, like the productions of the opposite party, under a fictitious signature. It is needless to conceal the fact that all this zeal in the incipiency of the enterprise was, more or less, prompted by an expectation of being a component part of the faculty at the outset." "As will always be the case," he writes further, "diverse views were advocated in respect to the contemplated new school, especially touching its cognomen, location, and the corporate powers under which it should be conducted. As the ball was rolled on, it increased in magnitude and importance, and many influential friends gave in their adhesion to its interests. The press teemed with essays pro and con, while the Legislature was invoked, by all the considerations that party zeal could adduce, to interfere so as to defeat the purpose of the adventurous aspirants who dared call in question the vested rights of a century" (t).

The time seemed ripe early in 1824 to begin the preliminary organization that should formulate these "diverse views" into a working plan. McClellan was about to fulfill the prophecy of Morgan concerning the University Medical School, that "it may give birth to other useful institutions of a similar nature," and, like Morgan, he proposed to launch his school under the charter of an institution of liberal culture, choosing for that purpose the well-known Washington County School, now Washington and Jefferson College, then called Jefferson College, and located at Canonsburg. In consequence, he joined Dr. Eberle, Dr. Joseph Klapp, and Mr. Jacob Green, a son of the Rev. Dr. Ashbel Green of Princeton, in formulating the following letter and proposition to the trustees of that institution on June 2nd: "The undersigned," the letter reads, "believing, upon mature consideration, that the establishment of a second Medical School in the city of Philadelphia would be

---

(t) It does not appear what "century" can be referred to, unless it is the abbreviated "century" of sixty years of University medical school's life.

advantageous to the public not less than to themselves, have formed themselves into a Medical Faculty, with the intention of establishing such a school; and they hereby offer to the trustees of Jefferson College to become connected with that institution on the conditions herewith submitted, subject to such modifications as on a full and free explanation shall be found satisfactory to the parties severally concerned. The undersigned beg leave to submit herewith the plan which they have devised for forming the faculty contemplated, and for conducting the concerns of the same, open to amendments and alterations in the manner already proposed." The result was the adoption by the trustees of the following resolutions, which were, no doubt, the plan already referred to. It embraces eleven points: "1st: That it is expedient to establish in the city of Philadelphia a Medical Faculty, as a constituent part of Jefferson College, to be styled the Jefferson Medical College. 2nd: That the Faculty of the Medical College shall consist of the following professorships: 1st, a professorship of Anatomy; 2nd, of Surgery; 3rd, of Theory and Practice of Medicine; 4th, of Materia Medica, Botany and the Institutes; 5th, of Chemistry, Mineralogy and Pharmacy; 6th, of Midwifery and the Diseases of Women and Children. 3rd: That whenever a vacancy occurs by death, resignation, or otherwise, it shall be filled by a gentleman who shall be nominated by the remaining professors, or a majority of them, and appointed by the trustees of the College. 4th: That a professor may be removed by the Board of Trustees, with the consent of the majority of the other medical professors, after a full and fair investigation of the alleged causes for the removal, but in no other way. 5th: That the medical school shall have no claims whatever on the funds of Jefferson College. 6th: That the medical professors shall make arrangements among themselves for the time and place of lecturing, for examinations, and for the general benefit of the school; that the time for conferring medical degrees shall be determined by the trustees, on the representation of the Medical Faculty. The same fee shall be paid to the President of the College by the graduates for degree as for a degree in the arts. 7th: That this college shall use all suitable influence to send medical pupils to the Medical School connected with it in Philadelphia; and the Medical Faculty shall promote in every way the interests and prosperity of the college. 8th: That the young men who have attended one course of lectures in any respectable medical institution shall be admitted to a standing in all respects equal to the one they had left. 9th: That ten indigent young men of talents, who shall bring to the Medical Faculty satisfactory testimonials and certificates, shall be annually admitted into the Medical School, receive its medical instruction, and be entitled to its honors without any charge. 10th: That the following persons, duly elected, be, and are hereby appointed, to the following professorships, viz.: Doctor George McClellan, Professor of Surgery; Dr. Joseph Klapp, Professor of Theory and Practice of Medicine; Dr. John Eberle, Professor of Materia Medica; Jacob Green, Esq., Professor of Chemistry, Mineralogy and Pharmacy. 11th: That the president of the board be, and is hereby, appointed to forward these resolutions to the professors elect, and to hold any necessary correspondence with them on the subject until the next meeting of the board."

This document was the beginning of the official existence of Jefferson Medical College, although the institution may really be said to date from the opening of McClellan's Walnut street lectures in 1821. Jefferson Medical College was, as yet, on paper, and its struggles just begun. Dr. Klapp resigned, and so great was the difficulty in completing a faculty that the project of opening the school in the following winter, 1824-5, was abandoned. During the next summer, 1825, the first real faculty of the institution was organized, and its announcements issued. It included the following members: John Eberle, M. D., in Theory and Practice; Benjamin Rush Rhees (u), M. D., in Materia Medica and Insti-

(u) Dr. Rhees was a young man of twenty-seven, of delicate constitution, but of an earnest and vigorous intellect. He was born in Beula, Pennsylvania, in 1798, of Welsh parentage, but on his father's death in 1804 came to Philadelphia. He was educated in the University of Pennsylvania, but some difficulty prevented his class from receiving their diplomas. Dr. James Rush was his preceptor. He was resident physician of the City Hospital for a time, and, after a period of foreign travel, settled in practice in the historic Loxley House of Philadelphia, where he gave private instruction, one of his students, Henry D. Smith, being the first matriculate of Jefferson Medical College. Dr. Rhees taught several subjects at

tutes; Jacob Green (v), in Chemistry; Nathan R. Smith (w), M. D., in Anatomy; Francis S. Beattie, M. D., in Midwifery; and George McClellan in Surgery. Of these, Drs. McClellan, Eberle, Rhees and Green were the forces that upheld the institution during its critical period of beginning. The faculty began prospecting for a building and chose the old Tivoli Theater, on the south side of Locust, then Prune street, below Sixth. One writer (x) happily describes the location from the point of view of old students revisiting it in later years. Starting at Ninth and Market, if they "turn their faces southward, they will see as they advance two stately buildings standing upon their right. At that early day the south building represented the greatest medical school of this country. If they now continue their walk to Walnut street, turn to the left and go eastward for two squares, they will have a fine park upon their right called Washington Square. This was once the Potters' Field, the receptacle of dead paupers and executed criminals. Continuing on until they arrive at Sixth street, turning southward, they will see on their left, opposite the square, a row of fine buildings. These occupy the spot of the Walnut street prison, a grim and ghastly structure, which extended to Prune street. Having arrived at Prune street, now Locust, turn to the left, walk eastward on the north side of Locust until you get opposite to No. 518; halt! right-about-face! and survey that structure. You see a very humble-looking building ornamented with inscriptions, such as 'Roussel's Mineral Water,'

---

various times, as emergency required, until his death in 1831, at the age of thirty-three years. He was "a man small in stature, with black, curly hair, with a dark blue eye and a most lively and expressive countenance. In temper he was ardent; in affection warm; in action impulsive; in friendship sincere. He was a man of varied acquisition. His inquisitiveness knew no limits. Whilst his powers were mainly devoted to his duties as a physician and as a professor, yet had he time to court the muses and to pursue his researches into the domains of theology and classical literature."

(v) Jacob Green, born in 1790 in Philadelphia, was a man of thirty-five. He was a classical graduate of the University and valedictorian of his class. He was made professor of Chemistry in Princeton in 1818, and later in Jefferson Medical College, the latter of which he held until his death, in 1841. He received his medical degree from Yale in 1827.

(w) Drs. Smith and Beattie only served for a short time.

(x) Dr. Washington L. Atlee, in an address before the Alumni in 1873.

'Manufactory of Soaps and Perfumery,' etc. As we survey it, it seems to exclaim—
> To what base uses have I come at last!

Now let us remove all these embellishments, that decorate or disfigure its walls, and replace the broken lights, and we will have returned it to its original condition, just as it appeared in the year 1826."

As the autumn approached, measures were taken to interest the new student arrivals, and McClellan, Eberle or Rhees, lectured every evening for the purpose, and with such effect that when school opened in November, its first class numbered one hundred and seven (y); while that of the University, for the same year, embraced four hundred and forty, an increase of sixteen over the second year preceding (z). The trustees secured an enlargement of their charter during the year, by which resident trustees for the medical school could be chosen. The head of this local board was the Rev. Dr. Ashbel Green, long president of the College of New Jersey, but then living in Philadelphia. The trustees of the University had been apprehensive of the effects of a new school, no doubt having in mind the unfortunate experiences with two schools at the close of the Revolution, and they even memorialized the Legislature on the ground "that the contemplated location of the Medical Department of Jefferson College is required by no public necessity, and will be followed by very injurious consequences." To this the faculty of the new school prepared a counter memorial, saying, among other things: "Were it ascertained that the organization of a second Medical School in the city of Philadelphia, would have the influence, apprehended by the Trustees, to diminish the respectability of an institution so honorable to the state and useful to the community; or, that it would prejudice the scientific character of the profession, then would we, at once, abandon so injurious an enterprise." They added reasons for another school, citing the large classes the University still had, the inconveniently large num-

---

(y) The faculty's memorial says 115.

(z) There were 487 in 1824-5, the largest attendance of any year in the University's history before 1848-9. The number of matriculates was but slightly affected for many years, and their graduates even increased very materially, so that it was soon evident that there was abundant room for two institutions.

ber of 550 students for one school, and the examples of London and New York. The result was that the power to confer degrees was not secured by the new school without resort to the Harrisburg courts, and as it had a class of twenty ready for their diplomas, Dr. McClellan acted with characteristic vigor. A vivid description of the occurrence is given by Dr. Atlee, then a student at Lancaster. "In the spring of 1826," he writes, "nearly half a century ago, four young medical students were assembled in the office of Dr. John L. Atlee, of Lancaster, for the purpose of forming a quizzing club. Quietly engaged in our deliberations, we were suddenly disturbed by a startling rap at the door. In a moment a young man, breathless and excited, bounded into our midst. He was a stranger to us, but our preceptor, soon entering, recognized him as a classmate and introduced us severally by name. His features were strongly marked, his gray, penetrating eyes deeply set, and his tongue and body were in constant motion. He seemed to be the embodiment of strong will, indomitable energy and determination, and every action of his small wiry frame bore the impress of a restless and vigorous brain. At the door stood a sulky with a sweating, panting horse, which he had driven without mercy over sixty miles that very day, having left Philadelphia the same morning. He *must* be in Harrisburg, thirty-six miles beyond, that night. His horse could go no further. He *must* have another. I never saw a better illustration of that passage in Shakespeare, where Richard the Third exclaims—

A horse! a horse! my kingdom for a horse!

My preceptor's horse and sulky were soon at the door and at his service. Hector, a noble animal, did his work well that momentous night, and before twenty-four hours had elapsed after he had left Philadelphia, this young M. D. (mad doctor) was hammering at the door of our legislature! His mission in Harrisburg was soon accomplished, and, as before, he arrived in Lancaster that night. It was very dark, yet, in spite of all remonstrances, he ordered out his horse and off he flew for Philadelphia. He had driven but a few miles, when, while dashing along, he upset in the highway. Here was a predicament from which he could not extricate himself without assistance. It was night, and the honest country people were in bed. After repeated halloos a farmer made his appearance with a lantern, which threw some light on the dismal scene. Quite naturally, the farmer began to inquire into all the particulars of the accident instead of at once attempting to right the difficulties. 'Come, come, good friend, that won't do. Let us put our shoulder to the wheel and leave explanations until another time.' Things were soon put into driving order, and next day the charter of the 'Medical Department of Jefferson College' was in the city of Philadelphia." "Need I say," he adds, "that this genius was young McClellan?"

The commencement was held on April 8th, and diplomas were awarded to the following graduates, whose respective theses are given: From Pennsylvania, George Baldwin, on "Cholera Infantum;" John B. Brinton, on "Cholera;" George Carll, on "Anthrax;" Charles Graeff, on "Rheumatism;" Charles M. Griffiths, on "Cholera Infantum;" Jesse W. Griffiths, on "Intermittent Fever;" Nathan L. Hatfield, on "Dysentery;" William Johnson, on "Extra-Uterine Pregnancy;" Thomas B. Maxwell, on "Lobelia Inflata;" Benjamin Shaw, on "Medical Practice;" J. Frederick Stadiger, on "Epilepsy;" from New Jersey, Peter Q. Beekman, on "Syphilis;" Ralph Glover, on "Hernia;" from New York, M. L. Knapp, on "Apocynum Canabinum;" from Kentucky, Atkinson Pelham, on "Mania a Potu;" from Massachusetts, James Swan, on "Scrofula;" from Vermont, Joel Foster, on "Neuroses;" from Ireland, John Graham, on "Epilepsy;" from Connecticut, Benjamin B. Coit, on "Tetanus;" and from South Carolina, Thomas M. Dick, on "Epidemics" (a).

The chief events of the next year, 1826-7, were the appointment of Dr. W. P. C. Barton to a chair of Materia Medica in June of '26, and Dr. John Barnes to occupy the vacated chair of Midwifery, over which there was a most unfortunate legal quarrel. Medical Jurisprudence was also added to the chair of Dr. Rhees,

---

(a) It is notable that among the twenty-five graduates of 1828, two years later, was a young Pennsylvanian, Samuel D. Gross, who was to add honors to his alma mater in later years. His thesis was on "Cataract." The first catalogue is that of 1829, issued by the dean, W. P. C. Barton, M. D.

and in the face of all obstacles the session closed with a smaller attendance, but an increased number in the graduating class, namely, thirty-four. These results plainly indicated the necessity of a permanent home for the institution, owned by its officers; but the school was yet too much of an experiment to warrant such an undertaking, unless there should arise some friend or friends, ready to provide the means. There had been enlisted in the membership of the Philadelphia contingent of the trustees, some of the most notable Presbyterians of the city, and among these was the Rev. Ezra Stiles Ely, D. D., pastor of the Third Presbyterian Church, who was secretary of the Board, and who proved to be the man of the hour. Dr. Ely proposed to the board to assume the entire responsibility of erecting a new building himself, and on March 22, 1827, the offer was given effect by the trustees deciding "that the additional trustees of Jefferson College, in their capacity as trustees, and not otherwise, do hereby agree with the Rev. Dr. Ely, that if he will cause to be erected a Medical Hall for the use of the Medical School, on such plan as shall be approved by this board, the additional trustees will rent the same of him and such persons, if any, as he may associate with him as proprietors of said hall, for a term of time not less than five years, at a rent of one thousand dollars a year, to be paid in the month of November in each of the said five years,—after said building shall be fitted for use." This money was to be provided by assessing the various chairs: those of Anatomy, Surgery, Materia Medica and Chemistry, two hundred and fifty dollars each, and smaller sums to the rest. The faculty agreed and, by May, a lot on Tenth street, between Juniper alley and George street, was secured and building plans adopted, so that, by August, 1828, "the very elegant and appropriately furnished new building in Tenth street" was ready for use.

Meanwhile, more difficulties arose in the faculty. The able professor of Anatomy resigned in October of '27, compelling Dr. McClellan to fill two chairs. In June following, a new trouble with the chair of Midwifery, then filled by Dr. Barnes, caused the trustees to vacate all the chairs and restore them on the 26th, with that of Midwifery unfilled and Dr. Robert M. Patterson in the chair of Anatomy. Dr. Patterson was called to the University of Virginia, however, and the chair was occupied, as before, with Dr. Samuel McClellan as assistant. Dr. Eberle lectured on Midwifery, and the year 1828-9 closed fairly well. The next year's prospects were modified by the withdrawal of Dr. Barton to New York in December, as naval surgeon, with his course to be finished by Dr. Rhees, and the promotion of Dr. Samuel McClellan (b) in January of 1830, to the chair of Anatomy. In February, Dr. Eberle resumed the chair of Materia Medica, with Midwifery attached, and Drs. James and William Rush were elected to his chair of Theory and Practice, William being named as adjunct. These gentlemen, however, declined, and Dr. Daniel Drake (c) of Cincinnati took the chair, and again, for the first time in three years, the faculty was complete. The year 1830-1 thus opened with the brightest of prospects; for Dr. Drake gave a new impetus to the school, and the influence of his teaching was felt in the city throughout the entire profession. Dr. Drake, however, was ambitious to found a great medical college in the West; at the close of the session he withdrew for that purpose, and, persuading Dr. Eberle to take like action, both went to Cincinnati in 1831. This was the hardest blow the Jefferson Medical School had yet received, but still another disaster followed in the death of Dr. Rhees. In consequence, the chair of Practice was filled by Dr. John Revere in 1831-2; the chair of Obstetrics by Dr. Usher Parsons, that of

---

(b) Dr. McClellan was a younger brother of the founder, born in 1800. He was educated chiefly in his brother's office, in the University, and in the medical department of Yale College, where he graduated in 1823. He spent three years in travel in Mexico, and in 1828 began his connection with the chair of Anatomy as Demonstrator. In 1832 he resigned his chair in favor of Dr. Granville S. Pattison, and he was chosen to the chair vacated by the death of Dr. Rhees. In 1836 the chair was divided, giving him that of Obstetrics and Diseases of Women, in which he was so successful that on the vacation of all the chairs in 1839, he was re-elected. He soon resigned, however, and retired to private practice. Dr. McClellan had a remarkable memory; he was "a quiet, unassuming man," beloved by all who knew him. He died in 1854.

(c) Dr. Drake's fame belongs to the West, and is well known to every student of American medicine. He was a native of New Jersey, born in 1785, and died in 1852, at the age of sixty-seven.

Materia Medica by Dr. Samuel Colhoun (d), that of Anatomy by Dr. Granville Sharpe Pattison, with Dr. Charles Davis as adjunct in the chair of Chemistry. Drs. Parsons and Davis resigned at the close of the year, and the misfortunes of the preceding year told heavily on the graduates.

The year 1832-3 began with Drs. Pattison, George and Samuel McClellan, Revere, Colhoun and Green as the faculty, and, excepting the addition in 1836 of Dr. Robley Dunglison to the chair of Institutes and Medical Jurisprudence, the institution had six years of freedom from change in its members. This was a period of such growth that the graduating classes, beginning with that of '34, rose yearly from fifty-two to fifty-eight, seventy-two, one hundred and twenty-five, and one hundred and eight. This was due in large measure to the qualities brought into the school by Drs. Pattison, Revere and Dunglison. Dr. Revere was a man of forty-four years, the son of Paul Revere of the Revolution. Born in 1787 in Boston, he graduated from Harvard in 1807 and four years later received his medical degree in Edinburgh. He soon established himself in Baltimore, and made some valuable discoveries in applied chemistry. In 1831 he was called to this chair in the new school. Here his excellent qualities as a physician and lecturer added greatly to the strength of the faculty during his ten years of service. He and Dr. Pattison both resigned in 1841 to take like chairs in the University of New York (e).

Dr. Pattison was a prominent figure in the Jefferson School during this period of ten years. He was a brilliant lecturer and teacher, but a man of intense feeling and strong prejudices. Years previous to his connection with this College his impetuous temperament, and some unfortunate experiences in Europe, combined to involve him in serious difficulties. He was of Scotch parentage,

(d) Dr. Colhoun was born in Chambersburg, Pennsylvania, in 1787, and died in 1841 at the age of fifty-four. He was a graduate of Princeton in 1804 and of the University Medical School in 1808. He settled in Philadelphia, and, after his nine years' service in Jefferson Medical College, joined the Drs. McClellan and others in a new school. He was a bachelor, learned and of genial, generous disposition.

(e) Dr. Revere died in New York in 1847, at the age of sixty years, one of the eminent men of the profession. Dr. Pattison died there four years later, at almost exactly the same age, and with equal eminence.

born in Glasgow in 1792, and at the age of seventeen began the study of medicine in the private school of Dr. Allan Burns. At nineteen he became demonstrator of Anatomy for his preceptor and two years of success led him to open a school of his own. Soon after he was appointed to a life position in the Andersonian Institute, but in the winter of 1818-19 removed to the United States, with the hope of succeeding Dr. Dorsey in the University of Pennsylvania. Not successful in this, he settled in Philadelphia and joined the movement for a new medical school, in which he took such aggressive measures as to print the Whildin thesis, before referred to, with its expunged passages retained and italicized. This engendered the most bitter feeling, and it was further increased by rumors of a Glasgow scandal, in which Dr. Pattison, although acquitted on trial, was believed by his opponents to be guilty. He attributed these rumors to Dr. Nathaniel Chapman, and in 1820 challenged the Doctor, thereby giving more publicity to the affair. In October of the same year, he entered upon the duties of the chair of Anatomy in the University of Maryland at Baltimore. Here his success as a teacher was repeated, but he afterwards returned to England and held the same chair in the University of London, recently organized. In the session of 1831-2 he came to Philadelphia to his position in Jefferson Medical College. "In the graduation in the spring of 1833," said he, in an introductory lecture six years afterwards, "the list of our graduates only numbered *sixteen!!* In four years afterwards, our list of graduates outnumbered that of our sister institution, the University of Pennsylvania—of that school with which we were accused of madness for attempting a competition. These facts are mentioned, gentlemen, not for the purpose of vaunting; but surely we are excusable in feeling an honest pride in a triumph so gratifying to ourselves and so honorable to our institution" (f).

A member of the faculty of this decade, 1831-41, who was the

(f) The University School had 405 students in 1837, the year referred to, and 162 graduates, by far the largest number in her history up to that date. According to one authority, Jefferson had 125 that year, the largest number up to that date in her own history. The records, however flattering to Jefferson's growth, do not quite confirm Dr. Pattison's statement for 1837, or even the total for four years, 1833-7. He may not have been correctly reported.

harbinger of greater days for Jefferson, and one who was to be the connecting link between the old and the new Jefferson Medical College, was Dr. Robley Dunglison, who joined the faculty in June, 1836. He was "no ordinary man," writes Dr. S. D. Gross over thirty years later; "indeed, in more than one sense of the term, he was an illustrious man; a great scholar, an accomplished teacher, a profound physiologist, an acute thinker, a facile writer, a lucid, erudite and abundant author." Dr. Dunglison was a man of forty years when he joined the young school; he was born in Keswick, England, in 1798, was educated at a well-known classical school, and began the study of medicine in his seventeenth year. After work in the universities at Edinburgh, London and Paris, he was licensed by the Royal College of Surgeons and began practice in 1819. In 1824 he received his degree from the University of Erlangen, became accoucheur to the Eastern Dispensary of London, and began lectures on Midwifery. Soon after, at the age of twenty-six, he received from the ex-President of the United States, Thomas Jefferson, an invitation to join the medical faculty of the University of Virginia, of which he was the founder. His teaching was to cover almost the whole field of medicine:—anatomy, physiology, surgery, materia medica, pharmacy, and the history of medicine. He not only accomplished it successfully for nine years, but also produced his great work on "Human Physiology" and his "Medical Dictionary," which has so well stood the test of time. In 1833 he was chosen for the chair of Materia Medica, Therapeutics, Hygiene and Medical Jurisprudence in the University of Maryland, where he wrote his work on "General Therapeutics," and in June, 1836, he accepted the chair of the Institutes of Medicine in Jefferson Medical College, which he held for thirty-two years, becoming emeritus professor only a year before his death, at the age of seventy-one. Dr. Dunglison was a man of the widest sympathies and interests, and one of the most prolific authors of his time. It is said that the total issue of his books aggregated about 155,000 volumes. He received the honorary degree of Doctor of Medicine from Yale and Doctor of Laws from Jefferson College. He was "a many-sided man, with a rare blending of mental qualities, an admirable symmetry of mind and character, a delicate and discriminative judgment, a capacious memory, a fervent love of truth, a keen insight into human nature, an amazing coolness and self-control, great powers of endurance, and a remarkable freedom from prejudice, eccentricity and exaggeration. These it was which fitted him for his peculiar stations in life, and made him what he was, a beacon light in the world of medical literature, and one of the foremost writers and teachers of his day." Dr. Dunglison was the element of conservative strength of this period, and was undoubtedly the leading influence in the reconstruction that was soon to come, and symbol of the order that was to spring from the chaotic years preceding 1841.

The changes that closed the old order began in the session of 1838-9, and these related to the building, the charter and the faculty. Classes were now so large that additions to the building became necessary, and as it was still the property of the Rev. Dr. Ely, and the charter granted no property rights, it was determined by the "additional trustees," who were the governing body of the medical school, to secure an independent charter. This was effected early in the spring of 1838, giving Jefferson Medical College of Philadelphia an independent existence, "with the same powers and restrictions as the University of Pennsylvania," and constituting the "additional trustees" its first board. On April 19, these trustees addressed a last communication in their old capacity, saying: *"Resolved,* that the President be directed to communicate to the mother board at Canonsburg, that, in accepting the charter which separates them from the Jefferson College at Canonsburg, the additional trustees are influenced by the conviction that such a separation is for the mutual benefit and convenience of both bodies, and desire it for no other reason; and that this board will retain a grateful sense of the kind and fostering care ever exhibited towards them by the parent institution, and will in their new capacity be always ready to acknowledge their past obligations, and to exchange, in every way in their power, kind offices with Jefferson College at Canonsburg."

Jefferson Medical College was destined to celebrate the first year of its independent existence by a faculty disagreement, which compelled it to vacate all the chairs in May, 1839, in order to remove the founder of the institution from the chair of Surgery, and, as it happened, from the school. The College, now firmly established, felt able to dispense with McClellan, its founder, and no longer needed the "fostering care" of the mother institution at Canonsburg. On July 10, 1839, the old faculty was re-elected, giving the chair of Surgery to Dr. Joseph Pancoast and Materia Medica to Dr. R. M. Huston; but as Dr. McClellan and Dr. Colhoun were soon followed by Dr. McClellan's brother, who resigned the chair of Midwifery, Dr. Huston was given that chair and Dr. Dunglison added Materia Medica to his. The new faculty was now composed of Drs. Pattison, Revere, Dunglison, Pancoast, Huston and Green. As a consequence of these measures, nearly half of the graduating class withdrew, preferring to sit under McClellan's teaching or to enter other schools in the year 1839-40. The class numbered only fifty-eight this year and sixty the next. The changes of the year following were still greater and resulted in entirely removing the original faculty. These changes began February 1, 1841, with the death of Dr. Green; on the 2nd of April, Drs. Pattison and Revere resigned to go to New York, and all the chairs were again vacated. Thus closed the first period of Jefferson's history, a stormy time that may be said, in reality, to cover the years since 1821, when young McClellan, at the age of twenty-five, began his lectures on Walnut street.

Dr. McClellan was forty-three when he left Jefferson. He "immediately conceived the project of a third medical school," writes a colleague (g), "and with characteristic buoyancy of spirit and determination of purpose, he went in person, accompanied by a single professional friend, to solicit a charter from the State Legislature." This time he attached his school to Pennsylvania College at Gettysburg, securing it full corporate privileges as the Medical Department of that institution (h). As a faculty he had

---

(g) Dr. S. G. Morton.
(h) The board created the department on September 18, 1839, in answer to the faculty's proposal of the 14th preceding. The legislative act was approved March 6, 1840.

secured, for the chair of Anatomy and Physiology, Dr. Samuel G. Morton (i); for the chair of Principles and Practice of Surgery, himself; Dr. Colhoun for the chair of Materia Medica and Pharmacy; Dr. Samuel McClellan for the chair of Obstetrics; Dr. William Rush for the chair of Theory and Practice of Physic; and Dr. Walter R. Johnson for the chair of Chemistry. They secured a building on Filbert street, above Eleventh; in November opened their session with a class of nearly one hundred students, and for four years the school maintained this average. The only change during this period was the succession of Dr. Robert M. Bird to the chair vacated by the death of Dr. Colhoun in 1841. Two years later, in 1843, the financial difficulties compelled the faculty to resign (j), and Dr. McClellan retired to private practice as the founder of two medical colleges. He survived but four years longer and died in 1847, in his fifty-first year. Dr. McClellan was eminently a bold and practical operative surgeon, although he was much more than that. He probably had greater pride in what he

---

(i) Dr. Morton was a native of Philadelphia, born in 1799, of Irish lineage. His father's death led to his mother's location in a Friends' community near New York, so that his early years were spent under its influence. He was left an orphan in 1817. A copy of Dr. Rush's lectures led him to study medicine; he joined the class under Dr. Parrish, and in 1820 graduated from the University Medical School. After extensive study in Europe he was graduated in 1823 at Edinburgh, and in 1826 settled in Philadelphia practice. He was a man of quiet, scholarly and scientific tastes, a voluminous writer of natural history, archæology and various allied lines of research. He died in 1851, at the age of fifty-two years.

(j) This institution had an independent existence of twenty years, until in 1859 it was merged with another school which sprang from the private anatomical school founded by Dr. James McClintock the same session that closed McClellan's connection with Jefferson. The faculty chosen to succeed McClellan's embraced Dr. William Darrach for Practice; Dr. H. S. Patterson for Materia Medica; Dr. W. R. Grant for Anatomy and Dr. John Wiltbank for Obstetrics. The next year Dr. Washington L. Atlee was given the chair of Chemistry, and in 1845 Dr. David Gilbert that of Surgery. Four years without change were succeeded by a new building, erected at Locust and Ninth streets, but no change occurred in the faculty for three years, when Dr. John J. Reese succeeded Atlee, Dr. J. M. Allen was given the chair of Anatomy, and Dr. Francis Gurrey Smith that of the Institutes. The next year Dr. Patterson's death gave his chair to Dr. John B. Biddle, and in 1854, Dr. Gilbert was chosen for the chair of Obstetrics, Dr. John Neil for that of Surgery, and Dr. Alfred Stillé for the chair of Practice. Anatomy went to Dr. T. G. Richardson in 1856, and two years later to Dr. John H. B. McClellan. In 1859, however, all the faculty resigned, and the faculty of the Philadelphia College of Medicine took their places, and thus merged the two schools, by closing the latter. This institution had a long legal controversy over the claims of Drs. Darrach and Wiltbank as successors to the original charter.

would have called the "practical" than in any other characteristic. "Recollect," said he, in 1836, to the class about to receive diplomas, "recollect what I have so often and so constantly urged on your attention, respecting the rules of inductive science. Be always governed by the observation of symptoms, and not by the imaginary causes of them. The whole science of nature consists in the classification of phenomena. We can do but very little in the way of theory, and nothing in the way of hypothesis. Be content, I beg of you, to follow the dictates of common sense in all cases and under all circumstances. Be satisfied with the opinions you can form from a plain and careful examination of the indications which nature holds up to your view; and reject all inquiry into the secret and undefinable causes of life and disease. You cannot imagine the advantages which you will gain by such a course of practice over those who are governed by the long-exploded precepts of the schoolmen—revived and repolished, as it must be confessed they have been, by the innovators of France. While they are balancing doubts and difficulties, and vibrating from one conjecture to another, you will be fortified by the calm and unchangeable dictates of sound reason and philosophy." Dr. McClellan's life was characterized by his love of Surgery and his ambition to found a medical school. There is no doubt that, in his affection, the highest place was always held by the school he founded first, Jefferson Medical College.

While the University, Jefferson, and the Medical Department of Pennsylvania College were growing along together from 1839, another private school was arising to form a fourth medical college. Dr. James McClintock, the originator of the Philadelphia School of Anatomy, or rather of the first school bearing that name, in 1838, as has been stated, had such success in his brilliant demonstrations in the western room of that building, that three years later he was called to the chair of Anatomy in a Vermont, and, subsequently, to a Massachusetts institution. He returned to Philadelphia in 1843, and again took charge of the western room, adding, the following year, lectures on Practice, by Dr. J. H. McCloskey, and on Materia Medica by Dr. Jackson Van Stavern.

Three years later, in the spring of 1847, he secured a charter for the Philadelphia College of Medicine, which proposed both summer and winter sessions, degrees to be conferred at the close of either session. Some of the lectures were given in the old western room of the School of Anatomy, and some in the school of Pharmacy, on Filbert, above Seventh street. In this faculty, he lectured on Anatomy, Physiology and Surgery; Dr. Jesse R. Burden on Materia Medica; Dr. Thomas D. Mitchell on Practice and Obstetrics, and Dr. William H. Allen on Chemistry. The first graduates numbered eighteen. In the autumn they moved to their new building on Fifth street, south of Walnut, where, during the session of 1847-8, they had an attendance of sixty-nine students, with thirteen graduates in March and twenty-one in July. The faculty in this year chose Dr. Henry Gibbons for the chair of the Institutes, Dr. C. A. Savory for the chair of Obstetrics, Dr. A. L. Kennedy for that of Chemistry and Dr. M. W. Dickerson for that of Comparative Anatomy. In 1849 Dr. Rush Van Dyke occupied the chair of Materia Medica and Dr. C. C. Cox that of Obstetrics. There were other changes during the first seven years, and yet during that time about four hundred were graduated. The institution was reorganized in 1854, adopted the national code of ethics, and had a faculty composed of Dr. George Hewston, lecturing on Anatomy; Dr. Henry Hartshorne on the Institutes, Dr. Isaac A. Pennypacker on Practice, Dr. James L. Tyson on Materia Medica, Dr. Joseph Parrish on Obstetrics, Dr. E. M. Tilden on Surgery, and Dr. B. Howard Rand on Chemistry. The next year Dr. Lewis D. Harlow lectured on Obstetrics. In 1856 Dr. A. T. King filled the chair of Practice and Dr. George Dock that of Surgery; the next year Dr. Hartshorne lectured on Practice, Dr. W. S. Halsey on Surgery, Dr. W. H. Taggart on Materia Medica, and Dr. James Aitken Meigs on the Institutes; in 1858, Dr. W. H. Gobrecht taught Anatomy. In 1859, in virtue of an agreement between the Philadelphia College of Medicine and the Pennsylvania Medical College (the Gettysburg School), the faculty of the latter resigned, and its chairs were taken possession of by the faculty of the former, composed of Drs. Rand, Hartshorne, Harlow, Halsey, Taggart, Meigs and Gobrecht.

The institution, which occupied the castellated structure on Ninth street, below Locust, lasted but two years, although it began prosperously and had, the first year, about forty graduates; for a combination of difficulties, due chiefly to the opening of the civil war of '61, caused the dissolution of the Medical Department of Pennsylvania College, which McClellan had founded.

If McClintock's College sprang out of the western room of the School of Anatomy in 1847, it may have been because some of the men connected with the eastern room had, the previous year, of January 28, 1846, secured a charter for Franklin Medical College, and opened it in the old building on Locust above Eleventh street, built for the school Chapman founded in 1817. Dr. John B. Biddle was its dean, and the faculty was composed of Dr. Paul B. Goddard for the chair of Anatomy, Dr. C. C. Van Wyck for the chair of Surgery, Dr. David H. Tucker for the chair of Medicine, Dr. Biddle for the chair of Materia Medica, Dr. William Byrd Page for the chair of Obstetrics, Dr. L. S. Jones for that of Physiology and Jurisprudence, and Dr. Robert Bridges for that of Chemistry. They began with a class of thirty-seven, and had five graduates in the commencement of '47. The institution survived only two sessions, and had the honor, during that period, of being the fifth of the regular medical colleges of Philadelphia. In these years, 1846-7 and '48, we find the largest number of regular medical schools for men in the city's history. The University School was at Ninth street, below Market; Jefferson, on Tenth street, below Chestnut; the Pennsylvania, on Filbert street, above Eleventh; the Philadelphia, on Filbert street, above Seventh, and the Franklin on Locust street, above Eleventh; while medical students were remarkably numerous, ranging from the University's 509 matriculates in 1848 down to Franklin's 37 enrolled (k).

This was not all. The greatest medical center in the land was not only productive of great medical activity on regular lines, but

---

(k) It is interesting to note that the following year, 1849, a medical society was organized at the house of Dr. James-Bryan at Tenth and Arch streets, called the Medico-Chirurgical College. It was only a medical society, not a College for lectures. Dr. Bryan had a private school, called The Surgical Institute, in the same building.

offered a fine field for experiments. So thought the German supporters of the first Homeopathic College in the United States, at Allentown, Pennsylvania. This institution had been opened in 1835, thirteen years before, to teach the doctrines of Samuel Hahnemann in the German tongue. The establishment of a similar one in Philadelphia had been discussed frequently in later years, but it was not until the members of the Central Bureau of the American Institute of Homeopathy held a meeting at the home of Dr. Jacob Jeans of Philadelphia, in February, 1848, that measures were decided upon. Dr. Constantine Hering and Dr. Walter Williamson were among those present, and plans were made for a petition to the Legislature for a charter. This was secured on April 8, following, and a faculty organized, composed of Dr. Jacob Jeans for the chair of Practice, Dr. Caleb B. Matthews for the chair of Materia Medica, Dr. Walter Williamson for the chair of Obstetrics, Dr. Francis Sims for the chair of Surgery, Dr. Samuel Freedley for the chair of Botany, Dr. Matthew Semple for that of Chemistry, Dr. W. A. Gardiner for that of Anatomy, and Dr. Alvan E. Small for that of Physiology and Pathology. On the 15th of October lectures were begun at 627 Arch street, in the rear of the building, and a dispensary was opened; but the next year, when the second McClellan school moved into new quarters, the Homeopathic Medical College of Philadelphia moved into the old Filbert street building, above Eleventh street. This institution brought a new element into the medical field that affected medical discussion more or less from that time on. Another institution, called Washington Medical College, was chartered four years later, though not organized. The first school struggled hard for existence and finally succumbed. It rose again to become the well-known Hahnemann Medical College and Hospital, on Broad street; but Homeopathy never gained so firm a foothold in Philadelphia as in many less conservative cities. As a contrast to this movement, there was chartered also in 1848 the Eclectic Medical College of Philadelphia, which existed for a time on Haines street, west of Sixth. Eclecticism suffered an even worse fate than Homeopathy, however, and the school was discontinued during the war.

This ferment of medical thought went beyond medical theory and opened the question of woman's entry into regular medicine. The subject was intimately associated with the various sociological movements of the day, and was only incidentally connected with the field of Obstetrics. It seemed chiefly to arise from the desire of women for a larger field of activity. The first woman to graduate in this country was Elizabeth Blackwell, a student of Dr. William Elder of Philadelphia, in 1848. She was allowed to graduate from Geneva Medical College, in the State of New York, as an experiment, but other women were refused the next year. Women then made application to the various institutions in Philadelphia in 1849, but without success. The demand was met by Dr. Henry Gibbons, Dr. J. A. Birkey, W. J. Mullen, Robert P. Kane and John Longstreth securing a charter on March 11, 1850, for the Female Medical College of Pennsylvania, with a Board of Trustees headed by the Rev. Albert Barnes. The faculty secured were Dr. N. R. Mosely for the chair of Anatomy, Dr. James F. X. McCloskey, dean, for the chair of Practice, Dr. C. W. Gleason for the chair of Surgery, Dr. Joseph P. Longshore for the chair of Obstetrics, Dr. W. W. Dickeson for the chair of Materia Medica, and Dr. A. D. Chaloner for the chair of Chemistry. They began their lectures on the 12th of October in the buildings at the rear of 627 Arch street (1), which the Homeopathists had occupied, and at once enrolled a class of forty students. From this number eight were graduated at the first commencement, which was held on December 30, 1851, at Musical Fund Hall; the names of these first graduates from the first woman's medical college in the world must always remain of the greatest historical interest. Six were from Pennsylvania, namely, Ann Preston, Susanna H. Ellis, Anna M. Longshore, Hannah E. Longshore, Phœbe M. Way and Frances G. Mitchell; one from New York, Angenette A. Hunt, and one from Massachusetts, Martha A. Sawin. Of these the most interesting to the city and the school was Ann Preston, a Friend, thirty-eight years of age, born in 1813 in West Grove, Chester County, Pennsylvania. She had already lectured to women on Physiology and Hygiene in various

---

(1) 229 Arch was its old numbering.

cities before entering this school, and, after receiving her medical degree, continued her studies. In 1852 she was called to the chair of Physiology and Hygiene, and thus became the first woman professor in a medical college in this country. The next year, there entered another student, Elizabeth Horton Cleveland, who was graduated in 1855, and took an advanced course of study in Europe in order to obtain clinical advantages for the proposed college hospital, which became a necessity on account of the difficulty women found in securing entry to Philadelphia hospitals. At the close of the session of 1856-7 she was chosen for the chair of Anatomy, with which she had been associated since the previous spring, and these two women, one the dauntless pioneer, and the other the skilled operator and administrator, carried the institution through its long period of struggle against obstacles within and without, and eventually brought it the success which is now historical (m). In that day, the woman's movement was considered almost as unpardonable an innovation as exclusive systems were, and indeed the followers of new medical theories were more favorable to woman than was the regular school of medicine. In consequence, some of the first friends of the woman's movement were among those who were not calculated to enhance its reputation. The woman's college strove to avoid this tendency and determined to raise the institution to the highest medical standard of the conservative schools and put it largely under the management of women. This soon resulted in a complete change in its faculty and management, and by 1853 Dr. Preston became the veritable founder of the conservative woman's college of to-day. In that year some of those founders of this school, who had withdrawn from it, conceived the plan of an institution that should solve all the difficulties of the times by teaching every system to both sexes. They secured a charter in 1853 under the name Penn Medical University (n), and opened

---

(m) Dr. Preston died in 1872 and Dr. Cleveland in 1878. Other notable names of later date are Dr. Rachael L. Bodley, Dr. Frances E. White, Dr. Anna E. Broomall, Dr. Clara Marshall, Dr. Anna M. Fullerton, and others. The name of the school became the Woman's Medical College in 1867.

(n) The charter of this school, and of the Eclectic, were bought some time later, and a "College" was started under the name Philadelphia University of Medicine and Surgery. Several institutions, with the same "University," later became involved in trouble about bogus diplomas, issued by one or two of them.

a course of lectures in a building on the north side of Market street, above Eleventh. It was the last effort of the period to create new medical colleges, and it had a spasmodic existence even down to the decade after the civil war. Its career serves to illustrate some of the extreme tendencies of that period, and the movements that were shifting and reshifting to settle the status of medical ethics, educational standards, woman in medicine and exclusive systems.

These movements were by no means peculiar to Philadelphia, although on account of her pre-eminence in medical education they were concentrated here. The bearing of all these elements on the question of medical ethics was first brought to the public attention of the profession as early as 1844 in the State Medical Society of New York, by which date the medical colleges of the land had almost doubled in number in little over a dozen years. The private school system, inaugurated by Dr. Chapman in 1817, while it had, in a measure, succeeded in supplying the deficiencies of the short courses of that day, had also opened a gate for an indiscriminate uprising of medical institutions of any sort or character. These great problems were of so important a nature that, in the New York Society of that year, Dr. N. S. Davis secured a motion to call a national convention to consider them. A preliminary convention was held in New York in 1846, of which Drs. John Bell and Alfred Stillé of Philadelphia were vice-president and secretary, respectively. Two of the most earnest advocates of the proposed national association, among Philadelphians, were Drs. Stillé and Samuel Jackson, although the only college in the city which responded to the invitation to join the preliminary organization in New York, was McClellan's second school, the Medical Department of Pennsylvania College. On the 5th of May, 1847, Dr. Isaac Hays, chairman of the Philadelphia Committee of Arrangements, welcomed at the old *Academy of Natural Sciences*, now a part of the Lafayette Hotel, representatives of forty medical societies and twenty-eight colleges, assembled to organize the *American Medical Association*. It is not the place here to enter into a history of the *Association*, but only to note those elements that bear upon the peculiar development of the profession of Philadelphia. The report on Medical Ethics was presented by Drs. Hays and Bell and adopted; higher educational standards were recommended to the colleges, and the constitution was so framed as to invariably secure a majority of the delegates from permanent state and county societies. The latter provision was intended to animate and encourage state and county organization, and ultimately limit the membership to such bodies. These were features that at once showed Philadelphia's leadership of the conservative element. Dr. Isaac Hays proposed a more exclusive form of organization, but it was defeated. The convention then resolved itself into the *American Medical Association*, with the venerable chief of the Medical Department of the University of Pennsylvania, Dr. Nathaniel Chapman, as president, Dr. Alfred Stillé as one of the two secretaries, and Dr. Isaac Hays as treasurer.

The effect of this gathering was to stimulate interest in all branches of medicine in Philadelphia, and especially in the purpose to elevate educational standards, the University being the first of the schools to begin the movement. The most marked result was the assembling of physicians of the city and county on December 11, 1848, in the Hall of the College of Pharmacy, with Dr. Samuel Jackson, late of Northumberland, as chairman, and Dr. D. Francis Condie as secretary, to form a county medical society. The old *Philadelphia Medical Society* had ceased to exist two years before, in 1846, and on January 16, 1849, it was replaced by the *Philadelphia County Medical Society*, and its first officers, then chosen, were Dr. Samuel Jackson (o), as president; Drs. John F. Lamb and Isaac Parrish, as vice-presidents; Dr. D. Francis Condie, recording secretary; Dr. Henry S. Patterson, corresponding secretary; Dr. William Byrd Page, treasurer, and Drs. Joseph Warrington, Thomas H. Yardley, William Mayburry, Wilson Jewell and Thomas F. Betton as censors. This society, on account of its connection with the state and national bodies, at once assumed a semi-official standing wholly unlike the old society, and in that respect more like the College of Physicians, although these two organizations had differ-

---

(o) Dr. Jackson was spoken of as "late of Northumberland," his former residence, in order to distinguish him from Dr. Samuel Jackson of the University.

ent aims. From this time onward these were the two great semi-official medical bodies in Philadelphia, the County Society the general one and the College of Physicians more limited in membership and representing the more conservative element, although membership was frequently held in both. It was in 1858 that the County Society first acted upon the question of woman in medicine. Owing to the general feeling on the subject, it was decided not to countenance women as regular physicians, and the following year secured the same action in the State Society. An interesting picture of the profession of that day and of the society's relation to it is given as follows:

"When the meetings of the society adjourned in 1848," says Dr. John B. Roberts, in his closing address to the County Medical Society in 1892, descriptive of the medical activity of that period, "the members trudged on foot to their homes in Mulberry, Sassafras or Schuylkill Eighth (p) streets, or possibly took an omnibus of the old style, since street cars were unknown. They doubtless felt secure, however late the adjournment, as they met on the corner an occasional watchman calling the hour of the night and the state of the weather. At this time the Penn squares, at Broad and Market streets, recently the site of the waterworks, had been laid out and were expected soon to become ornamental parks. Now the site of these expected parks is unknown to the children who exercise with roller skates on the pavement of the public buildings, and chase each other about the Reynolds statue. The Medical Department of the University of Pennsylvania had in its faculty Chapman, Hare, Gibson, Horner, Jackson, George B. Wood, H. L. Hodge, James B. Rogers and George W. Norris. This medical school had just increased its sessions to five and a half months, in order to elevate the standard of education and to show disapproval of the short four months' session, usual in the medical colleges of the United States. In the winter of 1849 and 1850 the course was made six months—from October 1st to the end of March; and in order to compensate for the increased expense to the students for board, the fees for lectures were reduced. Unfortunately this advance

---

(p) The former names for streets from Schuylkill to Broad.

was not adopted by other schools, and in 1852-3 the six months' session was discontinued and a shorter course adopted. The faculty of the Jefferson Medical College, at Tenth and Sansom streets, contained the well-known teachers—Dunglison, Huston, Joseph Pancoast, J. K. Mitchell, Mütter, Charles D. Meigs and Bache. This school, in 1848-9, increased its session from four months to four and a half months. The Pennsylvania Medical College, or the Medical Department of the Pennsylvania College, erected in 1849 the building now called Peabody Hotel, on the west side of Ninth street below Locust, which was subsequently occupied by one of the notorious institutions issuing bogus diplomas. Here were teaching at the time of the founding of our society, Drs. Darrach, Wiltbank, Patterson, Grant, David Gilbert and Washington L. Atlee. The Philadelphia College of Medicine, chartered in 1847, was, in 1848-9, situated on the west side of Fifth street below Walnut. The members of the faculty were James McClintock, Gibbons, Savory, Kennedy, Vandyke, Cox and W. W. Dickson. This school gave two courses in each year, graduating students not only in March, but also in the early part of July. At this time the Franklin Medical College was in operation on the north side of Locust street, above Eleventh, in a building erected originally by the Medical Institute, and torn down only two or three years ago for improvements in the neighborhood. Its faculty consisted of Goddard, Van Wyck, Tucker, John B. Biddle, Page, Jaynes and Bridges. The present Woman's Medical College of Pennsylvania was founded in 1849, with a charter from the Legislature similar to that of the Franklin Medical College. Its first course of lectures was given in 1850-51. It was situated on Arch street. The Homeopathic Medical College, the predecessor of the present Hahnemann Medical College, was instituted in 1846, and occupied, in the days of which we speak, a structure on the north side of Filbert street, above Eleventh, on part of the site now occupied by the Reading terminal station. The Eclectic Medical College of Pennsylvania was chartered in 1850, and in 1852 was situated on Haines street west of Sixth. The Philadelphia School of Anatomy was on College Avenue (later called Chant street, and running alongside of St. Stephen's Episcopal Church, between Market and Chestnut streets), east of Tenth. It was occupied as a private school of anatomy by Joseph M. Allen, who, in 1852, gave up the school. It was then occupied by Dr. D. Hayes Agnew, whose success as a teacher is well known to the present generation. Dr. Agnew was followed by Dr. Garretson, Dr. Andrews, Dr. Sutton and Dr. Keen. Dr. Keen relinquished the school in 1875 at the time the U. S. Postoffice took its rise from the old site of the demolished buildings of the University of Pennsylvania. Subsequently the school was revived by Dr. Boisnot in Hunter street, above Tenth, and between Market and Filbert streets. Here I subsequently became its proprietor, teaching anatomy and operative surgery. From the lectures given there by me and my associates was developed the post-graduate school on Lombard street, above Eighteenth, known to you as the Philadelphia Polyclinic and College for Graduates in Medicine. It is interesting to remember that at this time the Pennsylvania Hospital had an Obstetric Department, under the care of Drs. H. L. Hodge and Joseph Carson; that the Wills Eye Hospital, on Race street, the Blockley or Philadelphia Hospital, and St. Joseph's Hospital were in active operation; and that the Preston Retreat, recently built, was being used by the Foster Home because the funds of the Preston estate were not available, being in the Schuylkill Navigation Company's stock. The Friends' Asylum, on Walnut street below Fourth, was still in existence, but probably had very few patients, while the City Hospital at Bush Hill, Schuylkill Fourth and Coates streets, was a pest hospital, ever ready, but seldom occupied by patients. The College of Physicians was then holding its meetings in the so-called Picture House of the Pennsylvania Hospital, on Spruce street above Eighth, whence it removed in 1863 to Thirteenth and Locust streets, to the building in which we now meet. In April, 1851, a committee of the Philadelphia County Medical Society reported that the whole number of practitioners of all kinds in the county, so far as could be ascertained, was 582. Its report says: 'Of these 397 are physicians—regular practitioners, 42 homeopaths, 30 Thompsonians, 2 hydropaths, 32 advertising doctors, 37 practitioners of medicine and druggists, and 42 nondescripts or unascertained.'"

In the midst of the changes in the profession of Philadelphia the strong conservative elements behind them were the University faculty, headed by Chapman down to 1850, and the able Jefferson men, known as the faculty of 1841, both of which groups had long periods of freedom from change, the one for twelve years and the other for fifteen. The decade of the "forties" was a period of great and evenly balanced power in these two great schools, and if there were years of dominant good fortune in the University in the decade preceding this one, probably the same might be said for Jefferson in the decade following. For the University, the year 1835 was the beginning of her dozen years without change in the faculty. It included at that date Dr. Nathaniel Chapman in the chair of Practice, Dr. William Gibson in the chair of Surgery, Dr. William E. Horner in the chair of Anatomy, Dr. Samuel Jackson in the chair of the Institutes, Dr. George B. Wood in the chair of Materia Medica and Pharmacy, Dr. Hugh L. Hodge in the chair of Obstetrics, and Dr. Robert Hare in the chair of Chemistry. Most of these men had been connected with the faculty since as early as 1819, when Physick and Gibson took the chairs of Anatomy and Surgery. With them had been Dr. William P. Dewees, whom ill health, unfortunately for the institution, compelled to resign in the year 1835, when, as has been said above, began a long period of immunity from change. Many of the elements of strength were present before that time; but nothing takes the place of unity and *esprit de corps* in a faculty, and it is probable that these became strongest in 1835. This was also a period of literary activity; the text-books of the land were those produced by the faculties of the University and of Jefferson.

Dr. William P. Dewees, who resigned in 1835, was a Pennsylvanian of Swedish lineage, born in 1768, at Pottsgrove. He began the study of medicine at an early date with a practicing apothecary, and afterwards had Dr. William Smith of Philadelphia as his preceptor. He graduated from the University Medical School in 1789, and settled at Abington, about fourteen miles north of the city. He was drawn to Philadelphia practice by the needs of the fatal epidemic of 1793, and soon attracted the attention of Drs. Rush and Physick. Here he determined on Obstetrics as his especial field, began a private course of lectures on the subject, and was strongly recommended for that chair in 1810. Ill health compelled him to withdraw to country life for five years, and in 1817, when he returned, he soon became associated with Drs. Chapman and Horner in Chapman's private instruction. From this time he became an authority on Obstetrics. His "Practical Observations on Midwifery" became known over the world, and was followed by his systematic works. In 1825 he became adjunct professor to the chair of Obstetrics in the University, and on account of the ill health of Dr. James, he was the practical occupant of that chair for almost ten years, when he succeeded him. An accident in 1834 practically closed his career; he resigned in 1835, and, after travel and other means of restoration, died in 1841, at the advanced age of seventy-three.

With Dewees, in Dr. Chapman's private faculty, was another notable figure, who succeeded Physick as Dewees did James. This was Dr. William E. Horner, twenty-five years younger than Dewees, born at Warrenton, Virginia, in 1793. Dr. Horner was a man of intense intellectual life in a frail body; to his ardor and ambition was joined a faculty for details and mechanism that made Anatomy his choice. He came of English stock, was educated under a private tutor, the Rev. Charles O'Neill, a graduate of both Trinity College (Dublin) and Oxford. Under his direction Dr. Horner continued until 1809, when he began work in medicine under Dr. John Spence of Dumfries. With him he studied three years, and had two sessions in the University of Pennsylvania Medical School, when the war of 1812 led him to secure a commission as surgeon's mate in the Government service, July 3, 1813. After spending a short time at the University, early in 1814, in order to graduate, he had an extensive experience in Canada and in the hospitals at Buffalo, until the spring of 1815. Returning to Warrenton, he soon became satisfied that he was fitted for larger things than a country practice, and, no doubt, inspired by the successes of Virginians like Chapman and Hartshorne, he resolved to try his powers in the great medical metropolis of the continent. "The Rubicon is passed," he wrote in his journal. "I have forsaken my friends and my practice and am now on my way to Philadelphia to seek my fortunes. I have put all at hazard. Oh, thou Father everlasting, be propitious to my cause!" This was in 1816, and he was but twenty-three. The following spring he was fortunate enough to secure the office of dissector to Dr. Caspar Wistar, and aid to Dr. Chapman in his private work. He was successively assistant to both Wistar and Dorsey, and on the death of the latter, in 1819, became adjunct professor of Anatomy to Dr. Physick. His health was still poor, but his strong will upheld him until 1821, when he spent a year abroad. Returning much improved, he entered upon the most successful work of his life. Like Wistar, he made great use of models and other illustrative means, that became important additions to what is now known as the Wistar and Horner Museum of the University. After fifteen years, on Dr. Physick's death in 1837, he succeeded to the full chair. He had scarcely received this appointment when the great cholera epidemic of 1832 caused him to offer his services to take charge of a hospital." He published his work on Anatomy, made some anatomical discoveries, especially relating to the eye, and, although not a brilliant lecturer, was a most successful instructor of hundreds of appreciative students. His work continued, with some interruptions, almost until his death in March, 1853, the same year that Dr. Chapman died.

Two years later the faculty lost another of the Southern members of the old faculty. This was the gifted Baltimorean, Dr. William Gibson, LL. D., the successor of Physick in Surgery in 1819. He was but thirty-one when he was called from the chair of Surgery in the University of Maryland, of which he was one of the earliest promoters. Born in 1788, in Baltimore, he was educated at St. John's College, Annapolis, and later in Princeton. His medical studies were begun under Dr. John Owen of Baltimore, and after one course of lectures in the University of Pennsylvania, in 1806, he went to Edinburgh, where he attended lectures and studied under the direction of John Bell. Graduating in 1809, with a thesis on a phase of ethnology that attracted much attention, he went to London and had a most extensive acquaintance with prominent men and events, which were afterward described in a literary style that was one of his chief characteristics. Among these men were Sir Charles Bell, in whose family he was a private pupil, Abernethy and Sir Astley Cooper, to mention only medical names, and it was here that he had exceptional opportunities for observation of the wounded of Waterloo. He returned to Baltimore in 1810, and two years later joined the new medical staff of the University of Maryland in the chair of Surgery, where he at once distinguished himself. He also had experience in the war of 1812, as did his colleague, Dr. Horner. His service was that of surgeon in the militia of that state, in 1814, when the British made their attack on Baltimore. Seven years of brilliant work as a lecturer there, resulted in his being chosen successor to Dr. Physick, when, in 1819, the latter was transferred to the chair vacated by Dorsey's death. "As a lecturer," says one writer, "he was clear and emphatic; his voice was distinct and melodious; his language was well chosen, and his style of enunciation was attractive. His demonstrations of surgical anatomy were readily comprehended by the student; some of them especially, as those in connection with the neck, with hernia and with lithotomy, could not be surpassed in lucid exposition. For purposes of demonstration, Dr. Gibson had himself prepared and procured by purchase an ample collection of morbid structures, diseased and fractured, bones, models and casts, as well as pictures of large size, illustrative of disease, or of the anatomical parts of the body involved in operations. To these were added the approved mechanical appliances of the day. In this teaching he has set the example that has been followed extensively by other surgeons." Dr. Gibson had the unusual experience of successfully performing the Cæsarean section twice, and successfully, on the same person. His chief scientific publication was an outline work on surgery that was widely used, although his skillful pen was freely used aside from that. He was an extensive traveler and a man of varied accomplishments in music and other fine arts, and was one of those who easily win the friendship of the great men of the world. After thirty-six years of service in the chair made famous by Physick, he resigned in 1855, and became Emeritus Professor of Surgery, at the age of sixty-seven. He was a man of wealth and spent his remaining years in retirement, finally making his home in Savannah, Georgia, where he died in 1868, at the advanced age of eighty.

Dr. Robert Hare was called as Professor of Chemistry from a Virginia institution, in the same year that Gibson came from Baltimore. Dr. Hare was not a Southerner, however, as were Chapman, Horner and Gibson, but was born in Philadelphia in 1781, and early became interested in Chemistry, which he and Silliman studied under Dr. Woodhouse in the University. It was in 1801, at the age of twenty, that he invented the oxy-hydrogen blow-pipe, and won the Rumford medal of the American Academy of Arts and Sciences. Dr. Hare expected to succeed Woodhouse in 1809, but soon went to William and Mary College, Virginia, as professor of Chemistry, whence he was called ten years later to Philadelphia. Here he spent twenty-seven years of most notable work as a philosophical and practical chemist and instructor. Harvard had given him the honorary degree of Doctor of Medicine three years before, and his extensive researches and inventions in electrical and other fields made his name famous. Indeed, Faraday, after exhausting every experiment, finally adopted Dr. Hare's deflagrator, an electric heater also producing light, as the best that was possible at that date, 1835. The scientific apparatus invented by Hare was extensive and so valuable that it was presented to the Smithsonian Institution at his decease. Pharmacy and Toxicology are deeply indebted to his researches, as are many other fields of applied chemistry. He was brilliant in experiment and lecture, and had won an enviable position when he resigned in 1847, making a first break in the faculty of '35, after its twelve years of continuity. He died in 1858 at the age of seventy-seven, and if he had done nothing else, his contribution of the oxy-hydrogen instrument would have made his name one of the first in chemical annals.

The two new members of the faculty of '35 were Drs. George B. Wood and Hugh L. Hodge, who held chairs in the school for twenty-five and twenty-eight years respectively. Dr. Wood was a native of New Jersey, of Quaker parentage, born at Greenwich, in 1797, so that he was thirty-eight years of age when he entered the faculty. Educated in his preparatory work in New York, where he evinced signs of the remarkable ability through which he achieved such great distinction, he came to the University of Pennsylvania and graduated from the Collegiate Department with high honors in 1815. He at once began the study of medicine with Dr. Parrish, as has been noticed before, and graduated with such standing from the University Medical School in 1818 that Dr. Parrish secured him as assistant in his private medical school. Here he developed those enlightened views upon medical ethics and practice that became so important an influence in American medicine. He was a man of slow but sure growth, and his power as a lecturer on Chemistry was such that in 1821 he was called to that chair in the new College of Pharmacy, and the following year was transferred to the chair of Materia Medica. During nine years of work in that department, nine months of which were spent with Drs. Hewson and Bache in preparing the National Pharmacopœia for the press, Dr. Wood plainly became the man for the chair of Materia Medica in the University in 1835. It is one of the happy features of the histories of the University and Jefferson that work on this pharmacopœia ripened a professional friendship between their two great representatives, Wood of the faculty of '35 and Bache of the Jefferson faculty of '41, which resulted in that joint monument of the two men, the United States Dispensatory. During the next fifteen years Dr. Wood completely modernized his department. "His courses of lectures upon Materia Medica," writes Dr. Hartshorne, "may be truly said to have been splendid, almost magnificent; adorned as well as made complete for the students' information by the exhibition, from day to day, of living specimens of plants from all quarters of the world, grown in his own private conservatory and botanical garden, maintained for this special purpose. When such could not at the time be obtained, fine pictorial representations were placed before the class in their stead; and his cabinet of mineral and other crude and prepared specimens was correspondingly complete. A printed syllabus of the course of lectures, interleaved for note-taking, was furnished gratuitously by him to each student. It may be said, indeed, that no portion of the curriculum of the Medical Department of the University, able and renowned as have been the other members of its faculty, ever added more to the great reputation and large classes of that institution than this model course." His "Practice of Medicine," issued in 1847, was widely adopted as a text-book. He was the successor of Dr. Chapman in 1850, on the resignation of the latter. While in the chair of Practice, which he held for ten years, he also issued a treatise on Therapeutics and Pharmacology. Dr. Wood was a most erudite, fresh and balanced medical scholar. His mind was systematic and infused with the modern historical method. His local and larger historical works, such as the history of the University and the Pennsylvania Hospital, a history of Materia Medica, and others, are excellent illustrations of this quality. He was a leader in nearly all the learned, scientific and professional societies at home, and honored by many of those abroad. Princeton gave him the degree of Doctor of Laws, and in his varied travels abroad he was greatly honored, while he did much to further the scientific plans of societies in America. He died in 1879, nearly nineteen years after his resignation, at the ripe age of eighty-two, one of those of whom he himself said:

"Everywhere they sow
The seeds of truth, which, spirit-nurtured, grow
To a rich harvest."

Dr. Wood's colleague of '35, Dr. Hugh L. Hodge, came of one of the most distinguished Presbyterian families, his brother being the eminent theologian of Princeton, Dr. Charles Hodge. The founder of the family, a Scotch-Irish Presbyterian, settled on Water street in 1730, and it was his son, Dr. Hugh Hodge, who studied medicine under Dr. Thomas Cadwalader, and to whom was born, in 1796, a more famous son, Dr. Hugh L. Hodge. Educated at boarding-schools, he entered Princeton in 1811 as a sophomore, and in three years graduated with the highest honors. He was eighteen when he entered Dr. Caspar Wistar's office, and in four years received his medical diploma from the University. After two years as a ship's surgeon on East Indian voyages, he settled on Walnut street, and the following year was chosen by Dr. Horner to take his place in Dr. Chapman's Institute during a brief absence. In 1823 Chapman called him to lecture on Surgery, which he did with utmost success. His favorite studies, Surgery and Anatomy, he was led to give up for several reasons, chief among them being his weakened vision, so that he soon took the place of Dr. Dewees in Obstetrical lectures and joined the staff of that department in the Pennsylvania Hospital. Thus, in 1835, he was the successful candidate over so strong a man as Dr. Charles D. Meigs, to the chair made famous by Dewees. He was a successful lecturer, admired and beloved by students. His work in Obstetrics was especially notable for his inventions in forceps and pessaries, that were used the world over. His works on Diseases Peculiar to Women and on Obstetrics were published late in life, the latter in 1863, the year he resigned his professorship. The work was written by an amanuensis and with the aid of his son, Dr. H. Lenox Hodge, for his vision had become seriously impaired. In all things he was ruggedly original, conscientious, accurate and clear. His *alma mater* honored him, in 1871, with the degree of Doctor of Laws. He died in 1873 at the ripe age of seventy-seven, nearly forty years after he entered the faculty of 1835.

The last, and, in one way, the most remarkable member of the faculty of 1835, was Dr. Samuel Jackson, who was the first and most effective apostle of the methods and principles of Laenec, Louis and the French school of medicine that were the true sources of the scientific methods of to-day. Dr. Jackson was of an ardent, enthusiastic temperament, peculiarly open to conviction, active and inquiring in mind and earnest in public welfare. His teaching had great influence from its warm, fresh and attractive originality; and his keen appreciation of the pathological importance of new ideas regarding organism and vital force made him a leader in those directions. Dr. Jackson's training was somewhat like that of his friend and colleague, Dr. Wood. Born in 1787, in Philadelphia, the son of Dr. David Jackson, one of the University's first graduates of 1768, he received his education in the Collegiate

Department of the University, and studied medicine under Dr. James Hutchison, Jr., and chiefly under Dr. Caspar Wistar. After receiving his medical degree from the University in 1808, his thesis being on "Suspended Animation," the death of his father and elder brother compelled him to take charge of his father's drug business for a time. He soon began practice, however, and in 1812 joined the First Troop of City Cavalry and served in Maryland until the close of the war in 1815. His active service in promotion of public sanitation placed him at the head of the Board of Health early in 1820 and made him a great benefactor to the city in the yellow fever epidemic of that date. His account of that year's scourge is the most authoritative. He believed in its domestic origin and non-contagiousness, and, in consequence, had great influence in promoting present-day care for sanitary vigilance. The epidemic of 1820 is the last of any importance in the city. Dr. Jackson's experience in pharmacy led, in 1821, to his becoming one of two professors in the new College of Pharmacy, he lecturing on Materia Medica and his colleague, soon succeeded by Dr. Wood, on Chemistry. Here ripened the methods and friendship of these two remarkable men. Very soon Dr. Chapman chose Dr. Jackson to lecture in his private school, on Medical Chemistry, and, later, on Materia Medica and Therapeutics, a position which he held until 1844. The next year, 1822, he also became one of the Almshouse Hospital staff, where he and Gerhard, Pennock and others were to do so much to introduce and develop the methods and principles of the French school. Here he advanced the study of auscultation and percussion, the new methods of diagnosis. "A student as well as a teacher among students," says Dr. Carson, and some of the first results of his work were reported in 1824. His clinical lectures inspired large numbers of students, and the profession as well, to active study of the French methods in Pathology, and in 1827 Dr. Chapman secured his election as assistant to his University chair, to relieve him of the departments of Clinical Medicine and the Institutes, which had hardly been given adequate treatment since that giant in capacity, Rush, had died. He became interested in the doctrine of Broussais, "but," said he, "it is not all true, nor does it compass all truth," and his and Dr. Drake's opposing views in the Medical Society of 1830-1 were the chief features of its meetings. It was the pathological work of Louis, however, that most attracted him, and he inspired Gerhard, Pennock, Stillé and others to go to Paris and study under the great pathologist. In 1832 Dr. Jackson formulated the best exposition of the new methods in a work entitled "Principles of Medicine founded on the Structure and Functions of the Animal Organism," which was the first work of its kind published in the country. It was he, Dr. Charles D. Meigs and Dr. Richard Harlan who were chosen that year to investigate the treatment of cholera at Montreal, and on his return he had charge of Hospital No. 5, when the disease arose in Philadelphia. Dr. Jackson had acted as assistant to Dr. Chapman for eight years, when, in 1853, he accepted the new chair created for the Institutes and Clinical Medicine. For the next twenty-eight years he was a power among the young men of the profession; perhaps the extent of his influence has but recently been appreciated. His writings were numerous and bore almost wholly upon phases of the pathological work of which he was so able an expounder. Dr. Jackson resigned in 1863, and died nine years later at the age of eighty-five, when he had seen all the old faculty of '35 retired or deceased, and the principles of Louis widely accepted.

Another connected with the old faculty of 1835 is worthy of especial interest, not only as assistant to Dr. Jackson and head of the newly instituted system of dispensary clinics for the University, but chiefly for his contributions to the science of medicine in the discovery of the difference between typhus and typhoid fevers. This was Dr. William W. Gerhard, who became assistant to Dr. Jackson in 1838, and led in the institution of the dispensary clinics three years later (q). Dr. Gerhard came of German Reformed and Moravian ancestry of old Pennsylvania and New Jersey families. Born in 1809 in Philadelphia, he was educated at Dickinson College, and after his graduation in 1826, began the study of medicine

---

(q) Dr. Jacob Randolph was the first appointed clinical lecturer on Surgery for the University and the Pennsylvania Hospital in 1845, and Dr. George W. Norris succeeded him three years later.

under Dr. Joseph Parrish. Six years later he graduated at the University Medical School with a thesis on the endermic application of medicines, which showed the excellence of his pathological work in the Almshouse Hospital and attracted much attention. After graduation, he visited Europe, eventually going to Paris, where he came into close relation with Louis. His study there, in association with Pennock and other young Americans, was chiefly clinical and his investigations covered a large field, including smallpox, typhus and typhoid fevers, cerebral affections, cholera and many other maladies; his first papers, in conjunction with Pennock, being on Asiatic cholera.

Returning to Philadelphia he began practice, still pursuing his investigations at the Philadelphia or Almshouse Hospital. He also became resident at the Pennsylvania Hospital in 1834. Auscultation, percussion and systematic clinical work were carried on by him even more successfully than by Dr. Jackson. In 1836 he established the difference between typhus and typhoid fevers, and made himself a world-wide fame. Indeed he was the greatest American exponent of the new scientific pathological methods of France. In 1838 he became assistant to Dr. Jackson in the University, and here showed his commanding powers as a clinical teacher. During that year also he joined with Drs. Pennock, Stewardson, Norris, Stillé, Goddard, Grant, Pepper, Patterson, Biddle, Carson, Mütter and others in the formation of the Pathological Society of Philadelphia, of which he became the first president. This society paved the way for the more permanent one of to-day, which was founded in 1857 in the old "picture-house" of the Pennsylvania Hospital, and whose first officers were: President, Dr. S. D. Gross; vice-presidents, Drs. LaRoche and Stillé; treasurer, Dr. Addinell Hewson; secretary, Dr. J. M. Da Costa, and assistant secretary, Dr. T. G. Morton. These two societies have been thought by some to have had more general and far-reaching scientific influence than either the College of Physicians or the County Medical Society, and it must be admitted that at least in the field of the new Pathology they have been of the first importance. In 1841 Dr. Gerhard had succeeded in establishing dispensary clinics for the University in the Medical Institutes in associaton with Dr. W. P. Johnston, and in 1842 published his treatise on the diagnosis, pathology and treatment of the diseases of the chest. An attack of typhoid fever in 1837 had seriously impaired his health and interrupted his work, so that in 1843 he went to Europe for rest. His life was a busy one from that time on until about 1868, when he began to retire from active practice. He died in 1872 at the age of sixty-three, a genial, kindly, gentle clinical teacher, who must always be associated in Philadelphia with the introduction of the scientific methods of to-day (r).

While the University faculty of 1835 was enjoying its prosperity, as has been said, the chairs of Jefferson Medical College were vacated on April 2, 1841, when Drs. Pattison and Revere went to New York. Four days later the chairs were filled by men so able and so harmonious, that the régime has been since known as "the New Jefferson Medical College." Of this faculty one, Dr. Robley Dunglison, had been with the College five years in the chair of the Institutes; Dr. Joseph Pancoast of the Anatomical chair had been two years with it in the chair of Surgery, and Dr. R. M. Huston had been a like length of time in the chair of Materia Medica; but the merit of the new order consisted in the excellence of every chair, without exception. The new members were Dr. T. D. Mütter for the chair of Surgery, Dr. J. K. Mitchell for the chair of Practice, Dr. Charles D. Meigs for that of Obstetrics, and Dr. Franklin Bache for that of Chemistry. From that date on for fifteen years there followed a period of remarkable prosperity and growth. Even when change necessarily came on account of age, the addition was a man whose name soon gave Jefferson even more honor than she could confer on him. As a result, the last half of this period is the beginning of the golden age of the second great School of Medicine in Philadelphia. "During these years, the period of the true rise and healthy growth of the school," writes Dr. John H. Brinton,

---

(r) Dr. Caspar W. Pennock was a Philadelphian, born in 1801. He graduated in 1828 from the University, and was primarily an investigator by the new methods. He also studied under Louis in Paris and was intimately associated with Dr. Gerhard in his work, until attacked by paralysis, which afflicted him for more than twenty years. He died in 1867.

"the attitude of the faculty was one of harmony, nay, of unanimity. Many of these great advances in teaching were then effected which gave the stamp to the school, and helped not a little to bring about that prosperity which has lasted, unbroken, to the present day. Chief among these was the origination of the great system of Collegiate Clinics. The establishment of such a means of teaching had been in the minds of successive faculties from the very beginning of the institution. Indeed, an infirmary had been opened within the walls of the Jefferson College in May, 1825, in advance of its first session, and on the 9th of that month Dr. George McClellan performed the first surgical operation in the anatomical amphitheater. The system of practical teaching thus introduced was continued, with more or less regularity, down to the period of the reorganization. By the new faculty, the Collegiate Clinic—Medical as well as Surgical—was made a prominent feature in the weekly curriculum. To use the words of Professor Mitchell in his introductory of 1847, the clinic became 'the right arm of the College.' In addition to the clinics of the College, the class had access to the lectures at the Pennsylvania Hospital and at the Blockley Almshouse. To the latter they were carried twice a week in large omnibuses hired for the purpose, the students often crowding the top as well as interior of the vehicles. This disorderly transportation was an event of great delight to all small urchins on the route, and afforded in winter, as I well recollect, inestimable chances for snowballing and boyish sharp-shooting. The mode of instruction by Collegiate Clinics met at first with opposition; it was denounced and sneered at. It was said that it was imperfect and insufficient, that it conveyed false impressions and was calculated to mislead rather than instruct. It may be that at first it was imperfect. It undoubtedly was inferior in some respects to Hospital Clinics, nevertheless it was a great step in advance, and the defects in the system soon brought their own remedy." This remedy was, of course, the hospital, which grew from small beginnings about two or three years later.

The strength of Jefferson was in the personal power of its faculty, from the refined, scholarly Dunglison, whose career has been already noticed as the bond between the old and new, to the youngest of the new members. It is also interesting to note in this faculty the proportion which came from the South; this includes Drs. Huston, Mitchell and Mütter. Dr. Robert M. Huston was the wise, calm, clear-minded dean of the faculty for nearly the entire period, and became its first emeritus professor on his resignation in 1857. He was a Virginian, born in 1794, and studied medicine with such ability that in 1812, at the age of eighteen, he entered the government service as an assistant surgeon. He afterwards entered the Medical School of the University of Pennsylvania, where he graduated in 1825 at the age of thirty-one. Dr. Huston entered the old faculty in 1839, thirteen years later, to occupy the chair of Materia Medica, but was transferred to that of Obstetrics; and in the new organization he was chosen to the chair of Materia Medica and Therapeutics, the latter of these two subjects being his favorite branch of study. His convictions were in accord with the less heroic methods of treatment advocated during these years. As a lecturer he is said to have been characterized by simplicity and sincerity, and used manuscript entirely. Dr. Huston's business ability was of the utmost service to Jefferson, and when he died in 1864 the loss of his valuable counsel was deeply felt.

The member of the old faculty, who joined it in 1839, about the same time as Dr. Huston, was its famous surgeon, Dr. Joseph Pancoast, who succeeded the founder, until in the new order of '41 he was given the chair of Anatomy. Dr. Pancoast was only thirty-four when he entered upon the duties of a professor. He was a native of New Jersey, born in 1805, and on entering upon the study of medicine soon found his favorite field to be that of surgery. Attending the University of Pennsylvania Medical School, he graduated in 1828, at the age of twenty-three, and at once settled in practice. Three years later he began teaching Anatomy, in which he soon won an enviable reputation. "His great object," writes Dr. Brinton, "was to teach Anatomy, not the anatomy of the dead, but rather of the living. With him it was Anatomy applied—Medical Anatomy, Surgical Anatomy. In his hands the bones lost their dryness, they became, as it were, living exponents of injuries and diseases. Their growth, their size, their measurements served as themes for discourses of the most pregnant character. No zealous student could faithfully attend his lectures and fail to carry away with him a mass of practical information of inestimable value in his future professional life. Dr. Pancoast's consummate knowledge of human anatomy, and his vast surgical experience had so enriched his mind that his teachings were instructive and without effort. Versed himself in the learning of the books, the charm of his lectures lay in that unwritten surgery which ever fell from his lips. This it was, I think, more than anything else which has given that value to his anatomical discourses, which only those who have heard him can appreciate. No one contributed more than he to enhance the renown of the Jefferson College." His boldness and skill as an operator, his advocacy of original methods and appliances in surgery, were the true bases of his power as an instructor. His work in the Philadelphia Hospital was for years of the highest character. Before he had been six years in Jefferson he issued his "Treatise on Operative Surgery," which ran through several editions. He also remodeled Wistar and Horner's text-book on Anatomy, and was a contributor to medical journalism. He resigned and became emeritus professor in 1874, after about thirty-five years of eminent service, and was succeeded by his son, Dr. W. H. Pancoast. He survived eight years longer and died in 1882, in his seventy-seventh year.

His gifted colleague in the Surgical chair, Dr. Thomas D. Mütter, had a far shorter life, of only forty-eight years, and it was his resignation in 1856, followed by his decease three years later, that first broke the unity of the new faculty of '41. Dr. Mütter came of German and Scotch ancestors, who settled in North Carolina in ante-Revolution days and afterwards founded some of the leading families of Virginia. Dr. Mütter was born in Richmond in 1811, and was left an orphan at the age of eight. After his grandmother's death he was reared by a relative, Mr. Robert Carter, who educated him at Hampden Sidney College, and placed him under the direction of Dr. Simms of Alexandria to study medicine. He received his degree in 1831, from the University of Pennsylvania, and his health being poor, he accepted a position on a vessel bound for Europe, and proceeded to Paris, where he acquired some of his chief characteristics as a surgeon. He also visited London, but, says Dr. Pancoast, "it was from the brilliant Parisian school, however, that Dr. Mütter's surgical character got its early bias. His quick, active, appropriative mind was readily imbued with the spirit of his distinguished teachers; and from its natural sanguine disposition he was ready—perhaps a little too ready—to seize upon the novelties of operative surgery, which were then so freely produced by distinguished men, with promises of advantage that, in some instances, were hardly fulfilled." He was intensely interested in the field of plastic surgery, and on settling in Philadelphia in 1832, at the age of twenty-one, he attempted to draw about him a private class of students. He was greatly encouraged by Dr. Jackson of the University, and, by another year, joined Dr. Paul B. Goddard, with eminent success. In 1835 he was called to lecture in the Medical Institute founded by Chapman, and his reputation was established. He had a mingled gentleness, energy and enthusiasm, clear method, vivid demonstration and lively expression that won the hearts of the students and commanded their admiration. His practice was so large as to prevent his giving much time to literary work; but his industry and skill as a collector resulted in the surgical and medical museum that is now widely known and bears his name in connection with the College of Physicians, where it has a home. After twenty-four years of instruction, over half of which was spent in the chair of Surgery in Jefferson Medical College, he resigned on account of ill health in 1856, and was succeeded by Dr. S. D. Gross.

The loss of Huston followed in the next year, and in 1858 the chair of Practice, also, was made vacant by the death of another Virginian, eighteen years older than Mütter, Dr. John Kearsley Mitchell. His is a family devoted to medicine; he came of two generations of physicians and has left behind him a son, the eminent Dr. S. Weir Mitchell, and a grandson, who is also of the profession. He came of direct Scotch lineage, and was born in Sheppardstown, Virginia, in 1793. At the age of fourteen he was sent to Scotland to be educated in the University of Edinburgh, where he received his classical degree. In 1816, returning to America, he came to Philadelphia and began the study of medicine in the office of Dr. Chapman, attending the University and the Doctor's private school. He graduated in 1819, at the age of twenty-six. Dr. Mitchell's health then becoming impaired, he sailed, as physician, on a vessel bound for China. He made three voyages. On settling in Philadelphia as a practitioner, Dr. Mitchell's skill and graces of character soon opened the way to a large practice, and he was chosen to the lectureship on Medical Chemistry in Dr. Chapman's Medical Institute in 1823, a post he held for nearly ten years. In 1833 the Franklin Institute secured him to lecture on "Chemistry Applied to the Arts," in which position he spent five years. He was the first chemist in the city to solidify carbonic acid; he discovered a solvent of caoutchouc, and anticipated Graham in the theory of the penetrativeness of fluids. During this period he had published numerous articles on medical subjects, many of which were characterized by an originality of view that became one of the chief features of his development. He was among the first advocates of the germ theory of disease, and, indeed, anticipated, in suggestion, many of the accepted theories of the present day. Dr. Mitchell was forty-eight years old when he was called to the new Jefferson faculty of '41 to the chair of Practice. His lectures and other discourses "were marked by profound and original thought, deep learning and extensive research," says one before quoted. "A vein of poetic imagination ran through all his works, and served to give grace and interest to his studies and descriptions of the most technical subjects. In addition to his scientific writings he also published a volume of poems. In person, Dr. Mitchell was tall and portly, with a gentle, polished bearing. He was open-handed and hospitable, a charming companion, a man of genial manners, and yet of great dignity of character. He was greatly beloved by his classes, and their affection for him he strongly reciprocated. He was the students' friend. In sickness and trouble they turned to him and never sought his aid in vain. Many a poor young fellow, struggling in the vortex of a great city's temptation, has he sustained by his wise counsel and kindly sympathy. Many a needy student has he helped from his own purse, and none the wiser. In his college lectures he was exceedingly happy; his terseness, his power of illustration, his way of putting things, his anecdote and lively wit, made a favorable impression on the class, an impression strengthened by their personal love for their teacher. He died in harness, holding his professorship to the end. The last official act of his life was the Commencement reception of the graduating class of 1858 at his house. His health at that time was feeble, and the question arose whether the entertainment should not be given by one of his colleagues. He insisted, however, on giving it himself, saying that he would probably not live to give another. His misgivings were prophetic; in a month he had passed away, leaving behind him the reputation of a distinguished teacher, a zealous investigator, a most eminent practitioner and a blameless citizen." He was also greatly interested in public affairs, a member of many leading scientific, professional and other societies, before which he lectured on widely diversified themes. He died in the early part of 1858 at the age of sixty-five, the first of the faculty of '41 to be removed by death.

Three years later, another of this noble company of teachers died at nearly the age of seventy. He, too, was a Southern man by birth and education, enthusiastic, vivacious, original and imaginative. Dr. Charles D. Meigs was for over twenty years the incumbent of Jefferson's chair of Obstetrics. He was an eloquent lecturer and a cultured gentleman of linguistic and literary tastes, whose affability endeared him to his students. He was born in 1792 in the Bermudas, whither his father had gone from Connecticut as Proctor in the English Courts of Admiralty, but spent a part of his boyhood in Connecticut, where his father was subsequently a professor in Yale. After his ninth year he lived in Athens, Georgia, of whose University the elder Meigs became president in 1801. Educated under his father's direction, he received his diploma from the Georgia institution in 1809, and soon began the study of medicine. His health during those days not being of the best, he was advised to visit his uncle, who was an Indian agent a few miles away, and live in the open air, among the Cherokees and other tribes then in that region. This he did, to the great improvement of his physical condition. In 1812 he entered the University of Pennsylvania Medical School and was graduated in 1815, at the age of twenty-three, though he did not receive his degree until two years later, when he decided to settle in Philadelphia. Here his talents were appreciated, although he gained practice slowly, and in 1826, when the *Kappa Lambda* (s) Society of the United States founded the *North American Medical and Surgical Journal*, he was chosen one of its editors, with Drs. Bache, Coates, Hodge, LaRoche, and later Wood, Condie and Bell. That was the beginning of his extensive literary production, and it was about this time that, against his own inclination, but on account of an excellent opening, he chose Obstetrics as his chief field of work. He published a translation of Velpeau in 1831, and every few years thereafter some work in the line of his specialty was produced by him. Among these was his first original work, "The Philadelphia Practice of Midwifery," and his "Obstetrics, the Science and the Art." His style was rich and full. "His love for the beautiful," says Dr. John Bell, "was ingrained in his philosophy, and gave a coloring both to his written and spoken compositions." In 1830 he began teaching in the private "School of Medicine," started by Gibson, LaRoche, Randolph and others, and after five or six years expected to succeed Dr. Dewees. The contest was close, but although he was not successful, he was soon called to a chair which he made of equal honor, in the Jefferson faculty of '41. "Dr. Meigs' manner before the class was peculiar and singularly impressive," writes Dr. Brinton. "He was eminently a scholar, and always seemed to me to teach not only his branch, but something more. He loved to dwell upon the value of learning, and to inculcate above all things that the physician should be a cultured man, or, as he put it, a member of the great Scholar Class. He was forceful in expression, apt in illus-

---

(s) This Philadelphia branch of it was begun by Drs. LaRoche, Samuel Jackson, C. D. Meigs and Thomas Harris, and had harmony of the profession as one of its chief aims. Its influence was remarkably successful in this direction. These editors originated the medical club which lasted for thirty years, and was the mother of like clubs innumerable.

tration, a lover of the arts, and blessed with a poetic and fervid imagination. With the mummied bones of an Egyptian girl before him, I have heard him in an enraptured burst recall the glories of Egypt's ancient days. At his magic words the scene rose up. There stood the palace, there the temple, where trod the priests of Isis; yonder lay the brick fields, thronged with the Hebrew slaves; at his feet the Nile murmured; there along the tangled rushes floated the wicker basket, and for a moment Teacher and Class stood in the presence of Pharaoh's daughter. No member of his many classes will, I am sure, ever forget Dr. Meigs and the strange charm of his words; at times poetic, at times charged with quaint humor; now rising to the highest pitch of philosophic reasoning, now sinking to impress laboriously upon the student mind the beauties of Carus's curve. One characteristic of his teaching was his zealous effort to bring others, and notably his class, to think as he did. He was all earnestness, and, immovable in his own convictions, he sought to make all share them with him." After nearly twenty years of this successful work his failing health led him to resign in 1860, and become Professor Emeritus, although an emergency led to his giving one more course. After several years of retirement he died, in 1869, one of the most engaging personalities of the old faculty of ante-bellum days.

In striking contrast to Dr. Meigs was the remaining member of this faculty, who, when Meigs was teaching Obstetrics in the Parrish School on one side of the street, and he teaching Chemistry in the Gibson School on the other, agreed with the former that the students of the two schools should attend the lectures of both men. Dr. Franklin Bache was, to use the words of his friend Dr. Wood, "extremely methodical, clear in his explanations, because clear in his own conceptions, conscientiously precise in all his details, and leaving no dark spot in his subject unillumined." In short, he was a "plain, clear, truthful, conscientious and efficient, but not a showy, splendid or particularly attractive lecturer; one from whose prelections the student would retire with his thoughts more intent upon the subject taught than upon the teacher." This was precisely the kind of character one might expect in the great-grandson of Benjamin Franklin. Dr. Bache was the grandson of the only daughter of Franklin who married Richard Bache of England. His father, an accomplished editor, was one of the victims of yellow fever in 1798, when Dr. Bache was but six years old. The boy was prepared for college by the Rev. Dr. Samuel B. Wylie, and in 1810, at the age of eighteen, he was graduated from the Arts Department of the University as valedictorian. He at once entered the office of Dr. Benjamin Rush, but in the year of his preceptor's death, 1813, he joined the army as surgeon's mate, although he had attended the University so as to graduate in 1814. He became surgeon of a regiment and served until 1816, when he returned to Philadelphia and began practice. He had shown great talent for, and interest in, Chemistry, and had published an article on muriatic acid so early as his sixteenth year. His practice grew very slowly, and during those early years he published a treatise on chemistry. His own family got him to deliver them a course of chemical lectures in 1821, and Dr. T. T. Hewson soon after engaged him to repeat the course to his private school. In 1826 he was also called to a lectureship in Franklin Institute, which he held for six years, until his election to a chair in the College of Pharmacy. Meanwhile he had been chosen, in 1830, to lecture in the School of Medicine of Gibson and others, and from these positions he was honored by the call to the chair of Chemistry in the faculty of '41 in Jefferson Medical College, when he was forty-nine years of age. His was one of those sterling and solid moral natures that establish the standards of public opinion about them, and for the long period of twenty-three years, ceasing only with his death, in 1864, at the ripe age of seventy-two, Jefferson felt the influence of his wise, learned and quiet life, and his students held him in reverence. His other publications, which were numerous and valuable, are always eclipsed in public memory by his work, in connection with Drs. Hewson and Wood, in revising the National Pharmacopœia in 1829, and by the still greater United States Dispensatory, issued by Drs. Bache and Wood in 1833. In the scientific and professional societies he was a leader, and served as president or vice-president of most of them. He was president of the American Philosophical

Society for the full time-limit then allowed. He, too, was one of the apostles of harmony in the *Kappa Lambda* and its journal, and was one of the most powerful influences in the profession of those years. With his decease, in 1864, passed the famous faculty of '41, excepting Pancoast, who served ten years longer. Jefferson, with such men as Dunglison, Mütter, Pancoast, Huston, Mitchell, Meigs and Bache, had become such a Mecca for medical students that, by 1854, it had a class of 627 within its halls, a number that had never been equaled in medical schools before the war.

Allied to the great educational movement of this period was medical journalism, which, for the first time, received the consideration due to its importance. Its promoters, of course, included many of those men prominent in other branches of medicine, as has already been indicated, but there were two who, while also prominent in other departments, are so much better known in the literature and journalism of this period that their careers must be of especial interest. The oldest of these was Dr. René LaRoche, whose father was a physician who had been educated in Montpelier, France, and practiced medicine in St. Domingo; but he removed to Philadelphia, where he was living in 1795, when Dr. LaRoche junior was born. Here he was educated, and in the war of 1812 became a Captain of Volunteers in Colonel Chapman Biddle's regiment. He began the study of medicine, and, in 1820, was graduated from the Medical Department of the University. After entering upon practice he became connected with the Private School of Medicine, but his powers were at their best as a writer. "It is said," observes one recorder, "that he was always writing, almost up to the time of his death, and that his posthumous writings include material for several volumes upon Music and its Uses in Medicine, on Fevers, on the Plague at Athens, and on History of Schools from the revival of medicine to the present time." He was a prolific contributor to medical journals of the first order elsewhere, and was one of the chief powers in the editorial staff of the Kappa Lambda Society's journal. He is probably best known by his great work on Yellow Fever, which is a classic on that subject. He was a member of nearly all the leading medical and scientific societies of the city, and was one of the strong influences of this period. He died in 1872 at the age of seventy-seven.

Better known as an editor, although he was a writer, too, was Dr. Isaac Hays, who was the true creator of the famous journals of the leading medical publishers, among whom Mr. Isaac Lea was so prominent. Dr. Hays was the son of a wealthy Philadelphia merchant and was born in 1796, a year later than Dr. LaRoche. He was educated under the Rev. Dr. Samuel B. Wylie, and graduated from the Arts Department of the University in 1816. After private medical study under Dr. Chapman he entered the Medical Department of his *alma mater*, and was graduated in 1820. His tastes were so decidedly literary and scientific that when, in 1826, it became necessary for Dr. Chapman to have another editor to assist on the *Philadelphia Journal of the Medical and Physical Sciences*, which he had founded in 1820, he and Mr. Lea chose young Hays, who was then but thirty years of age. The choice was so happy that he became sole editor soon after, and in November, 1827, to secure a national charter for it, changed its name to the *American Journal of the Medical Sciences*. It had the benefit of his excellent taste for over a half century. In 1843 the quarterly was supplemented by a monthly called the *Medical News and Library* (t), which, in its field, fully equaled its more grave and dignified mother journal, and has been an organ of no small power in the profession. He was a prolific editor of scientific works also, and the author of original papers and treatises, both medical and scientific, from his edition of "Wilson's American Ornithology," in 1828, to his "Diseases of the Eye," and other works, in later years. In 1846 he was one of the most active members of the New York convention, and it was he who presented the resolutions proposing a National Medical Association for the better management of standards of ethics and education. These resolutions he attributed largely to Dr. Alfred Stillé, his colleague on that occasion. At the later meeting Dr. Hays presented for adoption the code of ethics, which has been the recognized code of the profession ever since. To him was also very largely due the

---

(t) These have become respectively monthly and weekly. The latter omits "and Library."

publication of the Transactions of the American Medical Association for several years, and his services as treasurer only ceased at his own declination of re-election. He was a member of numerous societies, both at home and abroad. He was secretary of the Kappa Lambda Society, and was one of that company of members of the American Philosophical Society who sought to perpetuate the Wistar parties after Wistar's decease. In 1869, when he reached his seventy-third year, he was succeeded on the journal by his son, Dr. I. Minis Hays, and ten years later the maker of "Chapman's and Hays' Journal," as it was popularly called, passed away at the advanced age of eighty-three. Dr. Hays was of a remarkably judicial mind, so that during all the years he managed the above mentioned journals they never became known as the organs of any party or clique of the profession. Speaking in 1876, Dr. John Billings said: "The ninety-seven volumes of this journal need no eulogy. They contain many original papers of the highest value; nearly all the real criticisms and reviews that we possess; and such carefully prepared summaries of the progress of medical science, and abstracts and notices of foreign works, that from this file alone, were all other productions of the press for the last fifty years destroyed, it would be possible to reproduce the great majority of the real contributions of the world to medical science during that period" (u).

The literature and journalism of the period were flourishing; the growth of the schools marvelous; but in the matter of hospital advantages to students, Philadelphia was sadly lacking.

"Philadelphia has a distinguished reputation as a seat of medical authority," said Dr. Alfred Stillé, in his closing address to the County Medical Society of Philadelphia in 1863. "For a long time, and until a very recent period, all other American schools bore no comparison with hers either in their number and excellence or in the proportion of native physicians whom they educated. During three-quarters of a century she stood *facile princeps* among American seats of learning and science, and her claims to prëeminence

---

(u) Among a large number of prominent men who died during this period were Dr. S. G. Morton, Dr. Jacob Randolph, Dr. J. B. Rogers, Dr. John C. Otto, Dr. Henry Bond, Dr. W. R. Grant, Dr. Jos. Nancrede and others.

were uncontested. But how is it now? Gradually, in other cities, and especially in the commercial metropolis, rivals have grown up which threaten to eclipse her medical institutions, and to draw away from her a large number of the young men who are pursuing the study of medicine. . . . . The scanty provision for hospital instruction in one of our public institutions, the absolute closure against us for a long while of the larger hospital, which had once afforded clinical experience to our students, and the sorry substitute for it which the colleges adopted, all combined to diminish the attractions of our city as a school of medicine, at the very time when our principal rival was opening one hospital after another to clinical teaching, and in two of them creating independent faculties of medicine. . . . . I need not here enumerate the instances during the last years in which discussions upon various important questions of medical science and practice have taken place in the societies of our sister city, discussions which neither in fullness of matter, nor skill of argument, will compare unfavorably with those held under similar circumstances in European capitals. In a word, these two cities, in their medical history, forcibly remind one of Edinburgh and London. While scholastic learning and didactic accomplishments in teaching were held in supreme regard, the former place enjoyed the greatest reputation abroad, and even at home her graduates rose to the highest honors in the metropolitan profession. But, within the last quarter of a century, the period, in other words, during which physics have been applied to medicine, and since auscultation, percussion and their kindred methods of investigation, microscopical, chemical and physiological, have laid the phenomena of life and of disease open to the senses, the hospitals of London have become the most abundant by far of all the sources from which the natural history of diseases is being composed. Thus, collectively, as a medical school, they have eclipsed their former rival and superior." One of the results of the civil war, then raging, was—temporarily and partially—to supply this need of hospital training. But with the rising movements associated with the national catastrophe, this notable educational period closes.

CHAPTER IV.

CIVIL WAR PERIOD.

Philadelphia, as has been said, had, in 1820, a population of 113,000. In 1860, the census returned 568,000. The city still spread along the Delaware River and had also advanced westward beyond Broad street. The medical population had increased even more rapidly in proportion. It will be remembered that the period between 1820 and 1825 was remarkable for the scarcity of physicians, and that there were only sixty or seventy to a population of over one hundred thousand. To be exact, there were sixty-nine doctors in 1825, according to the correct directory of the day, and there were nearly as many five years before; but during the next thirty-five or forty years the private medical schools proved so attractive that by 1860 there were 551 regular physicians to a population of over half a million. As to location, the tendency was more and more toward the scattered condition that prevails at present. A glance at a directory of that date is of curious interest as an illustration of the changes in that respect (a). Besides the regular

---

(a) According to McElroy's Directory of 1860, the physicians in Philadelphia were as follows: D. Hayes Agnew, 16 N. 11th street; Hugh Alexander, Market near Margaretta; J. G. Allen, 1241 Lombard; Jas. Anderson, 1103 Thompson; J. B. Ard, 1616 Arch; C. M. Arey, 236 N. 10th; M. J. Asch, 417 Spruce; H. H. Ash, 1712 Vine; H. St. Clair Ash, 261 N. 11th; W. Ashmead, Germantown; A. H. Ashton, 737 S. 9th; S. K. Ashton, 9th and Pine; Saml. Atkinson, 1137 N. 2nd; W. B. Atkinson, 215 Spruce; W. F. Atlee, 210 S. 13th; W. L. Atlee, 1408 Arch; T. F. Azpaff, 524 S. 3d; Franklin Bache, Spruce and Juniper; T. Hewson Bache, Spruce and Juniper; Jas. W. Bacon, 222 S. 9th; C. S. Baker, 623 Master; D. R. Bannan, 739 Spruce; J. Barker, Graff and 11th; Samuel Barrington, 112 S. 18th; T. S. Bartram, 256 N. 12th; Elizabeth P. Baugh, 1102 Mt. Vernon; M. M. Beach, 1122 Vine; Joseph Beale, 1805 Delancy; G. H. Beaumont, 812 Arch; Louis Beckedorff, 225 Brown; Carl Beeken, 411 Wood; Theo. Beesley, 10th and Arch; John Bell, 727 Spruce; H. D. Benner, 841 S. 3d; B. Berens, 909 Arch; Jos. Berens, 513 N. 6th; C. P. Bethell, 911 Franklin; J. J. G. Bias, 911 Lombard; Rufus Bicknell, Market near 38th; J. B. Biddle, 1117 Spruce; W. W. Bidlack, 2203 Vine; David Birch, 252 Girard avenue; J. F. Birch, 11th and Green; C. S. Bishop, 334 N. 10th; J. L. Bishop, 974 N. Front; Wm. Blackwood, 1602 Arch; M. Blon, 116 Union; Henry Bloom, 710

members of the profession there was a noticeable increase in adherents of exclusive systems: The followers of Hahnemann enrolled twenty-six and supported a school; the "Eclectics," seven in all, were also struggling to support a school; while the "Botanics" numbered four. The "cuppers and bleeders" had fallen from 25 in 1825 to 16 in 1860, showing that the reaction against heroic treatment had been far-reaching even at that date. The women, who at that period were catalogued with these non-regular representatives, were making a courageous endeavor to maintain them-

---

Sansom; L. D. Bodder, 920 Arch; J. E. Bodine, 227 Race; C. S. Boker, 1022 Chestnut; Robt. Bolling, 256 S. 12th; F. E. Bond, 1209 Filbert; Jas. Bond, 10th and Locust; H. Borland, 612 Richmond; Anthony Bournonville, 221 N. 4th; A. C. Bournonville, 427 N. 4th; D. G. Bowman, 1700 Green; D. P. Boyer, 1516 N. 4th; W. M. Breed, 1106 Vine; W. C. Bridges, 119 S. 20th; Saml. Brincklé, 1215 Chestnut; Wm. Brincklé, same; M. Brinkman, 628 Wood; John H. Brinton, 1007 Walnut; Peter Broes, 1713 Lombard; S. S. Brooks, 1320 Vine; David S. Brown, Front near Norris; R. H. Brown, 1229 Melon; S. Brown, 655 N. 10th; S. P. Brown, 633 N. 11th; Solomon Brown, 22d near Arch; Wm. Brown, 647 N. 10th; Felix Bruckner, 414 N. Front; John Brunet, 411 S. 2d; Jas. Bryan, 1305 Walnut; Jos. R. Bryan, 1124 Green; J. D. Bryant, 45 N. 17th; F. J. Buck, 1139 Pine; Lee W. Buffington, 2023 Arch; S. D. Burdett, 1004 Green; Jos. A. Burdick, 236 N. 8th; Geo. H. Burgin, Jr., 121 N. 18th; Francis Burleigh, 907 Christian; Robt. Burns, Frankford; D. Burpee, 326 S. 16th; Richard Burr, 604 Frankford av.; A. Busch, 116 Union; S. W. Butler, 1319 Chestnut; W. C. Byington, 1014 Spring Garden; M. Calkens, 1421 Chestnut; Elizabeth Calvin, 1302 Green; A. B. Campbell, 1419 Chestnut; Jos. Carson, 1120 Spruce; E. L. Carter, 9th and Pine; G. J. Chamberlain, 622 S. 11th; Saml. Chamberlaine, Spruce and 2d; M. Chambers, 502 Spruce; T. C. Chase, 1128 Vine; Andrew Cheeseman, 1336 Pine; H. T. Child, 510 Arch; C. W. Chipman, 320 N. 7th; J. C. Clark, 520 Buckley; Wm. Clendaniel, 133 Pine; Elizabeth Cline, 645 N. 9th; J. R. Coad, 334 S. 5th; B. H. Coates, 710 Arch; L. M. Coates, 534 S. 4th; M. W. Collett, 329 S. Broad; D. F. Condie, 237 Catherine; J. Conry, Manyunk; Thos. Conway, 540 N. 12th; C. C. Cooper, 52 N. 13th; J. C. Cooper, 139 Arch; Jas. Corse, 150 N. 10th; David Cowley, 124 S. 9th; John Cox, 1603 Arch; T. W. Craige, 329 N. 4th; T. S. Crowly, 2103 Chestnut; J. Cummiskey, 631 Spruce; Wm. Curran, 1314 Arch; L. Curtis, 624 Wood; J. Da Costa, 212 S. 11th; H. A. Daniels, Florida and Catherine; Jas. Darrach, 1205 Arch; Wm. Darrach, 1120 Arch; J. Davidson, 815 Walnut; Jonathan Davis (colored), 713 S. 11th; W. A. Davis, 1006 Coates; A. C. Denkyne, 782 S. 2d; J. S. De Benneville, 123 S. 7th; T. A. Demme, 523 N. 4th; S. J. Deputy, 234 Lombard; Philip De Young, 305 Callowhill; M. W. Dickeson, 211 Lombard; A. C. Dickinson, 44 N. 7th; Ernest Diese, 458 York av.; E. H. Dietrich, 315 N. 10th; Thos. Dillard, 1720 Pine; Edward Donnelly, 1308 N. 4th; Peter Doriot, 1025 Walnut; E. C. Daugherty, 744 S. 12th; E. F. Drayton, 1629 Filbert; H. E. Drayton, 924 Pine; Thos. M. Drysdale, 1705 Race; W. J. Duffee, 624 Catherine; Geo. Duhring, 614 Arch; R. J. Dunglison, 121 S. 10th; T. R. Dunglison, 1116 Girard; Wm. Dunton, 734 Pine; J. M. Eagleton, 1021 Mt. Vernon; J. Ebeling, 910 Race; D. Egbert, 221 S. 9th; A. Elliott, 904 Poplar; J. L. Elliott, 403 N. 12th; Susanna H. Ellis, 231 N. 10th; Gouverneur Emerson, 926 Walnut; J. V. Emlen, 531 N. 13th; I. Eshleman, 317 Spruce; Chas. Evans, 702 Race; Horace Evans, 635 Walnut; R. T. Evans, 343 N. 12th; Jos. Fabian, 130 Vine; A. Fellger, 240 S. 12th;

selves as, at least, physician-nurses, and were working out the problem of their true position in the profession in an effort to establish their college.

The College of Physicians, the County Medical Society, the Pathological Society and the Northern Medical Association were the professional organizations. The University on Ninth, and Jefferson on Tenth street, were the foci of the entire regular profession of the city, while the other institutions were making their final struggle for existence. Besides the Pennsylvania and Philadel-

Emil Fischer, 121 N. 9th; A. H. Fish, 1608 Vine; W. J. Fleming, 1911 Vine; John Flynn, 16 N. 19th; Wm. Flynn, 25 S. 19th; John Fondey, 1128 Vine; G. C. Foote, 215 Vine; W. S. Forbes, 257 S. 17th; D. M. Fort, 812 S. 9th; Robt. Foster, 1520 Vine; A. Foulke, 541 N. 7th; J. L. Foulke, 1034 Spring Garden; J. M. Fox, 134 S. 11th; Samuel Frudley, 549 Marshall; W. H. Freeman, 652 N. 11th; W. S. Frick, 821 N. 8th; Albert Frické, 235 N. 6th; J. J. Fullmer, 221 N. 5th; Edwin Fussell, 910 N. 5th; Wm. Gallaher, Haverford and 36th; Wm. Gardener, 1106 Poplar; C. S. Gaunt, 1713 Lombard; J. F. Gayley, 133 S. 18th; J. F. Geary, 25 S. 16th; L. H. Gebhard, 618 Race; C. F. Gebler, 1329 Coates; John Gegan, 601 S. Front; W. Gelb, 321 N. 11th; W. W. Gerhard, 1206 Spruce; A. S. Gibbs, 342 S. 16th; David Gilbert, 731 Arch; J. C. Gilbert, Chestnut Hill; W. K. Gilbert, 507 S. 9th; W. H. Gillingham, 1232 Chestnut; W. W. Glentworth, 817 Race; D. S. Glonginger, 305 N. 6th; W. H. Gobrecht, 818 Walnut; P. B. Goddard, 1322 Walnut; W. H. Gominger, 1135 Germantown av.; W. Georges, 1107 Arch; A. H. Graham, 1332 Lombard; Wm. Granger, 929 Spruce; C. E. Green, 1021 Race; F. F. Greene, 1237 Germantown avenue; Wm. Gregg, 130 Race; W. P. Grier, 1428 Spruce; E. Griffin, 727 N. 7th; A. W. Griffiths, 216 N. 12th; J. D. Griscom, 1028 Arch; S. D. and S. W. Gross, Walnut and 11th; W. Guersey, Frankford; B. B. Gumpert, 982 N. 6th; F. B. Hahn, 238 N. 9th; A. D. Hall, 828 Walnut; E. A. Hall, 1735 Wallace; John P. Hall, 1204 Locust; W. S. Halsey, 701 Pine; C. E. Hamerly, 3d and Federal; G. S. Hamil, 2242 Callowhill; George Hamilton, 1600 Summer; W. N. Handy, 932 N. 5th; M. A. Hanly, 639 Pine; W. H. Hanly, 263 N. 12th; J. J. Hare, 238 New; L. D. Harlow, 1023 Vine; I. N. Harper, 111 Race; Thos. Harper, 1811 Walnut; R. P. Harris, 1609 Spruce; Wm. Harris, same; B. Hart, 1214 Coates; Chas. Hartshorne, 120 S. 12th; Edward Hartshorne, 1439 Walnut; Henry Hartshorne, 1433 Arch; J. H. Haskell, 657 N. 10th; N. L. Hatfield, 501 Franklin; I. I. Hayes, 249 S. 10th; Isaac Hays, 1527 Locust; W. H. Hazard, 224 Pine; P. Heaney, 938 Christian; G. C. Heberton, 1509 Arch; S. Heine, 632 N. 8th; A. Helfenstein, 1008 Shackamaxon; J. S. Helfrich, 936 N. 4th; Henry Heller, 845 N. 4th; W. S. Helmuth, 312 S. 10th; Wm. Henry, 507 Pine; Jos. Heritage, 811 S. 3d; Daniel Hershey, 994 N. 5th; Addinell Hewson, 1005 Walnut; George Hewston, 100 N. 12th; H. F. Heyl, 2033 Summer; J. S. Hill, 831 N. 10th; C. Hine, 445 Shippen; A. G. B. Hinkle, 691 N. 13th; Sarah Hinkle, 254 N. 13th; R. Hitchcock, 21 N. 9th; J. N. Hobensack, 236 N. 2d; Hugh L. Hodge, 903 Walnut; J. M. Hoffman, 465 N. 4th; S. L. Hollingsworth, 1533 Spruce; J. F. Holt, 420 S. 18th; W. Hooper, 112 S. 13th; H. St. G. Hopkins, Chestnut Hill; Jos. Hopkinson, 1613 Walnut; E. T. Hornberger, 735 S. 2d; M. Horner, 134 Arch; S. H. Hornor, 1106 Walnut; Benj. Housekeeper, 610 Richmond; J. G. Howard, 702 Pine; G. W. Howell, 1111 Brown; W. D. Hoyt, 701 Spruce; J. S. Huckel, 6th and Catherine; I. W. Hughes, 40th and Chestnut; E. Hunt, 112 N. 9th; J. G. Hunt, 527 N. 4th; Wm. Hunt, 431 Arch; John Hunter, 44 N. 7th; Robt. M. Huston, 1208 Arch;

phia hospitals, there were the Charity Hospital, the St. Joseph's Hospital, the Protestant Episcopal Hospital, the Children's Hospital, the Philadelphia Lying-in Charity, the Wills Hospital, the Preston Retreat, the Howard Hospital, and several dispensaries and lying-in departments of other hospitals. Pharmacy and dentistry had also advanced and developed.

In 1860, Lincoln was elected, and the Confederacy formed in the South almost before the North realized what was happening. Philadelphia had become the great medical center of the land, and the

---

G. W. Hutchins, 326 N. 20th; E. B. Jackson, 211 N. 10th; E. O. Jackson, 1701 Lombard; Owen Jackson, 520 S. 12th; Saml. Jackson, 224 S. 8th; Samuel Jackson, 1237 Spruce; E. Jacoby, Chestnut Hill; B. W. James, 1013 Green; David James, same; F. Jaquett, 317 S. 6th; Jacob Jeanes, 519 Vine; James Jenkins, 1120 Mt. Vernon; Wilson Jewell, 420 N. 6th; A. C. Jones, 1442 S. 2d; Thos. Jones, 1169 S. 12th; Z. R. Jones, 318 N. 9th; O. A. Judson, 1135 Spruce; C. E. Kamerly, 3d and Federal; John K. Kane, 1027 Walnut; Jos. Kane, 812 S. 2d; Wm. Keating. 283 S. 4th; C. P. Keichline, 502 N. 4th; Henry Keim, Manyunk; Wm. Keller, 257 N. 6th; E. B. P. Kelley, 502 Shippen; John Kelly, 318 N. 8th; Robt. Kenderdine, 712 Buttonwood; A. L. Kenney, 2 S. Merrick; Mrs. Jos. Kenney, 1207 Pine; M. G. Kerr, 1351 Melon; A. R. Kinkelin, 303 Union; Thos. S. Kirkbride, Insane Dept. of Pennsylvania Hospital; J. L. Kite, 457 N. 5th; Jos. Klapp, 622 Pine; W. C. Kline, 1213 Germantown avenue; I. D. Knight, 1513 Green; J. K. Knorr, 910 N. Front; G. H. Kruger, 311 N. 6th; John Lachenmeyer, 425 N. 4th; Paul Lajus, 1334 Spruce; W. P. Lambert, 832 Franklin; S. M. Landis, 728 S. 10th; S. W. Langdon, 148 Richmond; Geo. Langolf, 214 Spruce; E. F. Leake, Frankford; W. B. Leary, 721 Sansom; C. C. Lee, Race and 18th; J. K. Lee, Market and 34th; R. H. Lee, 1609 Frankford avenue; C. A. Leech, 1222 Coates; Jos. Leidy, 908 Sansom; N. B. Leidy, 243 N. 6th; A. Leiper, 11th and Callowhill; J. M. Leon, 928 Race; J. Lessey, 303 N. 9th; W. A. Letterman, 208 S. 13th; J. J. Levick, 1109 Arch; M. M. Levis, 418 N. 6th; Richard Levis, 523 N. 6th; D. T. Lewis, 2004 Pine; E. Lewis, Jr., 1108 Chestnut; F. W. Lewis, 202 S. 11th; E. Lichau, 431 Race; A. Lippe, 1224 Walnut; Josiah Litch, 127 N. 11th; Squier Littell, 1232 Arch; Hannah E. Longshore, 1116 Callowhill; Jos. S. Longshore, 1430 N. 11th; F. E. Luckett, 113 S. 13th; J. L. Ludlow, 10 Merrick; G. B. Lummis, 145 Coates; L. M. Lyon, 506 N. 3d; J. C. Lyons, 1354 N. Front; C. A. McCall, 1354 N. Front; E. McClellan, 1441 Walnut; John McClellan, 1029 Walnut; Jas. McClintock, 150 N. 11th; J. R. McClurg, 1100 Walnut; W. F. McCurdy, 829 Race; W. McFadden, 863 N. 5th; H. D. McLean, 1315 Lombard; B. McLerney, 1336 Cherry; W. C. McMackin, 2nd and Reed; A. S. McMurray, 1306 Pine; B. A. McNeill, 421 S. 16th; T. A. McRean, 625 N. 7th; A. McWhinney, 1510 Vine; John Macavoy, 1235 N. 4th; I. MacBride, 1757 Frankford avenue; G. W. Malin, Germantown; W. H. Malin, Frankford; Benj. Malone, 658 N. 8th; R. S. Mansfield, 727 N. 10th; G. W. Mason, 1263 N. 10th; R. Maris, 239 S. 8th; N. Marselis, 4th and Lombard; Geo. Martin, 415 York avenue; J. A. Martin, 415 York avenue; J. K. Mason, 310 S. 15th; Wm. Mabury, 7th and Vine; C. D. Meigs, 1208 Walnut; J. A. Meigs, 1531 Lombard; J. F. Meigs, 1208 Walnut; David Merritt, Shippen near 15th; Wm. Metcalfe, 1219 N. 3d; C. H. Miller, 629 N. 12th; S. B. W. Mitchell, 1338 Coates; S. Wier Mitchell, 1226 Walnut; Jas. Moore, 1343 Lombard; J. W. Moore, 313 Spruce; Geo. Morehouse, 227 S. 9th; Caspar Morris, 1435 Spruce; J. Cheston Morris, 1435 Spruce; S. R. Morris, 659 Germantown avenue; Jas. Mor-

IN PHILADELPHIA. 217

large and important student population was mainly from the South. Besides the 551 regular physicians there were nearly three times as many medical students. The membership of Jefferson had eclipsed all the records of medical schools in any land or time, and in 1859-60 its matriculates numbered 630; the University reached its largest enrollment that year in an attendance of 528; these two alone reached a total of 1,158, and the other schools combined, together with private students not yet enrolled in graduating schools, probably brought the number of students up to the neigh-

rison, Manyunk; N. R. Moseley, 412 S. 11th; S. Moseley, 1715 Walnut; Wm. Moss, 1320 Walnut; J. D. Mundy, 616 Spruce; S. Murphy, 38 N. Broad; J. F. Musgrave, 12 S. 17th; J. V. Myers, 1116 Callowhill; E. Neal, 923 Chestnut; Ebenezer Neal, 651 N. 12th; Andrew Nebinger, 1018 S. 2d; C. Neff, 1901 Chestnut; John Neff, 1901 Chestnut; C. Neidhard, 124 S. 9th; John Neill, 1352 Spruce; C. Noble; 456 N. 3d; L. E. Nordman, 5th and Green; G. W. Norris, 1534 Locust; J. W. S. Norris, 1802 Spruce; W. Notson, 946 S. 5th; M. O'Hara, 43 S. 17th; Geo. P. Oliver, 544 Germantown avenue; L. Orlovski, 947 N. 3d; E. A. Page, 1415 Walnut; W. B. Page, 1012 Walnut; W. Paine, 120 N. 5th, H. C. Paist, 133 Callowhill; Jas. Palmer, 2021 Winter; Jos. Pancoast, 1032 Chestnut; R. M. Pancoast, 21 N. 10th; S. Pancoast, 910 Spring Garden; W. H. Pancoast, 1032 Chestnut; J. V. Patterson, 101 S. 13th; W. F. Patterson, 719 S. 8th; J. R. Paul, 1006 Pine; Edward Peace, 1602 Chestnut; J. G. Pehrson, 107 S. 10th; J. L. Pierce, 1138 Race; Amos Pennebacker, 37 N. 11th; Alexander Penrose, 1133 Spruce; Benj. Phister, Jr., 548 N. 12th; J. M. Piersol, 1110 Spring Garden; Minna E. Piersol, 1100 Spring Garden; W. A. Piper, 727 N. 5th; J. W. Pattinos, 431 Lombard; David Posey, 241 Chester; D. R. Posey, 1102 Callowhill; B. Price, 302 N. 9th; Henry Primrose, 604 S. 10th; B. H. Rand, 106 S. 9th; F. Rattemann, 874 N. 5th; T. D. Rea, 2027 Girard; T. S. Reed, 186 S. 2d; John Reese, 1836 Delancy; N. C. Reid, 4th and Catherine; T. A. Reilly, 714 N. Broad; Isaac Remington, 312 N. 6th; A. Rene, 120 S. 17th; R. Reyburn, 1145 S. 10th; R. B. Reynolds, 633 Vine; S. K. Reynolds, 623 Richmond; John Rhein, 1109 Callowhill; J. E. Rhoads, Germantown; R. W. Richie, 1935 Lombard; E. S. Rickards, 310 Federal; W. M. L. Rickards, 601 N. 17th; T. H. Ridgely, 1131 Spruce; R. E. Ridgway, 1324 Brown; H. W. Rihl, 814 N. Front; J. L. Rihl, 551 Frankford avenue; B. Ripperger, 804 Walnut; E. F. Rivinus, 1813 Spruce; M. Riser, 422 S. 7th; C. B. Roberts, 1336 N. 3d; G. H. Robinett, 1619 Arch; L. Rodman, 1127 Arch; John Rodgers, 730 Carpenter; R. E. Roger, 1121 Girard avenue; J. S. Roher, 1719 Chestnut; J. S. Rose, 805 Arch; J. W. Rowe, 245 Thompson; W. S. W. Ruschenberger, 1932 Chestnut; P. W. Russell, 1702 Chestnut; H. J. Sartain, 725 Sansom; J. D. Schoales, 1418 N. 11th; E. Scholfield, 322 S. 5th; J. Schrotz, 331 N. 8th; F. Scoffin, 901 Pine; J. H. Seltzer, 1120 Green; Matthew Semple, 802 N. Broad; M. Senderling, 227 Richmond; M C. Shallcross, 729 Walnut; E. R. Shapleigh, 440 N. 8th; J. T. Sharpless, 1227 Arch; R. C. and R. Q. Shelmerdine, 834 N. 10th; Edward Shippen, 1205 Walnut; Jos. Shippen, 225 S. 9th; Wm. Shippen, 1205 Walnut; Nathan Shoemaker, 830 Arch; F. Sims, 709 Pine; Jos. Sites, 128 Laurel; D. C. Skerrett, 917 Spruce; A. M. Slocum, 603 Spring Garden; J. H. Smaltz, 820 N. 6th; A. J. Smiley, 908 South; T. T. Smiley, 902 Pine; A. H. Smith, 253 S. 17th; C. J. Smith, 1719 Lombard; Francis Gurney Smith, 1505 Walnut; Henry H. Smith, 1029 Walnut; D. Y. Smith, 756 S. 10th; S. A. Smith, 39th and Market; W. F. Smith, 433 N. 4th; George Spackman, 1610 Vine; E. A. Spooner, 270 S. 16th; J. C. Stanton, Manyunk;

borhood of 1,300 (b). As the bulk of this number was in the two leading schools, what can be said of them will serve as illustration of the rest, and as Jefferson and the University differed in but one or two respects, as regarded their student contituency, these differences may be noticed, and then the largest, Jefferson, may for several reasons be taken as the example of the exodus. Notwithstanding Jefferson's growth and popularity, the University continued to draw the largest attendance from the State of Pennsylvania.

To take the year, 1860-61, when the attendance from Pennsylvania would have the fairest chance to show its preference, we find that the University had 222 from this State, while Jefferson had but 140. This shows Jefferson's gains to have been chiefly from the

C. G. Stees, 517 N. 12th; John Sterling, 514 Spruce; J. G. Stetler, 1321 Girard avenue; Franklin Stewart, 1212 Cherry; R. Stewart, 830 N. 19th; S. Stewart, 3d and Queen; Wm. Stiles, 633 N. 8th; Alfred Stillé, 1500 Walnut; A. Owen Stillé, 1033 Chestnut; A. E. Stocker, 1429 Walnut; Sam'l Stone, 1331 Pine; W. D. Stroud, 1102 Arch; Jas. Summerville, 1131 Filbert; Wm. Sutton, 923 N. 5th; H. Swayne, 8 N. 7th; W. H. Taggart, 1610 Chestnut; C. H. Taylor, 830 N. 4th; J. E. Taylor, 563 York avenue; W. T. Taylor, 1306 Girard avenue; A. R. Thomas, 1421 Chestnut; J. G. Thomas, 1522 Vine; R. P. Thomas, 144 N. 12th; J. W. Thompson, 313 S. 18th; Fred'k Thumm, 662 N. 7th; Henry Tiedemann, 445 N. 5th; D. M. Tindall, 205 Catherine; C. E. Toothaker, 805 Vine; R. H. Townsend, 1518 Arch; S. Townsend, 433 Richmond; S. N. Troth, 661 N. 11th; George Truman, 142 N. 7th; S. Tucker, 826 Walnut; L. L. Turnbull, 1208 Spruce; C. P. Turner, 235 S. 8th; T. J. Turner, 602 Frankford avenue; C. P. Tutt, 1004 S. 11th; J. C. Tyson, 953 N. 11th; Silas Updegrove, 418 Richmond; E. B. Vandyke, 1502 Pine; J. K. T. Van Pelt, 1031 Chestnut; C. C. Van Wyck, Walnut and 10th; C. B. Voight, 331 Lombard; Henry Wadsworth, 1343 N. Front; L. L. Walker, 731 Chestnut; Ellerslie Wallace, 277 S. 4th; D. G. Walton, 154 N. 7th; D. O. C. Ward, 156 N. 15th; E. H. Ward, 232 N. 16th; G. H. Waters, 478 N. 6th; Phoebe M. Way, 36 N. 16th; Wm. Weatherly, 1036 Spring Garden; Martin Weaver, Germantown; W. L. Wells, 216 S. 9th; F. West, 1512 Pine; H. West, 1524 Pine; J. A. Whartenby, 814 N. 8th; Alex. Wilcocks, 1003 Walnut; T. C. Williams, 567 N. 5th; W. S. Williams, 635 N. 5th; D. Williamson, 1032 Pine; Augustus Wilson, 1315 Locust; Ellwood Wilson, 1339 Arch; Jas. H. Wilson, 838 Lombard; John Wiltbank, 1105 Arch; G. Winkler, 913 Race; H. G. Winslow, 224 N. 10th; Wm. Winter, 850 Randolph; Caspar Wistar, 726 Arch; R. M. Wistar, 515 S. 12th; Owen J. Wistar, Germantown; W. Witfield, 500 Powell; C. Wittig, 480 N. 4th; S. Wolff, 1227 Walnut; Geo. B. Wood, 1117 Arch; S. W. Woodhouse, 823 Chestnut; C. S. Wurts, 1701 Walnut; T. H. Yardley, 1005 Arch; Wm. Young, 416 Spruce; W. Young, 1412 Walnut; Henry Zell, 821 S. 7th; G. J. Zeigler, 1512 Chestnut, and Jacob S. Zorns, 608 N. Front; also four "Botanics," seven Eclectics and twenty-six Homeopathists. This directory is only approximately complete, as some well-known names are omitted. There are also many cases of misspelling. In the main, however, it serves to show very fairly the ranks of regular medicine in 1860.

(b) In 1857-8 there were 1,139—Jefferson, 501; the University, 435; Pennsylvania College, 140; and Philadelphia College, 63. This omits women students and others not in graduating schools.

country at large, outside of Pennsylvania, and if those should prove to be mainly from the South, it will readily be seen that Jefferson would be the greater sufferer from the war. Before turning to Jefferson let a glance be taken at the constituency of the University in any ante-bellum year, say 1856-57, for example, in order to contrast the *personnel* of the two schools: In that year, with a total matriculation of 454, of whom 150 were from Pennsylvania, the state furnishing the next largest number of students was North Carolina with 65, followed by Virginia with 48, Tennessee with 27, Alabama with 26, Mississippi with 15, and Georgia with 14; excepting New Jersey with 24, there being no Northern State furnishing so many as a dozen. Thus it will be seen that even in the University school, the attendance was composed chiefly of Southern students and Pennsylvanians, the number given here alone aggregating nearly two hundred of the former from states which furnished 14 and over. So that, for the University, the civil war involved a loss of about one-half of her students, unless they were reinforced from the North. And so it proved, for in 1862-63, her lowest enrollment during the war was 319, the lowest since 1815; and the next year out of a total of 401, Pennsylvania's list increased to 267, and no purely Southern State sent so many as six.

Jefferson, however, affords the best example of the effect of the war. The college had received some of its most able teachers from the South and West, which fact accounts for the large number of students from those quarters. In 1859-60, before the war had affected the question of constituency at all, Jefferson had a total enrollment of 630. The largest single contribution to this from any one State was from Pennsylvania, but that was only 120, while Virginia came next with almost as many, namely, 94; Alabama followed with over half as many, 50; Mississippi with 49; Georgia and North Carolina with 44 from each; South Carolina furnished 36, Tennessee 35, Kentucky 22, and Maryland 15, before a single Northern State is reached. These figures alone, not counting smaller numbers, give 389—i. e., nearly 400 out of the 630 were from Southern States, each of whose quota did not fall below 15. Jefferson's large Southern element made it the center of a movement which sprang up early during this session, and had, for its object, the union of all Southern students in the city in a withdrawal to some institution in the Southern States, so that after graduation they might be counted among the resources of the South. It was, undoubtedly, a part of the general movement in which the preliminaries of the Confederacy were effected, but was started into action by the raid of John Brown (c). The first public meeting was held at 9 o'clock, Tuesday morning, on December 20, 1859, at the Assembly Building, and nearly all the Southern students of the city were present. Two gentlemen, Drs. Luckett and Maguire, who were popular "quizzers" among those students, were called upon to express the sentiments of the majority. The former read a telegram from Governor Wise, of Richmond, Virginia, offering cordial welcome to those who should come to the college in that city, and also offering to pay all necessary expenses of transport. Letters were read from other institutions in that State and in North Carolina and Georgia, offering inducements and welcome. Already large numbers had pledged themselves to take the step and names were read, which, with those added during this meeting, reached the large number of about two hundred students. Dr. Hunter Maguire made the motion providing for their leaving in a body on the next evening, and a committee was appointed to carry out the plans adopted. "Of two hundred seceders," says a writer in the American and Gazette of December 30, 1859, "only eighteen were from the University of Pennsylvania, and one from the Pennsylvania Medical College." The only reason assigned in their resolutions was expressed in the preamble as follows: "We have left our homes and congregated in this city with a view to prosecute our medical studies, and having become fully convinced that we have erred in taking this step, that our means should have been expended and our protection afforded to the maintenance and advancement of institutions existing in our own sections, and fostered by our own people," etc. They decided to secede and go, for the greater part, to the Medical College of Virginia, at Richmond. "This conduct of

(c) The feeling among the students grew so bitter in these years that collisions were numerous and on one occasion so serious that Dr. Gibson remarked that "The very devil seems to have got into the students."

the students," writes Dr. S. D. Gross, "caused great commotion in our school, as well as in the University of Pennsylvania, and in the city generally. I was anxious that the Faculty should take some formal notice of this agitation, and that the dean should be commissioned to discharge this function as a part of his official duties. He, however, had great doubt of the propriety of the measure, and when, at length, he addressed the class, it was evident that his remarks fell still-born upon the ears of that portion of it which they were especially designed to influence and benefit. A strong appeal at an early day might, I have always been of the opinion, have been of great service. The day before the exodus occurred" (which Dr. Gross says was on the evening of the 23d, although he by a slip of memory puts the event two years too late), "I devoted fifteen minutes to the consideration of the subject, in which I strongly urged upon the different students the importance of remaining to the end of the session in close attendance upon the lectures; but, although my address was well received, the most profound silence prevailing during the delivery, it failed of its object. Only a few of the Southern students had the good sense to complete their course of studies. While this émeute was in progress, letters were received from different Southern schools . . . as the Richmond, Augusta, Charleston and Atlanta, offering to receive the seceders with open arms, and to give them their tickets, at the same time promising to graduate such as might present themselves as candidates. Governor Henry A. Wise made them a long speech of welcome on their arrival at Richmond, in the college of which most of them enlisted."

This was only the first loss of students from the South. The next year, 1860-61, Jefferson enrolled but 443, of whom 140 were from Pennsylvania. There was still a considerable number from the South; indeed, North Carolina furnished 43, the next greatest number to Pennsylvania, Virginia followed third with 37, Georgia and Kentucky each with 21, before a Northern State is reached, while 57 more were sent from four other States of the Confederacy. This still gave Jefferson a total of 179—approximately half of her constituency—from the Confederate section; and the University suffered in proportion, so far as the number of Southern students is concerned. But the conflict was now begun, and the year 1861-62 saw the total enrollment of Jefferson fall to 238; 153 of these were from Pennsylvania, only 16 from the entire South, and these were from the border: Virginia—beyond the mountains, probably—Maryland and Kentucky. In 1862-63, 275 were enrolled, with none but Kentuckians from the South; in '63-4 there were 351 under like conditions; in 1864-65 there were 380, and still none from below the Mason and Dixon line, and it was not until 1865-66 that small recruits of a dozen or less began to represent the late Confederate commonwealths. In that year the University's enrollment was 520 and Jefferson's 425, which serves to show Jefferson's larger dependency on the South in those years, and her heavier loss when the Southern men withdrew. It soon became apparent that these experiences were increasing the representation of both schools in the North, and in the West, and the old conditions were never restored, so far as Southern students were concerned. The noticeable increase of names from Ohio was, no doubt, in some measure, due to Jefferson's intimate relations with medical schools in the Ohio Valley, where she had secured the great surgeon who attracted many students in the years immediately preceding the medical secession.

With the opening of the war all the other regular medical schools collapsed, although the Woman's College revived after a brief suspension. As the University and Jefferson faculties had greatly changed, it will be of interest to see what influences were governing Philadelphia medicine from the secession in 1860 to the International Congress of 1876, to which period this chapter is devoted.

The names of Chapman, Wood, Jackson, Bache, Dunglison and others had begun to give place to those of Gross, Leidy, Agnew, Stillé, Da Costa, Mitchell and many more which are still in the mind of the public. The changes in the University really began as far back as 1847, when Dr. Rogers succeeded Dr. Hare. Not long after, in 1850, Dr. Chapman resigned, and Dr. Wood, taking his place, made way for the election of Dr. Joseph Carson to the chair of Materia Medica. From that time on, the names began to alter.

Drs. Carson, the Rogers Brothers, Leidy, Pepper, Henry H. and Francis G. Smith, Penrose, Stillé and Agnew, were the active, influential University representatives of the chief part of the period. Some of these, for example Dr. Pepper and the elder Rogers, were in service but a short time; others, as Drs. Leidy and Agnew, were more fully identified with the period, and two of them, Drs. Stillé and Penrose, are still living.

The Rogers family, father and two sons, were eminent in chemistry, the father, Dr. Patrick K. Rogers, being the successor of Dr. Hare in the chair devoted to that subject in William and Mary College, Virginia, when Dr. Hare became a University professor. It was a curious coincidence that his sons should successively succeed Dr. Hare in Philadelphia in later years. Dr. James B. Rogers, the elder son, was born in Philadelphia in 1802, the eldest of four sons, all of whom were eminent in the natural sciences, notably in chemistry and geology. He was educated in Baltimore and in the college of William and Mary, where his father held the chair of Chemistry, and began his medical studies in the office of Dr. Thomas E. Bond. Entering the medical department of the University of Maryland, he graduated in 1822 and began his first practice in a small town in Lancaster County, Pennsylvania, but soon returned to Baltimore and began a varied career as professor in Washington Medical College, lecturer in the Mechanics' Institute, superintendent of chemical works, and chemist, with his brother William, in state geological surveys. He also served four years in the chair of Chemistry in the medical department of Cincinnati Medical College. Returning to Philadelphia in 1840, he was associated with his brother Henry in a state geological survey, and soon became an instructor and examiner of medical students. This led to his becoming a lecturer on Chemistry in the Medical Institute in 1841, and in Franklin Institute three years later. It was during this period that he and his brother, Robert E. Rogers, the chemist, compiled a volume on chemistry, which was published in 1846. The following year, when he was forty-five years of age, he was called to the University to succeed Dr. Hare, after having become Professor of Chemistry in Franklin Medical College, which flourished for a couple of years. He had become prominent in the scientific organizations and was one of the original members of the American Medical Association. The Rogers family were of delicate physical constitution, and Dr. James B. Rogers was one of the frailest of them all, so that when he came to the chair of the University in 1847, it was to begin a career of only five years, for he died in 1852 at the age of fifty-one. "Dr. Rogers was a popular teacher," says Dr. Carson, his colleague, "the full storehouse of his mind was drawn upon to instruct his pupils, and no pains or labor did he spare to make easy to their comprehension the important truths he taught. In one portion of his course he was especially interesting; this was organic chemistry. Of late years it has become a prominent department of medical science, and from the success with which it has been cultivated, will become ultimately so interwoven with medicine as to require a large share of attention from medical students. Physiology and pathology are not the only branches to which organic chemistry is essential; therapeutics is gradually becoming amenable to its disclosures. The development of the mode of action of medicines to which organic chemistry has led has dissipated much uncertainty, and explained many phenomena which, although seen, were not understood. By demonstrating the importance of research upon the subject, and creating an interest in them, Dr. Rogers bestowed important service, and it was apparent that, in its reaction upon other branches, his mode of teaching materially aided the exertions of his associates."

His youngest brother, Dr. Robert E. Rogers, who had collaborated with him in his first publication, was then a man of almost forty years, the occupant of a like chair in the University of Virginia, and was considered the natural successor to the vacancy. He had written to one of his brothers, during his twentieth year, "my private desire always has been, and I think always would be, to follow, if possible, in your career; to become an instructor." Born in Baltimore in 1813, he lost both parents while still a boy, and from the age of fifteen came largely under the directing influence of his brother William, who became a professor in both William and Mary College and the University of Virginia, and was director of the Geological Survey of that State. Robert E. Rogers was educated at William and Mary, and after an unsuccessful attempt at civil engineering, he entered upon the study of medicine under Dr. Hare, probably about 1833, and graduated from the medical department of the University in 1836. His thesis had the honor of publication in the *American Journal of Medical Sciences*. He had evidently found his proper field of work and was at once made chemist to the first Geological Survey of Pennsylvania, of which his brother Henry was director. He soon became a prominent member of the scentific societies, and made a name as a lecturer before the Franklin Institute, especially in electricity. It was in 1841 that he was called to the University of Virginia to deliver the course of chemical lectures, which was interrupted by what proved to be the fatal illness of the professor, Dr. John P. Emmet, whom, in the following year, he succeeded in the chair of Chemistry and Materia Medica. It was here that he spent ten years of successful work, becoming also widely known through his activity in the American Medical Association, and it was from this chair that he was called in 1852 to succeed his brother, Dr. John B. Rogers, in the University of Pennsylvania. In his new office he proved himself abundantly able to carry on the work of his elder brother, and he here resumed his prominence in scientific circles. He also made a reputation as a medico-legal expert in toxicology. Indeed, his mind was marvelously practical, inventive, many-sided and rich in resources. In 1862, he was made an acting assistant surgeon for service in the great military hospital in West Philadelphia, and lost his hand in overseeing a practical invention intended to facilitate the laundry work of that great institution. Two years later, he was chosen, with a colleague, to investigate the processes of refining silver at the Philadelphia mint, and his work was so effective that it led to extensive reforms, not only in this mint, but in that at San Francisco, and in the Assay Office at New York, all of which were executed under his direction. He also served on the Assay Commission for several years, and as chemist to the Philadelphia Gas Trust. In 1877, he had been twenty-five years in the chair made famous by Rush, Woodhouse, Hare, and his brother, when the

University undertook some far-reaching changes in its curriculum and general methods, which, excellent as they have since proved, were then regarded with disapproval by some, among whom was Dr. Rogers. During the lecture season he was offered the chair of Chemistry and Toxicology in Jefferson Medical College and accepted it. He was now sixty-four years of age and spent only seven years in his new position, so that his career is properly identified with the University. He died in 1884, in his seventy-second year, widely honored and beloved, a popular instructor, the idol of his large classes, genial and amiable; known for his integrity, courtesy, energy and gentleness. The year before his death he was honored by Dickinson College with the degree of Doctor of Laws.

Two years before Dr. Rogers' election to the Faculty of the University, namely, in 1850, Dr. Joseph Carson had become the successor of Dr. Wood in the chair of Materia Medica and Therapeutics, at the age of forty-two. Dr. Carson was essentially a learned man and of a peculiarly calm and judicial poise of mind, so that his style has the ordered solidity of a Supreme Court decision, and leaves one with a feeling of absolute confidence in both his mental processes and their result. He came of a line of Scotch Presbyterians and early Philadelphians prominent in the merchant-shipping interests. Born in Philadelphia in 1808, he was educated at two well-known local academies, and at the University, receiving his classical diploma in 1826, at the age of fifteen. While employed in the wholesale drug house of a Dr. Lowber, who was much interested in botany, young Carson became attracted to this and kindred sciences, and determined to study medicine. Meantime he had shown those talents for patient observation and research which characterized his entire life, and his enthusiasm for medical botany gave new scope for them. Dr. Thomas T. Hewson became his preceptor, and the University graduated him in 1830, at the age of twenty-two. He became resident physician in the old Philadelphia, or Almshouse Hospital, then at Tenth and Pine streets, with Gerhard, Norris and others as his colleagues; but before undertaking private practice concluded to ship for one year as surgeon on an East India vessel. This voyage produced results in the form of a carefully kept journal of scientific observation, which attracted some attention. In 1832, he began practice, and three years later was enrolled among the members of the Academy of National Sciences and the American Philosophical Society, in both of which bodies he was a highly valued member. In 1836, he was elected Professor of Materia Medica in the College of Pharmacy, and edited the *American Journal of Pharmacy*. In addition to this work he was, in 1844, associated with Gerhard, Goddard, the elder Rogers, Morris and others, in the Medical Institute, where he lectured on Materia Medica and Pharmacy; and it was from these positions that, in 1850, he was called to the chair made so popular by Dr. George B. Wood. For twenty-six years he filled this position with ability and success. He also held many important positions in the great scientific and professional organizations, and was one of the founders of the American Medical Association. His writings were numerous and varied, but his history of the medical department of the University must always cause his name to be thoroughly identified with that great institution. He resigned his chair in 1876, in his sixty-ninth year, and died before its close, when his native city had just celebrated the nation's centennial. Sixteen years of his life were devoted to the University.

In 1853, three years after Carson's election, another new member, destined to make a name equal to, if not more famous than that of any of his predecessors, came to the chair once occupied by Shippen, Wistar, Physick and Horner. This was Dr. Joseph Leidy, of whom an eminent colleague (d) could say years after, that he was "the profoundest and most consummate teacher that ever held the chair of Anatomy, and whose fame as a comparative anatomist, paleontologist, geologist, zoölogist and botanist, was not bounded by his native city or country, but was co-extensive with the civilized world." Long before this date Dr. Leidy had been a friend, assistant and co-laborer with several of the faculty, especially Drs. Hare, Rogers, Wood and Horner. He had supplied Dr. Horner's place the year before his death, so that it was a practically foregone conclusion that the amiable and learned naturalist should be Hor-

---

(d) Dr. Alfred Stillé.

ner's successor. From boyhood Dr. Leidy evinced a genius for scientific observation—though not for generalization. He was an original observer, investigator and discoverer in the fields both of gross and microscopic anatomy and biology, and his remarkable artistic power of depicting his observations added vastly to the effectiveness of his teachings and writings. Some of his drawings of the lower forms of life which are religiously preserved in the College of Physicians, are marvels of artistic skill.

One can never turn to Dr. Leidy's antecedents without recallnig his striking self-introduction to a Philadelphia audience on one occasion, when the introducer remarked to him that he was already better known than the introducer himself, whereupon he answered: "I will introduce myself." Stepping to the front he said: "My name is Joseph Leidy, Doctor of Medicine. I was born in this city on the 9th of September, 1823, and have lived here ever since. My father was Philip Leidy, the hatter, on Third street, above Vine. My mother was Catherine Mellick, but she died a few months after my birth. My father married her sister, Christina Mellick, and she was the mother I have known, who was all in all to me, the one to whom I owe all that I am. At an early age I took great delight in natural history and in noticing all natural objects. I have reason to think that I know a little of natural history, and a little of that little I propose to teach you to-night." Christina Mellick Leidy was one of those intelligent, thoughtful women with a tincture of the poetic temperament, who seem to have almost prophetic intuitions. Although the Leidys had been plain Rhenish-German Americans, from the time of Penn, she believed that a career more brilliant than that of his ancestors was in store for her step-son, and it was through her influence that he was thoroughly educated. He was accordingly entered as a pupil at the age of ten in a Classical Academy conducted by a Methodist minister. He had already shown a remarkable interest in plants and minerals and sought many a companion among both boys and men who happened to know more about them than he. One day a visiting lecturer at the school talked to the pupils on mineralogy, and, from that time, the subject of natural history became young Leidy's ruling passion, and prompted him to begin a more systematic course of study. Thereafter the glens of the Wassahickon, the Schuylkill, Bartram's Gardens, and the fields and rocks for miles around became his favorite schools. A small book of drawings of shells made by him in his tenth year, displayed the artistic power and keen observation that were ever after so marked a feature of his scientific work. In his sixteenth year, through his mother's influence, he was placed with an apothecary and rapidly became efficient enough to be left in charge of the shop. This determined his mother to permit him to study medicine, and in 1840, he began his medical curriculum with Dr. James McClintock, the founder of the private school of Anatomy. When that gentleman was called away in 1841, young Leidy entered the University and chose Dr. Paul B. Goddard, Demonstrator of Anatomy and assistant to Dr. Horner, as his preceptor. His thesis on his graduation in 1844, *The Comparative Anatomy of the Eye of Vertebrated Animals*, was remarkably indicative of the main features of his future life work, so far as the science of medicine was concerned. He was not destined for the practice of medicine, although he essayed it; he was born a scientist, and, on his graduation, became assistant to Dr. Hare and later to Dr. Rogers, the elder. In 1845, he became prosector to Dr. Horner, and the next year was demonstrator of Anatomy in Franklin Medical College. During this period he was also coroner's physician. Dr. Horner took him to Europe in 1848, to aid him in making models and drawings of specimens in various hospitals and elsewhere; as did also Dr. Wood, two years later. On his return, he was given two or three medical positions, one of which was that of lecturer in Dr. Chapman's Medical Institute, and he at once took prominent rank in the scientific and professional organizations of the city.

In 1852, when he was not yet thirty years of age, he was asked to supply Dr. Horner's course of lectures, and the following year became his successor. "My recollections of Dr. Leidy," writes Dr. J. J. Levick, "go back to the days when he occupied a room in the rear of Dr. Goddard's house on Ninth street, opposite the University, from which, a little later, he moved to a house on Sansom street, above Ninth. I was a student of medicine and knew him as a hard-working young physician, bent on supporting himself, and compelled to be content with doing it in a very moderate way. I heard him give his first lecture on Anatomy in the amphitheater of the University of Pennsylvania, in the place of Professor Horner, then unable, from ill health, to lecture. We were all on the *qui vive* to hear what he would say by way of introduction. I recall that there was a little nervous swing as he came in the lecture room. No words were wasted by way introduction, but plunging *in medias res* he gave a good, intelligent lecture with apparent self-possession. Many years later he told me that he had lain in a warm bath for an hour before the lecture to get his nervous system thoroughly calm for the effort." His success was assured from that moment. His scientific papers cover a wide range of subjects and have made his name immortal, but we are here concerned solely with his relations to medical science. In 1861, he published his *Elementary Treatise on Human Anatomy.* Some excellent work was done by him in 1862-65 as assistant surgeon in the great Satterlee Hospital, where he was commissioned to conduct and describe autopsies, the results of which form a valuable part of the Surgeon-General's reports. He also became chief surgeon of the state military department. This was merely somewhat incidental work, as was also his practice, which he soon abandoned entirely, to devote himself to his department in the University, which occupied him for the long period of thirty-eight years.

Great as was Dr. Leidy's work in the medical school, he was equally distinguished in the University proper as head of the Department of Biology, which was inaugurated under Provost Pepper in 1882; in which also he held the chair of Zoölogy and Comparative Anatomy, and was largely instrumental in the development of the whole biological scheme. This he considered almost as pastime. "To increase knowledge of natural things, animate or inanimate, gigantic or microscopic, seemed to be a ruling passion," to use the words of another, "and, like a true huntsman, he cared less for the capture than for the pleasure of pursuing his game." His most congenial alliance was with the Academy of Natural Sciences, and it is probable that his fame will rest chiefly on his work in that department. For more than forty-four years, it has been said, "he virtually directed and managed the affairs of the museum," as he was chairman of the board, and curator, librarian or president, from 1845, the first year of his membership, to the close of his life. His first important publication in the Proceedings of this body bore the title, *Special Anatomy of the Terrestrial Gasteropoda of the United States*. It was in 1847 that he discovered that *Trichina Spiralis* found entrance into the human body by the use of hog's flesh. He was the first to announce this fact, which may be considered one of his most valuable contributions to medical science. The medical interest attached to this discovery is so great that some details of the steps by which it was reached may be acceptable. Hilton of England, in 1832, first observed the encapsuled trichinæ in human muscle, but mistook them for cysticerci. Paget, at that time a medical student, next described them, and did so without knowledge of Hilton's observations. Owen, the celebrated anatomist, shortly afterward described them more fully and gave the parasite the name of *trichina spiralis*. Leidy was the first to detect the trichina in the hog and he recognized it as identical with a parasite which he had previously observed in human muscle. To Leidy, therefore, belongs the credit of having first detected the identity of "trichinosis" in man and in the hog, although it was not until 1860 that the clinical symptoms of the affection were described by Zenker of Dresden, Germany. In 1871, he was also made Professor of Natural History at Swarthmore College, and three years later Harvard called him to her anatomical chair, but he declined the latter appointment. He was extensively sought after and largely engaged in national geological and geographical surveys. In 1879, he published his famous work on *Rhizopods*. Princeton also gave him a call to her scientific post-graduate faculty, but in vain. The Wagner Free Institute of Science secured him as the head of its biological department. His numerous publications and his general work won him prizes on both continents and the degree of Doctor of Laws from two institutions, one of which was Harvard (1886). He was a large man, of powerful frame. "Joseph Leidy inherited excellent constitution of mind and body," said President Wharton of

Swarthmore, "he was transparently sincere and absolutely devoted to truth; he was remarkably devoid of selfishness in any form; he had persistent and life-long diligence; he was systematic in his expenditure and careful in his economy of time; he held firmly to whatever he undertook; his temper was cheerfully equable and his disposition affectionate." He died in 1891, nearly sixty-eight years of age, and without having made an enemy during that long period. "It makes a difference to the world when such a man passes away," said the Provost, Dr. Pepper, before the Congress of American Physicians in Washington. "At his birth nature gave him her accolade, and all his life long he was loyal to the holy quest of truth, which is the vow imposed on those whom she invests as her chosen knights." But, with all his great career as a naturalist, to him medicine had secondary interest. The question as to how he filled the chair of Wistar and of Physick may be answered in the following words: "Dr. Leidy taught pure anatomy," says Dr. Hunt, "others of us applied the knowledge he gave. This was all he said he would do or engage to do. I mention this for you who are not familiar with such matters. Think of this! could a man enjoy higher praise than to know that for thirty-eight years he filled without objection a practical chair in an essentially practical school, for science, and science alone? In all that time, no jealous aspirant even whispered, 'This chair must be practically filled.' The luster he threw about the University dimmed or quenched all jealousies by its brightness. Professors, students, and all, behold how they loved him!" Besides Leidy, another protégé of Dr. Horner, and also his son-in-law, joined the faculty in 1855, as the successor of Gibson, whom he had long assisted as a clinical lecturer. Like Leidy, too, he was, when elected, about forty years of age and was a Philadelphian. Dr. Henry H. Smith was born in 1815, the son of an eminent lawyer, James S. Smith, and received his early education in a well-known classical school. Graduating from the University of Pennsylvania in 1834, at the age of nineteen, he began the study of medicine under Dr. Horner's direction in the medical department, which gave him his diploma three years later. After two years' service as resident physician at the Pennsylvania Hospital, he went to Europe, where he spent eighteen months in extensive study in the great hospitals of London, Paris and Vienna, and in other institutions. In 1841, on his return, he published a translation of Civiale's work on the treatment of stone and gravel, which attracted attention and conduced to his success as a private lecturer on surgery. He published other works in the next few years, and his reputation as a surgeon soon led to his election to the staff of St. Joseph's, the Episcopal and the Philadelphia Hospitals. He joined the last mentioned institution in 1854, when clinical instruction had been forbidden in it for nine years. It was through his influence, together with that of Drs. Penrose, Ludlow, Reese and Agnew, that it was again temporarily restored in October of that year, and permanently in 1859. His book on the work of American surgeons was also well received. In 1855, he and Gerhard, Agnew, Henry, Penrose and Parrish revived a private school under the name Academy of Medicine, and it was in that year that he was called to the chair of Surgery in the University, to succeed Dr. Gibson. In 1863, he issued his Principles and Practice of Surgery, embracing the substance of his three treatises on Minor Surgery, Operative Surgery and the Practice of Surgery. This was his greatest work. Dr. Smith and Dr. Agnew were colleagues at the University, and the latter was occasionally asked to supply a lecture for him in emergencies, occasioned by the exigencies of surgical practice. At the opening of the war Governor Curtin appointed him Surgeon-General of Pennsylvania, to organize the State Hospital Department. In this capacity he inaugurated the removal of soldiers to large hospitals, and was, no doubt, influential in leading the hospital movement to Philadelphia. He resigned this position near the close of 1862, however, and, although largely engaged in military surgery, gave his chief attention to private practice and to his professorship, in which he is said to have been "quiet, fluent, self-possessed, systematic and thorough." He was a member of various scientific and professional organizations, and in later years became especially prominent in the county, state and national and international bodies, serving as chairman of the executive committee of the Ninth International Medical Congress of 1887, and president of the section on Naval and Military Surgery. He died at the age of seventy-five, after many years of active practice as a surgeon. The ability of Dr. Smith was somewhat less prominently before the public in the latter years of his life, probably because of the overshadowing fame of his great successor in the chair of Surgery. After sixteen years of active work as an instructor, during the trying and critical period of the civil war, circumstances, it is believed honorable to all concerned, led to his becoming emeritus professor in 1871, at the age of fifty-seven years, and to the choice of Dr. Agnew as his successor. That his eminent abilities have been recognized is indicated by the fact that in 1885 he was honored by Lafayette College with the degree of Doctor of Laws.

Long before 1871, however, it had become evident that a surgeon of remarkable ability was acting in the capacity of clinical assistant to both Drs. Leidy and Smith, his official titles in 1863 being Demonstrator of Anatomy and Assistant Lecturer on Clinical Surgery. This man had come out of the old School of Anatomy, which, under his able instruction, attained the greatest fame of its long career. Even the two great medical schools were conscious of the rivalry of this extra-mural institution, whose students, under Agnew, numbered nearly three hundred. Dr. D. Hayes Agnew was by no means a young man when he took charge of the School of Anatomy in 1852. Having been born in 1818, he was thirty-four years old when he began his notable work in Chant street. He began with nine students, and before many seasons the capacity of the school was taxed to its utmost limit. In 1854, he opened a School of Operative Surgery in the second story of the same building, and this achieved an equal success. Among his assistants were Drs. R. J. Barclay, J. R. Sanderson, R. J. Levis, William Flynn, J. K. Kane, M. J. Asch, D. R. Richardson, J. T. Darby, Robert Bolling, J. W. Lodge, S. W. Gross and James E. Garretson. "The lecture-room of the School of Anatomy," writes Dr. J. Howe Adams, "was built in imitation of the ordinary lecture-room of a medical college. It had tier above tier of benches, rising so abruptly above each other that the seventh, or highest row, was fully twenty feet above the arena. It may be interesting to those who have sat for hours upon the ordinary clinique-room bench, which seems always to be made of boards particularly unyielding in their texture, to know that these benches were covered with cushions. This unparalleled luxury was the only portion of the 'royal road to learning' reached by the embryo anatomist of Chant street. In the arena was a revolving table, on which the cadaver to be demonstrated could be placed. Over this was a series of lights, so arranged as to throw their illuminations over the lecturer and the subject. Hanging in mid-air, by a wire from the ceiling, was a skeleton, which could be lowered when needed. On a shelf back of the lecturer stood a number of statues, representing, classically, the human form. One was a representation of Hercules, another of Mercury, a third of Venus, and a fourth 'The Discus Thrower.'" Here it was that he, with his crowds of students, large numbers of them Southerners, attracted the attention of Dr. Smith. As early as 1858, he began assisting the latter in his clinics, and continued in the University in this unofficial capacity until his appointment as Demonstrator of Anatomy by Dr. Leidy in 1863. For seven years thereafter, having in the meantime sold his school to Dr. Garretson, he gave his attention to the University, which thus secured the popular head of the Chant street school and all his influence. In 1870, Dr. Agnew became a member of the faculty of the University in virtue of his election to the chair of Clinical Surgery. This position had been vacant since its resignation by Dr. George W. Norris in 1857, but was revived in order to make Dr. Agnew a full member of the faculty. The following year Dr. Smith resigned and was made emeritus professor, and Dr. Agnew was chosen his successor. Agnew was now in his fifty-third year, a fact that shows unusual patience, in so able a man, in waiting for full recognition of his services. This, however, was not needed to add to his prestige, for his talents as a surgeon and instructor were already widely recognized.

The early life of Dr. Agnew was uneventful. The Agnew, or Agneaux, family is of Scotch lineage, and one of the oldest Pennsylvania families of Franklin County. Dr. Robert Agnew, the father of D. Hayes, had been educated under Dr. Thomas C. James, and after serving as surgeon in the United States navy, settled in Lancaster County, where he married the widow of an eminent Presbyterian divine, Rev. Ebenezer Henderson, and spent the greater part of his life. It was there that their only son, D. Hayes Agnew, was born, in 1818, and grew up with a marked inclination and love for the profession of his father. He was educated at a classical academy, Jefferson College, at Cannonsburg, and at Newark College, in Delaware, but did not graduate. After studying medicine under his father, he entered the University of Pennsylvania Medical School in 1836, when it was beginning to undergo the great revival under the faculty of '35. His talent for anatomy was evident during his entire course, and his industry equaled it. Graduating in 1838, with the thesis "Medical Science and the Responsibility of Medical Character," he returned to assist his father in Noblesville. Late in 1841, he was married to a daughter of Samuel Irwin of the Pleasant Garden Iron Works, in Chester County, and, after Mr. Irwin's death in 1842, was induced to abandon medicine and enter the firm of which his father-in-law had been a member. This he did in 1843, but the depression of the iron trade, during the years succeeding the panic of '37, was such that after three years of struggle the firm was obliged to assign, and Dr. Agnew resumed his profession with the intention of paying all the obligations incurred in his unhappy business venture. He settled in Cochranville, Chester County, and began private anatomical study, with the view of devoting himself solely to surgery. One of his customs was that of putting his "subjects" in a pond full of eels, which cleaned their bones most thoroughly. It so happened, however, that the favorite eel-seller of the region secretly caught his eels in this same pond, and the result was an unsavory reputation for Dr. Agnew. Circumstances finally led to his permanent location in Philadelphia, on Eleventh street, near the School of Anatomy, in 1848, in which he at once became a private student, and four years later took sole charge of it, as has been described.

During the next ten years his practice grew rapidly, and his consultation work became extensive, so that by the opening years

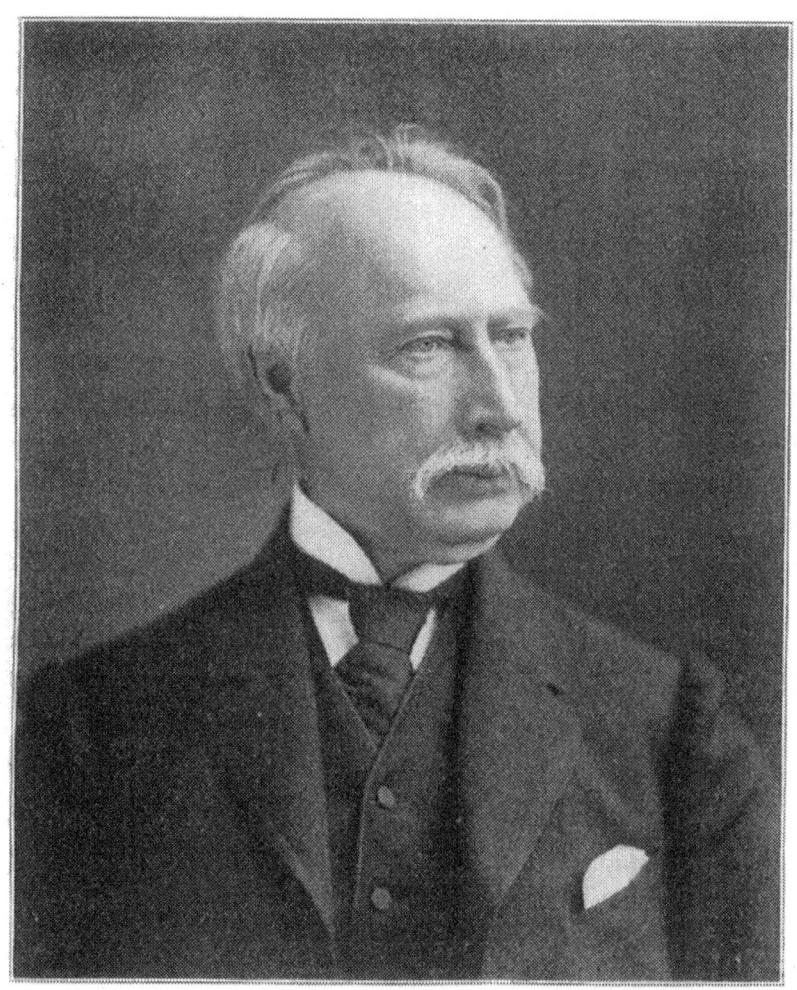

D. HAYES AGNEW.

of the war he was generally acknowledged one of the first surgeons of Philadelphia. Various hospital positions came to him, and he published some works of importance, his "Practical Anatomy" being one of them. In 1862, he entered the military hospital service, and had duties at Satterlee, Hestonville, Mower and in the volunteer service, the most of his work being performed at Satterlee and Mower. At Hestonville he was surgeon-in-charge. This extensive experience made him an authority on gunshot wounds, and by reason of it he was consulted by some of the most distinguished officers of the army. Among these was General Hancock, whom he cared for after the battle of Gettysburg, and who, as a result, became his personal friend. Many years later (in 1880) his services were demanded for a still more prominent citizen—President Garfield, in whose case Agnew was the principal consultant. During his war service came his University appointment, both of which occupied him to the fullest extent. Soon after the close of the war he joined Drs. T. G. Morton, H. E. Goodman and S. W. Gross in founding the Orthopædic Hospital, which was opened for patients in February, 1868. These gentlemen, with Drs. S. D. Gross and G. W. Norris, as consultants, constituted the first medical staff.

When he became full Professor of Surgery in 1871 he infused new life into his department, the facilities of which were greatly increased by the new developments attending the removal of the University to West Philadelphia in 1874. Dr. John Neill, and later Dr. John Ashhurst, Jr., were associated with him, and he took part in all the progress of that period. "Dr. Agnew's powerful personality," said the Provost, "made itself felt in the work and development of the Medical School of the University of Pennsylvania, from the beginning of his connection with it down to the last days of his life. . . . . It was most fortunate that in Agnew, Leidy and Stillé, the medical faculty contained men whose names and characters were towers of strength during these years of struggle." Princeton honored him with the degree of Doctor of Laws in 1874, not only for his vigorous work as a surgeon, but also for his contributions to surgical literature, which culminated in 1878 in his greatest work, "The Principles and Practice of Surgery," in three volumes. This work displays the readiness with which he appreciated the wonderful possibilities of asepsis, which was then revolutionizing surgery, although this was but one of its elements of greatness. Great as were Agnew's writings, however, the influence of his kindly personality, that led to his being called the "Dear Old Man," a title conferred upon him by the younger Gross, was probably even greater, and was constantly manifested during his ten years of service in the School of Anatomy, and for over a quarter of a century in his work as Demonstrator of Anatomy and Professor of Surgery in the University, of which he became emeritus professor in 1889. And yet, one thinks of Agnew, not as made greater by his University appointments or by his writings, or merely as a great operative and consulting surgeon, but as a great character, whose benign personality, clear mind, sound judgment, precision of operation and absolute confidence in his opinion, gave him the force of character of a chief justice in medicine. Someone has compared him to Sir Astley Cooper, of whom it has been written: "His influence did not arise from his published works, nor from his being a lecturer, nor, indeed, from any public situation which he held, although each of these circumstances had its share in producing the result; but it seemed to originate more from his innate love of his profession, his extreme zeal in all that concerned it, and his honest desire, as well as great power, to communicate his knowledge to another, without at the same time exposing the ignorance of his listener on the subject, even to himself. This must be looked upon as one great cause why his public character became so much diffused by his professional brethren, for he owed little of his advancement in life to patronage. Another peculiar quality, which proved always a great source of advantage to him, was his thorough confidence in respect to his professional knowledge, so that after he had once examined a case he cared but little who was to give a further surgical opinion upon it. This must inevitably have instilled an equal degree of confidence in those consulting him." Dr. J. William White has said that the following is equally descriptive of both Leidy and Agnew: "Appreciation of his rare intellectual gifts was forgotten in admiration of his sincere, sweet-tempered, loving nature. Retiring and unassuming, genial and kindly in spirit and manner, the friend of all, the enemy of none, as approachable as a child, ready at all times and with evident pleasure to give the benefit of his knowledge to all who sought it, his death will be mourned wherever science is valued throughout the earth; but we especially will miss his kindly face, his ready hand, his cordial greeting and his noble example of industry, integrity and manly character." His rugged constitution began to show its first signs of failure in 1888, and his last illness came in the spring of 1892, causing his death on March 22, at the age of seventy-four years. His was a life almost contemporaneous with the development of modern surgery, and his prime was reached at a time when his long training in Chant street had prepared him for the fullest benefit of that greater school—the hospitals of the war of secession; furthermore his sedulous training and his marvelous capacity made him a combination of specialists, such as is scarcely possible under present developments of the various branches of medicine and surgery" (e).

Three years before Agnew's subordinate appointment, the chair of Chapman and Wood received a new occupant in the person of Dr. William Pepper, Sr., whose brief career of four years, as Professor of Theory and Practice, terminated in the spring of 1864 and was followed by his decease in the succeeding autumn. Dr. Pepper was one of that band of University students who were attracted by the new methods of Louis and the French school, and through them and his own personal talents he had become one of the ablest and most conscientious diagnosticians in the city, some time before he was called to his University work. It was the general opinion of the profession of his day that nothing but a sturdy constitution was wanting to render his incumbency of the chair of Practice at least as brilliant as that of his more robust predecessors. He was fifty years old when he assumed the duties of his

---

(e) Dr. Agnew's relations with various scientific and professional organizations were extensive, though they are overshadowed by his greater influence in more individual action. He was president of the College of Physicians, the first surgeon to hold the office since Hewson.

professional chair. Born in 1810, in Philadelphia, he was educated in Princeton, where he distinguished himself and received his degree in 1828. Soon after, he entered upon the study of medicine under Dr. T. T. Hewson, and a year later began his course in the University of Pennsylvania. Graduating in 1832, Dr. Pepper took a most active part in the fight against the epidemic of Asiatic cholera of that year, and spent most of the summer in Bush Hill Hospital. Late in the year he departed for Europe to study in Paris, and there did excellent work under the various great leaders, particularly Louis and Dupuytren, who became his personal friends. It was here that ill health first threatened to disturb his plans and obliged him to spend a winter in the south of Europe. After two years in the French capital, he returned to Philadelphia in 1834, and, beginning practice, assumed charge of one of the dispensary districts, where his able and conscientious work soon drew attention to him as a skillful diagnostician and physician. He rapidly rose in professional estimation, joined the various medical and scientific societies, and was elected to several hospital staffs, among them that of the Pennsylvania Hospital, where he distinguished himself as a lecturer on clinical medicine, and prepared the reputation that gave him the University chair in 1860. "Dr. Pepper had a remarkable faculty in inspiring the confidence of his patients," writes Dr. Kirkbride. "Exceedingly careful in his preliminary examination, when he did express an opinion it seemed very generally to carry absolute conviction of its soundness to those to whom it was addressed. The general accuracy of his diagnosis, the extreme rarity, certainly, of grave errors of this description, fully justified their confidence. In the later years of his life his consultation practice was exceedingly large, and his professional brethren, who so often sought the benefit of his great skill, I am sure will bear me out in saying that his ability in the investigation of obscure diseases was of no ordinary kind, and the subsequent complete verification of his opinions in such doubtful cases very often excited surprise, as it could not fail to inspire confidence." These qualities could not fail to render him an impressive teacher and to secure for him that confidence on the part of his pupils without which the work of the teacher is wasted.

The year before his death the chairs of Drs. Hodge and Jackson were filled by the election of Drs. R. A. F. Penrose, who is still living, and Dr. Francis Gurney Smith, respectively. This was in 1863, the year Dr. Agnew became assistant to Drs. Leidy and Henry H. Smith; so that this may be considered the date at which the new period was inaugurated in the University. Dr. Francis Gurney Smith, like Gerhard, Pennock, Pepper, Stillé and others, was one of the disciples of Louis and the French school, and was chosen to his chair over competitors, among whom was Dr. Brown-Séquard. He was well advanced in life when he attained this position, being forty-five years of age. Dr. Smith was a worthy successor of Jackson, and has the honor of having established the first physiological laboratory in the University. He was the son of the eminent Philadelphia merchant of the same name, and was born in 1818. Educationally he was the child of the University, having received his classical degree in 1837 and his medical diploma three years later, after studying under the preceptorship of his brother, Dr. Thomas M. K. Smith of Brandywine, near Wilmington, Delaware. After serving as resident physician at the Insane Department of the Pennsylvania Hospital, and also as assistant to his brother, he began practice in Philadelphia, and in 1842 became one of the lecturers of the "Medical Association." From the beginning of his career he was especially interested in physiology and obstetrics, but this tendency to specialism did not prevent his becoming one of the most successful general practitioners of his day. By 1844, he was an editor of the *Medical Examiner*, a position he held for ten years. He joined Dr. J. M. Allen in his school of private instruction, which was one of the most successful of the period, and from this school both these gentlemen were chosen, in 1852, to the new faculty of the Medical Department of Pennsylvania College, Dr. Smith taking the chair of Physiology. This position he held for eleven years with such signal success that, on the declining health of Dr. Jackson in 1863, Dr. Smith was chosen to fill his place in the chair of the Institutes of Medicine. In 1859, he was elected visiting physician to the Pennsylvania Hospital, and there exhibited the qualities of a good clinical lecturer. He was one of the first staff of the Protestant Episcopal Hospital. When the war opened he was also on the staff of two other city hospitals, and was called to direct the military hospital on Christian street, a position he held until 1863, when he was assigned the medical care of wounded officers. Dr. Smith had also become prominent in professional and scientific societies to an unusual extent. He served as the first president of the Obstetrical Society of Philadelphia, and vice-president of the American Medical Association, and was a member of numerous other medical societies of this and other states.

It will thus be seen that Dr. Francis Gurney Smith led an extremely active life, and that his acquaintances, both professional and lay, must have been numerous, and his influence widespread. He was an experienced teacher of physiology when he succeeded Samuel Jackson at the University in 1863. "As a lecturer," writes Dr. Charles B. Nancrede, "he possessed that preëminent qualification, the power of arresting and retaining the interest of his hearers. Clear and lucid in his explanations, he was yet ever ready to explain again. Not satisfied, as so many men would have been after years of lecturing, to trust to their memory and knowledge, up to the very last, every lecture had devoted to it hours of thought and reading. He delivered his lecture extemporaneously, only resorting to his notes for long quotations, etc. . . . . He was, without exception, the most conscientious lecturer I have ever known; nothing was left to chance. Every experiment was tried over and over until there was no room for peradventure." This testimony of one who assisted Dr. Smith in his numerous class demonstrations is of great interest and coincides completely with that of others who acted as his assistants. As a result of his conscientious preparation, his lectures were marked features of the University medical course, and were crowded with the most attentive listeners. He was a cultured, courteous gentleman, and receptive of new knowledge from all quarters. He is said to have been the first to introduce hypodermic medication in this city. His extensive practice was among the most cultivated classes of

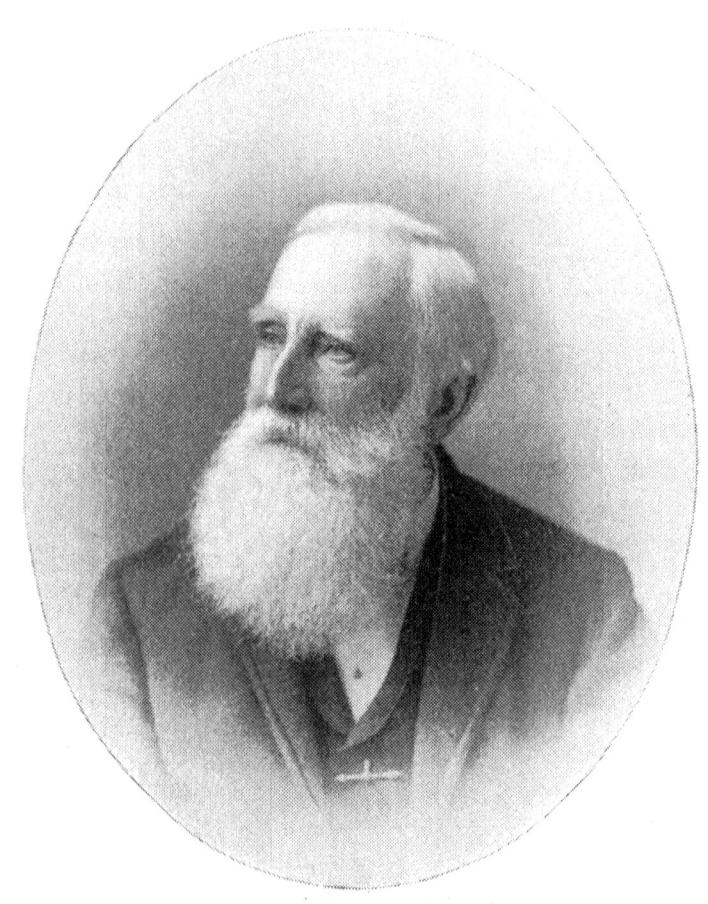

Philadelphia. His retirement, in 1877, was followed the next year by his death, at the age of sixty years, an event that was undoubtedly precipitated by long-continued over-exertion.

One of F. G. Smith's colleagues in the faculty of the University was Alfred Stillé, whose part in Philadelphia medicine, once so active, has been converted by the infirmities of age into the comparatively passive rôle of an interested and critical spectator of current events. The chair that Dr. Smith held, had, under Jackson, been the propagandist of French methods in medicine, and it may be said that it was the elder Pepper and Stillé who remodeled the chair of Theory and Practice according to those methods. Dr. Smith took his chair in '63; Dr. Pepper died in 1864, and early in that year Dr. Alfred Stillé became his successor. The active University men of that time were Rogers, Carson, Leidy, F. G. Smith, Agnew, Penrose and Stillé, all of whom were teachers in the old building on Ninth street, as well as in the present Medical Hall. The following were members of the auxiliary faculty: Drs. Harrison Allen, Horatio C. Wood, F. V. Hayden, Henry Hartshorne and John J. Reese. Dr. Stillé is now an octogenarian, so that in 1864, when he assumed the duties of the chair of Rush and Chapman, he was over fifty years of age, and had acquired, by his writings, an international reputation. Probably he has been a more logical successor of Jackson than any of those who were influenced by that interesting personality. What Gerhard was as an investigator in French methods, it could probably be said that Stillé has been in the philosophical application and expression of them. Dr. Stillé has been both aggressive and progressive, and has, therefore, been actively concerned, from the time of his student days in Paris to the present, in every subject connected with medical progress. It is not purposed here to give any account of his later life; but it may be of interest here to refer to so much of his early career as will show his relation to the period described in this chapter. Dr. Stillé's lineage can be traced much farther back than that of most Americans. As has already been noticed in the earliest pages of this volume, he is a descendant on the father's side of one of the first Swedish colonies on the Schuylkill and Delaware, back in the days of the barber-surgeon, Jan Petersen; while on his mother's side, his ancestry can be traced back to Chancellor Wagner of the University of Tübingen, in the middle of the seventeenth century. He was born in this city in 1813, and was educated both in the classics and in medicine in the University of Pennsylvania. On receiving his degree of Bachelor of Arts, in 1832, he began the study of medicine under Dr. Thomas Harris, and entered the University, where he came under the influence of Dr. Jackson. Graduating in 1836, at the age of twenty-three, he served as resident in the Philadelphia Hospital, and then went to Paris. Here he studied under Louis and others for two years and a half, and visited other hospital centers, returning in 1839. He at once entered the Pennsylvania Hospital as resident, and after two years' service began general practice. He was now twenty-eight years of age. In the next few years he found time to publish, with Dr. J. F. Meigs, a translation of Andral's "Pathological Hæmatology," and the following year, 1845, he became lecturer on General Pathology and the Practice of Medicine in the Philadelphia Association for Medical Instruction. It was during these years that he became an influential factor in the movement for extending the term of medical instruction and for the general elevation of medical education, which culminated in the organization of the American Medical Association. His activity and prominence in this body have been mentioned elsewhere in these pages. Some of his public addresses attracted widespread attention, and, in 1848, his "Elements of General Pathology" served still further to enhance his reputation. He was one of the first staff of St. Joseph's Hospital, in 1849, and five years later was called to the chair of Theory and Practice of Medicine in the Medical Department of Pennsylvania College, a position he continued to hold up to the year of the great student secession of 1859. In 1860, he issued his great work on Materia Medica and Therapeutics, in two volumes, which passed through several editions within two decades. When the war opened he became one of the staff of the great "Satterlee" Hospital, and other honors came in rapid succession, until they culminated in his election to the chair of Theory and Practice of Medicine in the University of Pennsylvania in 1864. The highest honors of the profession have since been awarded him, nearly all the leading societies having given him the office of chief executive. In his career, nothing has been recognized so fully as his active, and even aggressive, sympathy with all that he considered a helpful and vital part of general medical development. In consequence, he has been identified with almost every movement that is now a part of the most valuable conditions of present-day medicine. Such was his character when, in 1859, the period under consideration was ushered in by the great student secession that introduced the civil war to Philadelphia medical circles.

While the old names of the University faculty had been somewhat rapidly replaced by those of the Rogers, Carson, the Smiths, Penrose, Pepper, Agnew, Leidy and Stillé, the old names of Jefferson, by which she conjured such wonderfully large bodies of students, much more slowly gave place to new ones; indeed, it may be said that, if Dr. Gross be regarded as a member of the old faculty, he and Pancoast, in Surgery and Anatomy, were still the towering figures of the new faculty during all the changes incident to the accessions of Drs. T. D. Mitchell, S. H. Dickson, Ellerslie Wallace, B. Howard Rand, John B. Biddle, J. A. Meigs, J. M. Da Costa (f), and the younger Pancoast. These changes occurred during the twenty years from 1856 to the close of this period. Gross, in particular, was the great dominant influence, and undoubtedly was the chief factor in developing a western and northern constituency to replace the great losses from the South, occasioned by the exodus of students from that section, from 1859 to the opening of the war. The old faculty, however, continued virtually in existence down into the civil war period, for besides Gross and Pancoast, both Mitchell and Dickson had joined it before '62, when Dr. Wallace took the chair of Obstetrics, in place of Meigs. So that it may be said that the period was divided between the old and new faculties, with Gross and Pancoast as the dominant and uniting elements. As Pancoast and the members of the old order have been considered elsewhere, it will be necessary, in order to a proper

---

(f) Dr. Da Costa's full professorship came so late in this period as 1872.

appreciation of the influence at work in Jefferson, and through her, on the profession of the period, to gain some idea of the characters of the members of her faculty, and especially of the character of the most conspicuous among them, Prof. S. D. Gross. Gross was considerably older than most of his eminent contemporaries, who are generally associated with him in the mind of the public (g). He was more than a dozen years older than Agnew, eighteen years in advance of Leidy, and eight years the senior of Stillé. At the time of his death, he was on the verge of being an octogenarian, and his mental and physical powers were well maintained until very near his end. In other words, his personal influence, always remarkable, was also unusually protracted.

It must be admitted that the operations of surgery appeal more powerfully to the imagination of the public than the processes of induction by which the physician arrives at his diagnosis and determines his treatment. When the surgeon combines with a profound knowledge of his art, a majestic presence and courtly manners, he is almost deified by his patients and worshiped by his pupils. Dr. Gross was a man of this type, and, doubtless, partly because of the physical gifts so richly bestowed upon him by nature, he has been regarded as the greatest exponent of American Surgery. His elevation of mind and catholicity of view were contagious, and imparted themselves directly to his immediate acquaintance, and indirectly to those who only knew him through his writings. They inspired students and associates alike, and because of his long career as a teacher, writer and surgeon, in both the West and the East, his influence on American physicians and surgeons was probably more powerful than that of any member of the profession since the time of Rush. In consequence of his position in American medicine, the old world universities showered upon him honors such as have been conferred upon but one other American, while the profession at home has given him a recognition so far accorded to no other physician—a national statue (h). Such were

---

(g) Gross and Pancoast were of the same age.
(h) The statue to Dr. J. Marion Sims in New York, erected in 1894, is more local than national. It is worth remarking, too, that Dr. Sims and Dr. Gross were both Jefferson graduates.

the characteristics of Dr. Gross when, at the age of fifty years, he came out of the West, where, as he proudly said: "I left an empire of Surgery behind me"—and he was its emperor—and came to the largest medical school in existence up to 1856. "Conscious of his powers as a teacher," writes Dr. Da Costa, "in the prime of life and of vigor, ambitious to connect his name forever with that of the college where he had been educated, and which a band of men had made so flourishing," he "accepted the task without misgivings, and the result was unmixed success for himself and great benefit to the institution." It is said by an eminent editor: "Dr. Gross' majestic form and dignified presence, his broad brow and intelligent eye, his deep, mellow voice and benignant smile, his genial manner and cordial greeting remain indelibly impressed upon the memory of all who knew him."

In returning to Jefferson and the East, Dr. Gross came back to his own, in more senses than one. He was a native of Pennsylvania, born of German-American lineage at the home of his father, Philip Gross, near Easton, in the year 1805. It is said that his ambition to become a physician was evident before the age of six years, and when, with ordinary school advantages, his seventeenth year approached, he entered a physician's office. Feeling the deficiencies of his preliminary training, he determined to supplement them, and interrupting his medical course, he entered as a student at Wilkesbarre Academy, and Lawrenceville High School, for two years, and at the age of nineteen, went to Easton, where he entered the office of Dr. Joseph K. Swift. One day his eye fell upon the following sentence in Dorsey's *Surgery:* "In June last he applied to Dr. Irwin of Easton, the place of his residence, who instantly apprised him of the nature and importance of his complaint, and advised him *to go to Philadelphia.*" As he meditated upon the significance of the phrase here italicized, he formed the resolution that he should so master his profession that it should never be necessary to send his patients to anyone else; he should be a master himself. Among other books he studied were Wistar's Anatomy, and Chapman's *Materia Medica and Therapeutics.* His preceptor desired him to enter the University of Pennsylvania, and in 1826, the year of his majority, he went to Philadelphia with letters to Drs. Dewees and Horner; but he had heard a great deal of the brilliant work of Dr. George McClellan in the "new school," as Jefferson was then called, and, after visiting him, concluded to become his private pupil and to matriculate in that institution. "McClellan," he writes in his autobiography, "was an enthusiast, and I was not long in sharing his feelings." Gross had a splendid constitution and prodigious capacity for study, as well as unusual ability in self-instruction, for there is no doubt that, at this period, his education was scarcely inferior to that afforded by the liberal colleges of that day. He graduated at the end of the third session, in the year 1828, and very soon opened an office on Fifth street, opposite Independence Square. He at once began the translation of a French work on Anatomy, which brought him some of his first earnings. Other translations followed, and an original work on the Bones and Joints, in 1830. After spending eighteen months in the vain effort to secure a practice, he returned to Easton, where success awaited him, and where he also entered upon special studies in anatomy and in various lines of original research. His reputation increased so rapidly that, by 1833, he was offered the chair of Chemistry in Lafayette College, but chose rather to accept the position of Demonstrator of Anatomy in the Medical College of Ohio at Cincinnati. His work in that institution was so satisfactory that in 1835 he was called to the chair of Pathological Anatomy in the Medical Department of the Cincinnati College, where he laid the foundations of his great work on Pathological Anatomy, which for him won the admiration and friendship of Virchow and other eminent European authorities. His fame was now so extended that in 1839 he was called to both the Universities of Virginia and Louisiana, but, declining these appointments, accepted the following year a call to the institution in Kentucky, made famous by Daniel Drake and others, which soon became the University of Louisville, and in which he increased the fame, already great, of its chair of Surgery. Here he found full scope for his abilities, and continued his work of original research in various lines. Soon after Gross' accession to this school the number of its students was nearly doubled. Nearly ten years passed, and, in 1849, in consequence of litigation for the control of the school, he accepted a call to the chair of Surgery in the University of New York, where he was associated with Draper, Patterson, Bedford, Payne and Bartlett for one session. The attack on the Louisville trustees having failed before the session closed, Dr. Gross was importuned to return, his successor, Dr. Paul F. Eve, joining in the request, agreeing to resign if he would resume his former position. His New York residence was really but an episode in his long Ohio Valley career of over twenty years, for he resumed his old place, and in 1854 produced another original work on Foreign Bodies in the Air Passages, of which Sir Morrell Mackenzie said: "It is doubtful whether it will ever be improved upon." His writings and addresses had now made him an acknowledged leader in the medical world, and his extensive practice kept pace with his reputation.

In 1855, Dr. René La Roche urged him to become a candidate for Gibson's chair in the University of Pennsylvania, but he declined, and, he writes in his autobiography, "when it became known that I was inexorable, I wrote, at the request of Dr. D. Hayes Agnew, a warm testimonial in favor of Dr. Henry H. Smith, who was finally elected." But Dr. Dunglison had also written to him, pressing the claims of his *alma mater* and urging him to accept the chair vacated by Dr. Mütter. He consented, and it was undoubtedly a sense of duty that induced him, at the age of fifty, to break up a home replete with tender associations, and begin a new career. Dr. Gross arrived in Philadelphia in September, 1856, and in a few days began his duties by delivering the introductory lecture to the great classes of Jefferson. "After his graduation," writes Dr. I. M. Hays, "the great ambition of Dr. Gross was to become a teacher. His first effort in this direction was as Demonstrator of Anatomy in the Medical College of Ohio, in which, as previously stated, he delivered three lectures a week for two years. In the Cincinnati College he lectured for four years on Pathological Anatomy, after which he taught surgery for forty-two years. During all this time he invariably spoke extemporaneously, with the aid of a few brief headings; but he never appeared before his class without previous study and meditation and a thorough comprehension of his subject. Order and system were among his more important attributes as a teacher. Those who have heard him will never forget his enthusiasm, the marked interest he felt in what he was saying and doing, and the evidence of the feeling that he had a solemn duty to perform, and that upon what he uttered might depend the happiness or misery of thousands of human beings. The opening portion of his course on surgery was devoted to the discussion of the principles, the topics discussed having been inflammation and its consequences, syphilis, struma, tumors and wounds. These topics being disposed of, he took up the diseases and injuries of particular regions, organs and tissues, confining himself as much as possible to matters of fact, and not indulging in hypotheses, conjecture or speculation. His knowledge of pathological anatomy was of immense benefit to him in these exercises, and he freely availed himself of it as a means of illustrating every subject that he had occasion to discuss. Indeed, he always asserted that whatever reputation he possessed as a teacher and writer was in great degree due to his familiarity with morbid anatomy. What added greatly to his charm as a lecturer were his admirable diction, his commanding presence, and a resonant and well-modulated voice." Dr. Gross added to his teaching the founding and editing of a new journal, the *North American Medico-Chirurgical Review*, a journal which, in association with Dr. T. S. Richardson, he had already conducted in Louisville. He limited his local practice to office and consultation work, in order that he might have time to write his greatest work, the *System of Surgery*. "I had long contemplated such a work," he writes, "and I knew that unless I changed my residence I should never be able to fulfill an object which lay so near my heart, and was so intimately interwoven with my ambition and the great purposes of my professional life. Accordingly, upon my arrival in Philadelphia, I confined myself strictly to office and consultation business, to patients from a distance and to surgical operations. . . . . I had commenced the composition of my Surgery several years before I left Kentucky, and I now set vigorously to work to complete it. . . . . I had determined to do my best to make it, if possible, the most elaborate, if not the most complete, treatise in the English language, and I therefore gave myself ample time for the labor. . . . . I have often been told that I have simplified Surgery. A higher compliment could not be paid me." Elsewhere he says of it: "During all the period (forty-two years) I was unceasingly devoted to the duties of an arduous practice, both private and public; to the study of the great masters of the art and science of medicine and surgery, and to the composition of various monographs which had a direct bearing upon a number of the subjects discussed in these columns. The work should, therefore, be regarded as embodying the results of a large personal, as well as of a ripe, experience, of extensive reading and of much reflection; in a word, as exhibiting surgery as I myself understand it, and as I, for so many years, taught it." It appeared in 1859, and its great success is well known. The estimate of it which most appealed to him was that of a Dublin editor: "His work is cosmopolitan, the surgery of the world being fully represented in it. The work, in fact, is so historically unprejudiced and so eminently practical that it is almost a false compliment to say we believe it to be destined to occupy a foremost place as a work of reference, while a system of surgery, like the present system of surgery, is the practice of surgeons."

His life was prolific in other ways. In 1857, he and Dr. J. M. Da Costa, who joined him in many of his favorite projects, founded a new Pathological Society, which has already been mentioned in connection with an earlier one founded by Gerhard. When the war opened he endeavored to stem the tide of the students' secession, and headed one of the first public meetings, composed of Kentuckians then in the city. In the course of nine days he prepared a *Manual of Military Surgery*, which was widely used in both armies. In 1862, he was offered the direction of the George Street Military Hospital, but secured the position for Dr. L. D. Harlow, and himself took charge of the surgical ward. His membership in medical societies was too numerous to be here detailed, embracing many of the leading medical organizations of the world, and of most of those of his own state he served as president. He founded the Philadelphia Academy of Surgery in 1879, and the American Surgical Association in 1880, and was honored as president of the International Medical Congress of 1876. Jefferson College, at Cannonsburg, honored him with the degree of Doctor of Laws, in 1861; Oxford gave him that of Doctor of Civil Law, in 1872; Cambridge that of Doctor of Laws, eight years later; and the Universities of Pennsylvania and Edinburgh conferred upon him similar titles before his death in 1884. Dr. Gross was seventy-nine years old— almost an octogenarian—when the end came. He was entitled, if ever surgeon was, to be called "great," and this fact was universally recognized during his life. He realized his youthful ideals, for he became a master surgeon, a great writer, and, above all things, an eloquent teacher. Common consent has assigned him a lofty place in surgical annals, and it was scarcely a dozen years after his death, when, headed by the alumni of Jefferson, the medical profession placed his statue in the national capitol. Gross was the second physician for whom that honor was proposed, the first to actually receive it. This event occurred but a few months over forty years after that day in 1856, when he came to fill the first vacant chair of the old faculty of '41.

The next year, 1858, an older physician, born in the latter part of the preceding century and trained in the school of Rush, succeeded Dr. Huston in the chair of Materia Medica. Dr. Thomas Mitchell was of an old Philadelphia family, and was educated in the old Carson Academy, the Friends' Academy and the University of Pennsylvania, in the days when Rush was the dominant figure. Intending to study medicine, his preceptor, Dr. Parrish, advised him to spend six months in the drug store and chemical laboratory of Dr. Adam Seybert. He followed this advice, and, in 1809, began his medical course, graduating in 1812, the year before Rush died. Almost immediately he was chosen instructor in Physiology in St. John's College in Race street, where he won some reputation as a writer. A year later he was made lazaretto physician, and, in 1819, published a volume on medical chemistry. Meanwhile, he began practice in the city and suburbs; was honored by Princeton with the Master's degree, and, in 1831, joined Drs. Drake and Eberle in their college projects in Cincinnati, where he occupied the chair of Chemistry. He there published other works on chemistry and was associated with Eberle in conducting a medical journal. In the various changes that took place, he was finally, in 1837, elected to the faculty of Transylvania University, where, two years later, he filled the chair of Materia Medica; and, although he filled other chairs, he was identified with this one for the longest period—ten years. Soon after the Philadelphia College of Medicine was organized, he was called to its chair of Theory and Practice, and in 1857, when well advanced in years, he accepted the chair of Materia Medica in Jefferson Medical College, and held it until his death in 1865, eight years later.

In 1858, Dr. J. K. Mitchell was succeeded by another Southern man, sixty years of age, who had been trained under Wistar, Physick, Dorsey and Chapman, and had been, with Ramsay, one of the founders of the Medical College of South Carolina. Dr. Samuel H. Dickson was born in 1798, in Charleston, and was graduated from Yale College in 1814, at the age of sixteen years. He began the study of medicine under a preceptor in his native city, and had much experience with yellow fever, even as a student. In 1819, he was graduated from the Medical Department of the University of Pennsylvania, and again encountered the fever in Charleston. It was a few years later, in 1824, that he joined Drs. Ramsay and Frost in founding the Medical College of South Carolina, he, himself, taking the chair of Institutes and Practice. After twenty-two years in this institution, he was persuaded to accept a call to the University of New York, in 1847, to succeed Dr. Revere; but, in 1850, the Charlestonians brought influence enough to bear upon him to secure his return, the New York institution showing their regard for his services by giving him the degree of Doctor of Laws in the following year. Eight years later, in the year preceding the great exodus of Southern students, he was called to the chair of Practice in Jefferson Medical College, and spent the fourteen closing years of his life in that position, dying at the age of seventy-four, in 1872. Dr. Dickson, during his long service in the school he had founded, was one of the most influential men of South Carolina, not only in medical, but in literary and philanthropic circles, and his medical works were standards in their day, his most notable one being, probably, his "Elements of Pathology and Practice." It is noticeable that both he and Dr. T. D. Mitchell were well-advanced in years when they came to take the places of members of the faculty of '41. Dr. Dickson's chair during this period of severe trial to Jefferson must be associated with his successor, Dr. J. M. Da Costa, who, for several years, had been an influential instructor in the institution, and who, during the four closing years of this period (1872-1876), gave abundant evidence of the exceptional ability that has always marked his teachings. From the above it will be seen that when Dr. Dickson joined the faculty, in the last of the antebellum years, it was characterized by men of remarkable ability, while the number of students, on account of the secession of those from the South, was unusually small.

The next change came in 1862, when Charles D. Meigs retired from the chair of Obstetrics and gave place to Dr. Ellerslie Wallace. Dr. Wallace was a comparatively young man, and had been a successful instructor in the institution for some time previously. His work as a class teacher had been so brilliant as to attract especial interest and attention. He was but forty-three years old when he succeeded to the Obstetrical chair, as he was born in Philadelphia in 1813. He was of Scotch lineage, and was educated at Bristol for civil engineering, but was attracted to medicine by his brother, Dr. Joshua Wallace, who was then Demonstrator of Anatomy at Jefferson Medical College. He entered the college in the first classes of the faculty of '41, and received his degree in 1843. Dr. Wallace then began practice in this city, and soon became resident physician at the Pennsylvania Hospital. Three years later he resigned this position in order to become Demonstrator of Anatomy at Jefferson, and, for sixteen years, he performed the duties of this office with satisfaction to all concerned. His call to the chair of Obstetrics was a deserved promotion, and his career of over twenty years, as its occupant, made him widely recognized as one of the ablest teachers of Obstetrics in the country.

He resigned in 1883, and died early in 1885, at the age of sixty-five years.

Two years after Wallace's accession (i. e., in 1864) Dr. B. Howard Rand, secretary of the Academy of Natural Sciences, was elected Professor of Chemistry, at the age of thirty-seven years. The year before he had published his "Elements of Medical Chemistry," the outgrowth of several years as a teacher of that subject. Dr. Rand was a Philadelphian, born in 1827. He began the study of medicine under Dr. Huston, and received his degree from Jefferson in 1848, after having been clinical assistant to Drs. Mütter and Pancoast for two years. In 1850, he began his connection with the Academy of Natural Sciences, and, about the same time, he was chosen Lecturer on Chemistry to the Franklin Institute. He also had a similar chair in the Philadelphia College of Medicine until its existence ceased at the opening of the war. He was essentially a teacher of chemistry, and, as such, was chosen to the Jefferson chair in 1864. Dr. Rand was a member of various societies, and after thirteen years in his new position was compelled to resign on account of ill health in 1877, six years before his decease.

Dr. Mitchell died the year after Rand took the chair of Chemistry, and his successor, like himself, was drawn from the ranks of one of the recently extinct colleges. Dr. John B. Biddle was fifty years of age in 1865, when he was called to the chair of Materia Medica. He was a member of an old and distinguished Philadelphia family, and was born in 1815. He received a thorough education in well-known local academies and in St. Mary's College, Baltimore, where he received his classical degree. After a short time spent in the study of law, he entered Dr. Chapman's office, and also began his course in the University Medical School, from which he received his degree soon after his twenty-first birthday. The next year, or more, he spent in Europe, particularly in France, in further pursuit of his studies, and on his return established himself in practice. In 1838, he and Dr. Meredith Clymer founded *The Medical Examiner*, with which he and Gerhard and Francis Gurney Smith were so long and so successfully connected. He had a very pleasing style that was characteristic of both his oral and written discourse. In 1846, he joined Drs. James B. Rogers, Van Wick, Tucker, Goddard, Clymer and Leidy, in the organization of Franklin Medical College, Biddle taking the chair of Materia Medica, and continuing to occupy it until the college closed. In 1852, he published his textbook on Materia Medica, which was very successful, and the following year was called to teach that branch in the Medical Department of Pennsylvania College, which also closed with the opening years of the war. His success as a teacher made him the natural successor of Dr. T. D. Mitchell, in 1865, in Jefferson, where he began his best period of work. He has been described in the lecture-room as follows: "His erect person and manly, dignified presence, with an agreeable manner, combined to make him a graceful speaker, who won the attention of all who listened to him. He was always clear and impressive, and not unfrequently, when warmed by his subject, eloquent. He has been termed, in a recent notice of him, 'a medical orator.'" He also held the office of dean for a time, and with eminent success, for he was endowed with exceptional administrative ability. Dr. Biddle was a member of the Jefferson faculty for thirteen years, and at the close of his career the number of students had almost reached the high figure of the ante-bellum days. In 1878, his health began to fail, and he died the following winter, in January, at the age of sixty-four years. He had been connected with many public institutions, in both professional and other capacities, and was widely mourned. The Jefferson class numbered 572 at that time, and by way of testifying their regard for his memory, sent to his bier a chair of flowers, significant by its vacancy. But two other changes were made in the faculty during this period: the succession of the younger Pancoast to his father's chair, and the choice of Dr. James Aitkin Meigs for the chair of the Institutes of Medicine and Medical Jurisprudence in 1868. The latter event occurred three years after Dr. Biddle's election. As Dr. W. H. Pancoast is more fully identified with a later institution, notice of him will be more appropriate in connection with it, and this account of Jefferson's *civil war* faculty may close with some consideration of Dr. Meigs, whose decease occurred the same year as that of Dr. Biddle. Dr. Meigs was one of the younger men, indeed the youngest, in the faculty, excepting Rand. He was also one of those who were promoted to Jefferson from other local colleges, Jefferson or the University being the goal of every young and ambitious medical instructor. As a rule the Medical Department of Pennsylvania College was the stepping-stone to the portals of the greater institutions. Dr. Meigs was also a native Philadelphian, born in 1829, of a family of Scotch, English and German ancestry. He was one of the most learned men of the faculty, indeed, of the profession, and, although he died at the comparatively early age of fifty, he left behind him a permanent fame, both as a physiologist and an ethnologist. At the age of nineteen he graduated from the Central High School, and soon began the study of medicine under Dr. Francis Gurney Smith. He was graduated from the Jefferson Medical College in 1851, the subject of his thesis being "The Hygiene and Therapeutics of Temperament." He at once began practice, and very soon became a lecturer in the Franklin Institute, and a member of the Academy of Natural Sciences. In the latter institution he long served effectively as librarian. His chief subjects of study were Physiology and Ethnology, and soon he became widely known as a lecturer upon these subjects. In 1857, he was elected to the chair of the Institutes of Medicine in the Philadelphia College of Medicine, and continued to occupy it until 1859, when the school was merged into the Medical Department of the Pennsylvania College. In the same year he succeeded Dr. Smith, his former preceptor, in the same chair of Physiology in the last-named institution. This school closed with the opening of the war, so that Dr. Meigs was solely occupied with his hospital and private practice, until 1866, when he joined the summer faculty of his *alma mater*, and two years later succeeded to the chair of Professor Dunglison, who was the last but one of the old faculty. For thirteen years Dr. Meigs' connection with Jefferson was attended with the most happy results. "As a lecturer," writes Dr. H. C. Chapman, "Dr. Meigs was most eloquent, always interesting and holding the interest of his class. Speaking without notes, his excellent memory never failing him, and gifted with great command of language, he invariably succeeded in inspiring his students with his own enthusiasm." Again he says: "Dr. Meigs' knowledge of physiology, as shown in his lectures, was encyclopædical, as far as that expression may be applicable to any one person." Experimental demonstrations were prominent features of his course of lectures, although he believed that "the progressive or historical method is undoubtedly the best calculated to interest the student and give him a comprehensive and profound view of physiological science." Dr. Meigs was widely known, both at home and abroad, among men of science, and more than a dozen professional and scientific societies in all parts of the world enrolled him as a member. His loss and that of Dr. Biddle, in 1879 (i), together with other changes, were prominent events in the closing of the period, which began twenty years before in the secession of Southern students from Jefferson and the University.

While the most conspicuous figures in the medical profession of this period are those of the faculties in Ninth and Tenth streets, there are many other names that will at once occur to the student of recent medical history as belonging to men as able and influential as those connected with the schools. At the same time, while this is true, it must be admitted that the dominant influences of the profession of the period had their chief expression in the combined strength of the two faculties; and it is the course of such influences that an attempt is here made to follow. It would be interesting to consider the careers of some of those above alluded to, did space permit, but as able men become more numerous, groups of men, rather than individuals, as a rule, give topography to the field of medical history. Among the many able physicians and surgeons not connected with the two great schools were Dr. Washington L. Atlee, 1808-78, a graduate of Jefferson, and eminent as a gynecologist and obstetrician; in fact, a man far ahead of his time; Dr. T. S. Kirkbride, whose name is almost synonymous with that of the great Pennsylvania Hospital for the Insane; Dr. D. F. Condie, Dr. G. W. Norris, Dr. W. S. W. Ruschenberger, Dr. J. F. Meigs, Dr. Paul B.

(i) The summer session, which became fully established in 1870 in Jefferson, brought some new names to the school, among them being Drs. W. H. Pancoast, John H. Brinton, R. J. Levis, F. F. Maury, W. W. Keen, W. S. Gross, J. Solis Cohen, I. Ray, F. H. Getchell, J. E. Laughlin, and R. M. Townsend.

Goddard, Dr. J. Rhea Barton, Dr. Caspar Morris, Dr. John Neill, Dr. J. J. Reese, Dr. W. V. Keating, Dr. James Darrach, Dr. J. L. Ludlow, Dr. James E. Garretson, and Dr. Ellwood Wilson. There are many others still living, the foundations of whose fame were laid during this period. Of these, the most eminent are Dr. J. M. Da Costa and Dr. S. Weir Mitchell. Many more would be mentioned if we were dealing with current events, but, in accordance with the plan of this chapter, they must be omitted.

With these facts in mind as to the general personal influences centering about Ninth and Tenth streets, when the John Brown raid caused the secession of students in December, 1859, one is prepared to understand the rapid movement of events in medical circles during the great conflict that followed. Dr. S. D. Gross, as previously stated, presided at a meeting of Kentuckians on January 29, 1861, the earliest public event of this period in which a physician was prominent; and the earliest organization of ladies as nurses for the war hospitals was the Philadelphia Nurses' Corps, formed April 22d of the same year. The first military hospital was the Christian Street Hospital, between Ninth and Tenth streets, which opened with one patient on May 6, in Moyamensing Hall. Dr. John Neill was medical director, with Drs. Francis Gurney Smith, S. S. Hollingsworth, John H. B. McClellan and Ebenezer Wallace as aides, and Drs. John H. Brinton, John H. Packard, George C. Harlan and F. W. Lewis as assistant surgeons, and Dr. C. H. Boardman as resident physician. This was the only hospital found necessary for several months—indeed, until the general movements of the Army of the Potomac in 1862. In June some of the earliest regiments were fully organized, among them being the Pennsylvania Regiment of Independent Riflemen, of which Dr. H. Ernest Goodman was surgeon and Dr. David G. Bowman assistant; Col. Small's regiment, with Dr. John W. Mintzer as assistant surgeon; the Philadelphia Light Artillery Regiment, with Dr. H. Heller as surgeon and Dr. M. Heller as assistant, and the Keystone Regiment, with Dr. John H. Packard as surgeon. It is worthy of notice that it was the son of the founder of Jefferson, Gen. George Brinton McClellan, who was appointed commander of the Army of the Potomac. The volunteer service was the first to draw largely from the ranks of the profession, and the following list gives the names of the Philadelphia surgeons who served in it, in so far as such a list is attainable: In the cavalry were Dr. W. H. Taggart in the 2d Regiment (59th Volunteers); Dr. Daniel D. Swift in the 2d Provisional Cavalry; Dr. T. H. Sherwood in the 3d Regiment; Dr. N. R. Lynch in the 3d Provisional Cavalry; Drs. Thomas J. and Henry C. Yarrow in the 5th Regiment (65th Volunteers); Dr. William Moss and Dr. Swift (j) in the 6th Regiment; Drs. S. B. W. Mitchell and J. R. Wells in the 8th Regiment; Drs. George C. Harlan and A. R. Nebinger in the 11th; Drs. J. C. Schoales, J. C. Allen and R. B. Cruice in the 12th; Dr. William Ellershaw in the 16th; Dr. James B. Moore in the 17th; Dr. A. G. Reed in the 19th; and Drs. W. C. Phelps and Dr. Lynch in the 22d Cavalry. In the artillery were: Drs. John Graham and R. H. Wevill in the 2d Heavy Artillery, and Dr. Edward Shippen in the 1st Light Artillery. In the infantry were far the larger number: Drs. Thomas B. Reed and John W. Lodge in the 2d Reserves; Drs. James Collins and George L. Pancoast in the 3d Reserves; Drs. Benjamin Rohrer and Benjamin Barr in the 10th Reserves; Dr. William Lyon in the 11th Reserves; Dr. Phelps in the 11th Infantry; Drs. S. W. Gross and John McGrath in the 23d Infantry; Drs. William Craig, Mintzer and H. S. Gross in the 26th Infantry; Drs. Heller, Sherwood and W. H. H. Ginkinger in the 27th; Drs. Goodman and W. M. Borland in the 28th; Drs. Lewis H. Adler in the 47th; Dr. W. R. D. Blackwood in the 48th; Dr. W. H. Gobrecht in the 49th; Dr. Rufus Sargent in the 52d; Drs. David Merritt and J. S. Ramsey in the 55th; Dr. Joseph T. Shoemaker in the 56th; Dr. Thomas A. Downs in the 57th; Dr. Joseph F. Wilson in the 62d; Drs. James McFadden, Gerald D. O. Farrell and Z. Ring Jones in the 63d; Dr. W. C. Todd in the 66th; Dr. James W. Petinos in the 67th; Dr. James Shaw in the 58th; Drs. Henry A. Wadsworth and Fred F. Burmeister in the 69th; Drs. Martin Rizer and Richard Burr in the 72d; Drs. William Gunkle, George Rex, Burmeister

---

(j) When initials are not given, the name is a repetition, as reorganization transferred many surgeons to other regiments than the one they first joined.

and Isaac A. D. Blake in the 73d; Drs. F. B. Morris and McGrath in the 78th; Dr. John C. Norris in the 81st; Drs. J. R. Richardson, D. D. Clarke and Louis M. Emanuel in the 82d; Dr. W. S. Stewart in the 83d; Drs. John H. Seltzer, M. B. McAlear and George H. Mitchell in the 88th; Dr. A. Owen Stillé in the 90th, who died in 1862; Drs. W. G. Kier and C. W. Houghton in the 91st; Dr. G. W. Mays in the 93d; Drs. J. M. Boisnot and George P. Oliver in the 98th; Drs. B. F. Butcher, Silas Updegrove, David P. Boyer in the 99th; Drs. James C. Card and F. H. Gross in the 100th Infantry; Dr. William McPherson in the 101st; Drs. McAlear, W. T. Robinson and W. Scott Hendrie in the 104th; Dr. Philip Leidy in the 106th; Dr. J. H. Hassenplug in the 108th; Dr. Oliver in the 111th; Dr. T. L. Bartram in the 115th; Dr. Leidy in the 119th; Dr. Charles E. Cady in the 121st; Dr. Stewart in the 123d; Dr. Houghton in the 124th; Dr. Swift in the 126th; Dr. Ramsey in the 130th; Drs. C. D. Hottenstein and Kier in the 135th; Dr. Elisha E. Eaton in the 136th; Dr. McPherson in the 137th; Dr. Cady in the 138th; Dr. J. Stiles Whildin in the 145th; Drs. Blackwood and Graham in the 149th; Dr. Michael O'Hara in the 150th; Dr. Updegrove in the 157th; Dr. Nebinger in the 158th; Dr. Lynch in the 176th; Drs. George H. B. Swayze and Mays in the 178th; Dr. W. S. Frick in the 179th; Dr. Lyons in the 191st; Dr. Jones in the 195th; Dr. Barr in the 199th; Dr. Alonzo H. Boyer in the 200th; Dr. Whildin in the 208th; Dr. Houghton in the 214th, and Dr. Farrell in the 215th. These, so far as known, constitute the representatives in the volunteer service. There were also several in the regular army and navy, a branch to which Philadelphia has always contributed liberally. Dr. John H. Brinton did eminent service as brigade surgeon and as surgeon of the United States Volunteers. Yet, many as she sent into the field, Philadelphia's largest contribution to the medical service of the war was expended within her own limits.

The first military hospital in Philadelphia, as we have said, was organized on Christian street, on May 6, 1861, almost at the same time as the very first one of the civil war was opened at Washington. It was in December of that year, when plans for the spring campaign of the Army of the Potomac were making, that preparations were begun for large hospitals in cities near the field of action. Philadelphia, for several reasons, became chosen as the largest hospital center next to Washington in the East. Six buildings, including the Christian street hall, were secured as the Military Hospital of Philadelphia, with the old railway depot at Broad and Cherry streets as headquarters, and the rest as wards. The whole was under one management, that of Dr. John Neill. The Christian street building was a commissioners' hall; that at Fifth and Buttonwood had been a coach factory; the one at Sixteenth and Filbert, made famous by Dr. S. Weir Mitchell's novel, "In War Time," was an old arsenal, and the fifth, at South and Twenty-fourth streets, an old silk factory. Early in January, 1862, the Medical Department underwent various changes. Drs. Francis Gurney Smith, John H. B. McClellan and Alfred Stillé were active in its work of reorganization, one result being the separation of the various hospitals so as to make them independent of each other. The Broad and Cherry Hospital was of medium capacity, with 580 beds for patients and 40 for attendants, arranged on three floors, the most of them being on the second and third floors. The fact that it was a railway depot made it one of the chief distributing hospitals in the city. By February, three of these hospitals had their staffs complete: Dr. John Neill, as surgeon-in-charge, at Broad and Cherry, with Drs. Yarrow, Woodhouse, Harrison Allen and H. M. Bellows as assistants, and with George W. Shields, E. R. and J. W. Corson, James Tyson and W. R. D. Blackwood as medical cadets; at Fifth and Buttonwood, Dr. Meredith Clymer was surgeon-in-charge, with Drs. R. J. Dunglison and W. M. Breed as assistants, J. A. McArthur and C. M. King as medical cadets; at Christian and Tenth, Dr. J. J. Reese was surgeon-in-charge, with two medical cadets, R. Kelly and Edward Brooks. These medical cadets were students who were largely in attendance at all the hospitals during the war. In May, 1862, 716 sick and wounded soldiers arrived, and, the accommodations proving inadequate, other hospitals were built or adapted. In March of that year (1862) the Summit House Hospital, a remodeled suburban hotel, out on the Darby road about four miles, had been opened. It was a three-story structure, 65 feet by 50 feet and had arrangements for pavilions, sheds and tents, in emergency. The pavilion system was adopted at the suggestion of the Sanitary Commission. This hospital had two pavilions on one side of the hotel and one on the other, the regular capacity being 353 beds for patients, not counting emergency beds. Another which adopted this plan was Cuyler Hospital at Germantown, an old three-story town hall, with a row of pavilions extending from a corridor, seven on one side and two on the other.

In May the greatest of all the hospitals, not only of Philadelphia, but of the entire country, was begun in West Philadelphia, at Forty-fourth and Spruce streets, under the direction of Surgeon I. I. Hayes of the United States Volunteers. This was nearly a thousand beds larger than any in Washington, and more than a hundred larger than the next largest one, that at Fortress Monroe. It was begun on May 1st, and was ready for use in seven weeks, by June 6th. It was wholly on the pavilion plan, a long double corridor, with parallel pavilions extending at right angles on both sides, and an administration building in the center. To give an idea of its immensity, a short description by Surgeon Hayes may be of interest: "The building," he writes in October of that year, "was originally intended to accommodate one thousand patients. It is built upon the pavilion plan, and is found to be healthy and convenient of management. The administration building, in the center, is 71x63 feet and two stories high. The lower floor has a hall running through it, on one side of which there are three rooms; the central one is used as a surgery or dispensary, the others as mess-rooms for the officers. The central room on the opposite side of the hall is the reception-room; this is divided by a railing, behind which is the office of the assistant executive officer. Next to this room is the office of the surgeon-in-charge and of the executive officer; on the opposite side of the reception room is the office of the resident surgeons, and back of that the donation-room. On the second floor of the administration building are twelve rooms, which are used as quarters for the officers; in addition to these there are for the same purpose, two one-story buildings on the east front, each 75x14 feet and each containing five rooms.

The administration building stands between and is attached to two corridors, 71 feet apart, which are 14 feet wide and 13 feet high, and originally 560 feet long. These and the wards are only one story high. The corridors run east and west and are parallel with each other. The wards stand at right angles to them, and each is 167 feet long, 24 feet wide and 13 feet high; the roof has a pitch of six feet, and hence the height of the ward to the peak is 19 feet; there is no ceiling; the wards are twenty-one feet apart. In the original plan there were twenty wards—ten on each side. Soon after the original building was completed, four wards were added on either side, making twenty-eight in all, and the corridors were lengthened to 740 feet. These corridors terminate at the eastern end in a store-house, which is two stories high; the second story furnishes quarters for the Sisters of Charity. At the other end the corridors terminate in a smoking-room, 28x25 feet, for the patients. Over the smoking-room are quarters, on one side for the clerks, and on the other for druggists. A small wing, running off from each corner, midway between the smoking-rooms and the administration building, furnishes, on one side, a room for the chief ward master and, on the other, a mess-room for clerk and druggists. Two wings, of the same dimensions as the wards, and running parallel with them, at the eastern end of the corridors, are used as kitchens and laundries, the one-half of each being appropriated to either purpose. The hospital thus consists of a central administration building, two attached corridors used as dining-rooms, and on either side fifteen wings." The appointments and supplies for this immense hospital were a village in themselves. The buildings formed a parallelogram 815 feet long by 433 feet wide, and over eight acres in area, one-half being covered by hospital floors. The largest number this hospital was intended to accommodate was 2,000, but before October, 2,458 were actually cared for at one time, and before the war closed it had a capacity of over 3,500. The name of this institution was Satterlee Hospital. In October, it had a medical staff of thirty-five, exclusive of eighteen cadets. The thirty-six hospital and tent wards had each a surgeon, a sister of charity, ward master, three nurses, and, generally, a medical cadet; there being as many as forty-one cadets at one period. It was to hospitals like these that most of the greatest physicians and surgeons of Philadelphia gave their services.

Next in size to Satterlee, and only exceeded elsewhere in the United States by the hospital at Fortress Monroe, was Mower Hospital, at Chestnut Hill, opened in December of that year (1862). It occupied four blocks, between Abington and Springfield avenues, and the Chestnut Hill Railway and the County Line road, with the entrance from Willow Grove avenue. Its map gives the appearance of a necklace, with long pendants, thrown into the shape of a square, with rounded corners, the necklace proper being the corridor, 2,400 feet by 16 feet, and the pendants projecting from it forming the 50 pavilions or wards. The space surrounded by the corridor contained a field of seven acres, in the center of which was the administration building, connected with the long sides by a transverse corridor, and with the railway entrance by another corridor. The other necessary buildings were in the enclosure, while the pavilions all extended, as has been said, from the outside of the encircling corridor. This, it will be seen, was nearly equal in capacity to Satterlee, each of them being almost three times as large as any of the dozen other military hospitals in the city and suburbs. Its capacity was about 400 below that of Satterlee.

About two months later, February, 1863, another hospital was established about four miles from Philadelphia on the Germantown turnpike, near Nicetown, and given the name of McClellan Hospital. Its form was after the Mower plan, except that the corridor map would look rather like a boat with rounded ends and parallel sides, the pavilion wards, 18 in number, projecting from its outside. Its capacity was nearly 1,100 beds. Two other hospitals, somewhat larger than this, were those at Haddington and Summit House, the former with 1,329 beds and the latter with 1,204. Next in size to McClellan's Hospital was the Convalescent Hospital, with 766 beds; Cuyler Hospital, with 646; the Broad Street Hospital, with 525; the South Street Hospital, with 288; the Turner's Lane Hospital with 285; the Citizens' Voluntary Hospital, with 236; the Officers'

Hospital, and that of Camac's Woods, with 92; and the Islington Hospital, with 60. Another large suburban hospital was at White Hall, with 1,369 beds. This made fifteen military hospitals, in and about Philadelphia in December, 1864. At this date, there were patients in them as follows, the officer in charge and bed capacity being given with each: At Satterlee, surgeon I. I. Hayes (bed capacity 3,519), were 2,464; at Mower, surgeon J. Hopkinson (3,100), were 2,311; at White Hall, assistant surgeon W. H. Forwood (1,369), were 776; at Haddington, surgeon W. S. Gross (1,329), were 970; at Summit House, surgeon J. H. Taylor (1,204), were 845; at McClellan, surgeon L. Taylor (1,089), the beds were full, 1,089; at the Convalescent, surgeon T. B. Reed (766), were 590; at Cuyler, assistant-surgeon H. I. Shell (646), were 380; at Broad Street, assistant surgeon T. C. Brainerd (525), were 441; at South Street, acting-assistant surgeon R. J. Levis (288), were the full number 288; at Turner's Lane, surgeon R. A. Christian (285), were 211; at the Citizens' Voluntary, surgeon R. S. Kenderdine (236), were 48; at the Officers, assistant surgeon S. A. Storrow (92), were 20; and at Islington, acting-assistant surgeon J. V. Patterson (60), were 15. This gives a total bed capacity of 14,508, with 8,638 patients in the fifteen hospitals in 1864. It will thus be seen that Philadelphia was an enormous hospital center during the entire war.

A few facts will show how Philadelphia compared in this respect with other parts of the United States. In the whole Union there were 16 hospital departments, with a total bed capacity of 118,057. The largest of these departments was that of Washington, with 21,426 beds, while Philadelphia came next, with 18,709. The next largest was almost 4,000 beds smaller in capacity, and no others are to be compared with it. The Department of Pennsylvania was situated between two departments whose centers were Baltimore and New York, and embraced the hospitals in this state and one at Beverly, New Jersey. Outside of Philadelphia and its suburbs in the state were hospitals at Chester, York and Pittsburg, which, with the one at Beverly, had a combined bed capacity of only 4,201, so that Philadelphia and its environs, with 14,508 out of the total 18,709 bed capacity, almost constituted the department. Thus, it may be said that Philadelphia nearly constituted the second largest department in the United States, and that it contained the largest and third largest of the hospitals—Satterlee and Mower. In addition to this fact, Philadelphia and New York furnished by far the largest part of the medical supplies for the entire army. At Philadelphia the Government established a laboratory, one of three, for the manufacture of medicines, and its record for economy and service by far surpassed both the others.

In these hospitals nearly all of the most skillful physicians and surgeons of Philadelphia saw more or less of service during all the years of the war, adding greatly thereby to their usefulness and to their fame. It is a misfortune that the records of these hospitals are withheld from the public by the War Department by the orders of February 23, 1879 (m), for although partial lists of some hospitals and even complete lists of a few are accessible, no complete list of all has been found attainable. It is safe to say, however, that, with hardly an exception, all the best known members of the profession who were citizens of Philadelphia at that time, served in some of these great hospitals for a longer or shorter period.

With the close of the war and the renewed activity in medical circles, there arose a number of serious questions connected with the founding of new colleges. Some of these institutions had a brief but legitimate career, and some others had an equal brevity, but not so much can be said for their legitimacy. The general purpose of the class of schools referred to, was to have a place where "all systems of medicine" could be studied by both sexes. They were neither pure Eclectic nor Homeopathic, and can only be described as "irregular." The Eclectics never obtained a footing of any consequence in Philadelphia, although the Homeopathic school has won itself a place. The institutions referred to were made up largely of free lances from all quarters of medi-

(m) These orders say: "Compilations or statements relative to individual officers, enlisted men or organizations, will not be furnished from the records on file in the Record and Pension Office, for historical, memorial or statistical purposes, or for publication, or to complete the records of states, societies, or associations.

cine. Those among which the great bogus-diploma scandal occurred had assumed names and titles containing the word "University," ostensibly because of their "universal" aims, but, as some believed, really as a means of trading on the prestige of the University of Pennsylvania. There were four chartered schools beside the University, which contained this name in their title: The American University of Philadelphia; the Philadelphia University of Free Medicine; Penn Medical University, and the Philadelphia University of Medicine and Surgery. The two at the end of the list became merged under the title of the one last named. Soon after the war closed it was rumored that these institutions were selling bogus diplomas, and that the chief offenders were named Paine and Buchanan. The University of Pennsylvania led in an attack on all these institutions and secured a legislative investigation in 1872. The fight was long and bitter, extending over a dozen years, but resulted in the disappearance of all these institutions, although some of them strongly defended their legitimacy.

Of all the new colleges that arose during this period or of the old ones which revived, but one became permanent, and that was the Woman's Medical College, which resumed its lectures in its new building in October, 1862. The event was a most important one in the history of the entrance of women into the profession of medicine, and this institution undoubtedly had the honor of bearing the brunt of the fight, and of winning the cause. The most important part of the struggle fell within these years. The adoption of medicine as a career for women has always met with strong opposition or as ardent approval; partisan feeling seeming inseparable from any consideration of the question. The movement grew out of the demand for larger feminine privileges in all walks of life, and has now amply justified its claims; but readjustments are seldom accomplished without friction, and some peculiar difficulties arose, one of which concerned the supposed necessity of young men and women attending the same courses on anatomy together. It was on this latter point that a most serious outbreak occurred during the progress of the cause in Philadelphia. This outbreak is evidence of the fact that any innovation must go through the process of evolving its proper place and sphere. No one, probably, but would admit that the innovation in question is still in course of evolution; if anything were needed to remind one of the fact, it is that many medical schools and societies do not admit women, and, that the Woman's Medical College does not admit men, except in its faculty. On the other hand, it is also granted by all, that a clearly defined and rightful—even admirable—position is already recognized for women as trained nurses, or nurse-physicians, and for women physicians proper. The story, so far as Philadelphia and the Woman's College are concerned, comprises the events beginning with the action of the County Medical Society in 1859 against the recognition of women as practitioners, and culminating in 1871 with the practical admission of a representative of the Woman's Medical College into the American Medical Association, although the formal admission of a woman into both the National and County societies came some years later.

From the time when Dr. Elizabeth Blackwell, who had been a student of Dr. William Elder of Philadelphia, was the first graduated woman physician in the world (in 1848), to the time that the first woman's medical college, that at Philadelphia, graduated its first class of seven young women (in 1851), was but three years. From that time, when two of these graduates, Dr. Ann Preston and Dr. Hannah Longshore, a relative of one of the professors, began practice, to November 10, 1858, when medical women had become so numerous and aggressive that the first public action concerning them was taken by the County Medical Society, was but a little over seven years. It must be remembered, too, that this growth was parallel with the extension of those schools for teaching "all systems of medicine" to both sexes, and that the medical education of women became almost inextricably confused in the public and professional mind with irregular schools and irregular members of the profession. Indeed, some of the earlier friends and professors of the Woman's College itself were thought of in the profession at large as identified with or leaning toward some of the medical heresies so rife in that day. So extended was this feeling that the women themselves took measures to secure entire control of the college, and soon succeeded in making it a regular woman's school of a high order, by women and for women.

The action of the County Medical Society, in 1858, was taken long before these changes were so fully effected as to be clearly and unequivocally understood in the entire profession. This resolution, signed by the secretaries of the Censors and the Society, Drs. D. Francis Condie and R. J. Levis, was as follows: "In reply to the proposition embraced in the resolutions submitted for their opinion, the Censors respectfully report that they would recommend the members of the regular profession to withhold from the faculties and graduates of female medical colleges, all countenance and support, and that they cannot, consistently with sound medical ethics, consult or hold medical intercourse with their professors or alumni." This resolution was carried up to the State Society the next year, 1859, where the action was confirmed, without objection. In the Montgomery County Society, however, was Dr. Hiram Corson and others, who did object later on, in 1860, and who secured the coöperation of that society in a contest for the recognition of women. Dr. Corson, whose niece was the second woman graduate, to whose progress his aid had been rendered, from his conviction that there was a true place for the woman physician, led the fight in the State Society in vain. After the close of the civil war, the authorities of the Female Medical College of Pennsylvania (n), in 1866, appealed to the State Society, asking it not to refuse them recognition any longer, as the college standard was now high and its professors equal to the best. Drs. Ann Preston and Emeline H. Cleveland had been the chief instruments in this improvement. The appeal was in vain that year, and the next. In 1870, the fight was renewed, partly because of a counter-action in the Philadelphia County Society the year before, when some city physicians, Drs. Alfred Stillé, Washington L. Atlee and others, did consult professionally with such physicians as Dr. Emeline Cleveland, holding that the code of ethics was not concerned with sex. The result was that the action of 1860 was repealed; the State Society removed its ban on the recognition of

---

(n) Its present name, "Woman's," was not taken until 1867.

women in practice, and the Philadelphia Society followed this action three years later. In 1871, the Woman's Medical College secured recognition for its graduates in consultation. The question had been one of the chronic disturbances of the County, State and National bodies for almost as long as slavery had troubled Congress. In 1869, both the Philadelphia and Pennsylvania Hospitals had opened their clinical lectures to women, and it was in the latter that the revolt of the male students occurred; while from the faculties of the two colleges and from the staff of the hospitals came a vigorous remonstrance against the attendance of both sexes. In 1871, the latter hospital reaffirmed its determination to admit women on some basis, although it was many years before it was satisfactory to the women students in either hospital. Other hospitals followed this example, and soon after the close of this period (in 1878) the service of female physicians on the staffs of public institutions began with the appointment of Dr. Cleveland as gynecologist to the Department for the Insane in the Pennsylvania Hospital. It will thus be seen that the previous efforts gave confidence for the renewal of the fight in the national organization. In the meeting of that body, the year before, namely, 1870, Drs. Henry Hartshorne and Charles H. Thomas (o), delegates from the Woman's College and Hospital in this city, were, after much curious parliamentary skirmishing, refused admittance as representatives, but were admitted in a personal capacity. In 1871, Dr. Thomas became enrolled as a delegate, by a parliamentary error, and the point was practically and favorably settled. The whole question was shelved at the next meeting by the development of another most important question in Philadelphia medicine: the limiting of representation to county societies. This transferred the contention to the County Society, so far as Philadelphia women were concerned; for a Chicago woman, the first to be received, was admitted in the national meeting of 1876, in Philadelphia. The fight in the County Society continued for many years and has to do with the next period.

(o) Both gentlemen were members of the faculty of the Woman's College, the first being also on the lecture staff of the University Medical School.

The years 1871-72 were marked by disasters as well as victories. The period of the Revolution and War of 1812 might be characterized as the Yellow Fever Period, so far as epidemics are concerned, and the ante-Civil War decades, as the Cholera Period; the one now under consideration could, with equal propriety, be called the Smallpox Period, and the next one, possibly, the Typhoid Period. In general terms it may be said that the yellow fever ceased to be a recurring epidemic in 1820. The years that might be properly called yellow fever years were those of 1793, '94, '95, '96, '97, '98 and '99, when the losses from that disease were largest; and the years of decline: 1802, '03, '05, '19 and '20, the deaths ranging from 20 to 93, respectively, in 1819 and 1820, to the appalling figures of 1793 and 1798, which have been given elsewhere in detailed accounts. Twelve years after the yellow fever had practically disappeared, came the worst scourge of cholera the city ever experienced. This was in 1832. The first case appeared on July 5th; the culmination was reached on the 27th and 28th of the same month, and the final reports were made on October 4th. Some put the beginning of the epidemic as early as the 24th of June. This was a year when cholera was epidemic also in Quebec, Montreal and New York, Philadelphia suffering less than any of these cities in number of cases and in deaths; the latter reaching only 935, about one-third as many as in New York. The disease prevailed more extensively in Moyamensing and Southwark than in any other portion of the city. The next serious cholera year was in 1849, when 1,049 deaths occurred, which, considering the difference in population was considerably less disastrous, in proportion, than that of 1832. These are practically the only visitations from cholera with which the city has had to contend, the last one of any importance being in 1866. Cases of smallpox were formerly not infrequent; indeed, there is abundant evidence that its ravages have been felt more or less from the very first settlement, but it was only during 1871-72 that it became epidemic in Philadelphia. For instance, there were 145 deaths in 1808, and from that time down to the great scourge of 1871-72 there were but seven years when no deaths from smallpox were recorded. These were the years 1812-13-14-15 and 1820-21-22. Of the other years, those in which the deaths reached above 300, were 1824 with 325 deaths, 1852 with 427, 1861 with 758, 1865 with 524. Then came the fatal season of the winter of 1871-72, when the death-rate reached a total of 4464, since which time it has never, to any extent, been epidemic. In ratio of deaths to the thousand of population these years show some interesting facts: the only years that rose above two per thousand were 1824 and the season of 1871-72; the former being 2.37 and the last being, respectively, 2.78 for 1871, and 3.83 for 1872, or over six per thousand for the entire epidemic. "If a powder magazine," said one of the first public papers of the State Board of Health many years later, "had exploded in the heart of Philadelphia on the 1st of January, 1872, this calamity, frightful as it would have been, would not have caused a tithe as many deaths, would not have produced a hundredth part as much suffering, would not have affected an approach to as great a pecuniary loss as did the epidemic of smallpox, which was then raging. Thousands of lives, tens of thousands of maimed, disfigured or invalided persons, millions of money—such was the cost of that explosion of disease." There was about one death a week during all of July, 1871, but it was the last week of September before the rate went above a half dozen. The first week in October it rose to 23, and steadily increased until it was above 100 the second week in November. It reached its highest record, 233, for the week ending December 2, and kept well up near that figure for about two months; indeed the figures fell so slowly that it was the third week in March, 1872, before they went below a hundred a week, and not until May before fifty a week was reached. Even in June there was an average of twenty deaths weekly, and it was September before a month passed without at least a score of smallpox fatalities. No part of the city was exempt from its ravages, but it was most fatal in the Nineteenth, Twenty-sixth, Seventeenth, Second, First, Fourth, Seventh, Sixteenth, Eighteenth and Twenty-fifth wards (p).

(p) Scarlet fever was remarkably fatal during this period also, particularly in 1861, 1865 and 1870.

Typhoid fever became alarmingly frequent during the next decade. Even before, in 1865 and 1876, it had been almost as prevalent as in the worst epidemic year of that disease, 1888, which may be largely accounted for by the increased crowds during the war and during the Centennial celebration.

Present freedom from epidemics is due, first to quarantine measures, and, later, to increased application of the great and rapidly developing science of hygiene and sanitation through city and state boards of health; and it was largely out of the experiences of this period that the first measures were taken to secure the capstone of the sanitary system, the State Board of Health (q). Epidemics came, it was assumed, by the vessels of the port, and so early as 1700, as has been said, an act was passed to provide for inspection of vessels, and in 1720 Dr. Patrick Baird became physician of the port. Following him came Dr. Thomas Graeme and Dr. Lloyd Zachary, appointed in 1728; Dr. Thomas Bond in 1841; Dr. James Hutchinson, consultant, and Dr. Benjamin Rush, resident, in 1790; Dr. James Mease, resident, in 1795; Dr. James Duffield, consultant, in 1795; Dr. J. Redman Coxe, 1798; Dr. James Hall, 1799; Dr. Samuel Duffield, 1800; Dr. John Syng Dorsey, 1813; Dr. Alexander Knight, 1814; Dr. Josiah Steward, 1827; Dr. William C. Brewster, 1831; Dr. John A. Elkinton, 1836; Dr. Isaac N. Marselis, 1839; Dr. Henry Dietrich, 1845; Dr. William Henry, 1848; Dr. David Gilbert, 1852; Dr. J. Howard Taylor, 1855; Dr. Eliab Ward, 1856; Dr. S. P. Brown, 1858; Dr. John F. Trenchard, 1861; Dr. H. Ernest Goodman, 1867; Dr. Walter A. Hoffman, 1873; Dr. Philip Leidy, 1874; Dr. Robert H. Alison, 1883; Dr. Henry Leffmann, 1884; Dr. William H. Randle, 1887; Dr. Henry Leffmann, 1891; Dr. Edward O. Shakespeare, 1892; Dr. Henry C. Boenning, 1893. This ceased to be a state office in 1893, and the office of Lazaretto Physician was also changed to that of Quarantine Physician, Dr. Boenning becoming the appointee. This office at the quaran-

---

(q) The first suggestion of a State Board came at the close of this period by way of the national and state medical societies, but an act was not secured until June 3, 1885. Its first meeting occurred on July 2, four of the six members being Philadelphia physicians; Dr. Pemberton Dudley, chairman; Dr. Benjamin Lee, Dr. J. F. Edwards and Mr. Rudolph Hering.

tine station began in 1800 with the appointment of Dr. Mitchell Leib. Province or State Island, at the west side of the mouth of the Schuylkill, had been secured as a lazaretto in 1742-43 (old style), and by 1793-94 all vessels were ordered to anchor there for examination by quarantine masters, none of whom, by the way, were physicians. In 1794, a Board of Health was created and one of its first acts was the recommendation of measures to be observed at the quarantine station. This led, in 1800, to the creation of the office of Quarantine Master, which lasted ninety-three years; but as he was not a physician, professional interest attaches only to the successors to Dr. Leib, who was appointed at the same date. There were Dr. Nathan Dorsey, appointed in 1805; Dr. George Buchanan, 1806; Dr. Edward Lowber, 1808; Dr. Isaac Hiester, 1809; Dr. Thomas Mitchell, 1813; Dr. Joel B. Sutherland, 1816; Dr. George F. Lehman, 1817; Dr. Joshua W. Ash, 1836; Dr. Wilmer Worthington, 1839; Dr. Jesse W. Griffiths, 1842; Dr. Joshua Y. Jones, 1845; Dr. James S. Rich, 1848; Dr. T. J. P. Stokes, 1854; Dr. Henry Pleasants, 1855; Dr. J. Howard Taylor, 1856; Dr. L. S. Gilbert, 1858; Dr. D. K. Shoemaker, 1861; Dr. Thomas Stewardson, 1864; Dr. George W. Fairlamb, 1865; Dr. William S. Thompson, 1867; Dr. J. Howard Taylor, 1870; Dr. D. K. Shoemaker, 1873; Dr. W. T. Robinson, 1878; Dr. F. S. Wilson, 1884; Dr. H. B. Brusstar, 1887; Dr. Edwin M. Herbst, 1891, and Dr. Boenning as Quarantine Physician in 1893.

The lazaretto, or quarantine station, was, for various reasons, forced farther down the river, and in February, 1801, it was opened on Tinicum Island, where it fulfilled its duties for nearly a century; when it was, in 1895, removed to its present location, farther down the river at Marcus Hook. The most serious suffering at the lazaretto in recent years was experienced in 1870, during the effort of the officers to prevent yellow fever from entering the city.

While preventive measures were taken at the lazaretto, the Board of Health, amidst all its changes since its formation in 1894, has steadily improved the sanitary and hygienic conditions within the city, and, probably, made its most important advances during this period, due in no small measure to the fatal experiences of 1871-72, and the influences brought to bear through the American Medical Association. No better view of its progress has been given than in the following excerpts from an account of it recently prepared by the late President of the Board, Dr. W. H. Ford, by whose permission his advanced sheets have been used (r).

Dr. William H. Ford, whose History of the Board of Health is so prominent a feature of this chapter, died shortly after he completed it. The following obituary of this distinguished sanitarian is taken from the Medical Record of October 30, 1897: Dr. William H. Ford, president of the Philadelphia Board of Health, died suddenly of heart disease at his summer home at Belmar, N. J., on October 18th, at the age of fifty-eight years. He was graduated from Princeton College in 1860 and from Jefferson Medical College in 1863. He was, in 1862, appointed acting medical cadet in the United States army, being stationed at the Wood Street United States Army General Hospital in Philadelphia. Later, he was detailed as medical officer on board the hospital steamer Whilldin in the Pamunkey River, where he continued in service for a short time, when he was again stationed at the Wood Street Hospital, remaining there until the spring of 1863. In the following summer he was appointed assistant surgeon of the Forty-fourth Regiment, Pennsylvania Volunteers, and soon afterward he was made surgeon. He remained with his regiment until the defeat of General Lee, after the battle of Gettysburg, when he was mustered out of service. In 1863 he was elected resident physician in the Philadelphia Hospital, and in the following year he was reëlected. In 1865 he went abroad and spent three years in general and medical study. In 1868 he began the practice of medicine in private, and from 1869 to 1871 he was Assistant Demonstrator of Anatomy in the Philadelphia School of Anatomy. During the Centennial Exposition in 1876 he was a member of the Centennial Medical Commission of Philadelphia, being also chairman of the committee of this body on sanitary science. In the same year he was a delegate to the International Medical Congress, held at Philadelphia. In

---

(r) It was prepared as a souvenir of a meeting of the American Public Health Association.

1871 Dr. Ford became a member of the Philadelphia Board of Health, in 1875 its secretary, and in 1877 its president, continuing in the latter office until his death. During his connection with this board he planned and had issued a weekly bulletin of vital statistics of Philadelphia. He was largely instrumental in organizing the odorless system of cleaning wells, the public collection of garbage, and in establishing a department for regulating house drainage in Philadelphia. The organization of a department of milk inspection was also due to his efforts. In 1893 Dr. Ford planned and supervised for the Board of Health the construction and fitting up with all modern appliances of a large pavilion hospital for the treatment of cholera and contagious diseases, in conjunction with the Municipal Hospital. He took an active interest in the construction of a large and complete disinfection plant at the lazaretto, and proposed the erection of a hospital for tuberculosis at this station. In 1876 Dr. Ford was elected physician to the Foster Home. In 1879 he was made a member of the Board of Managers of the Sanitarium Association of Philadelphia, and in the same year he became a member of the Board of Directors of the Tenth Ward Charity Society and was elected chairman. Dr. Ford was the author of a thesis on "Gunshot Wounds of the Chest," founded upon his experience in military hospital wards. From 1872 to 1876 he edited the reports of the Board of Health, and from 1872 to 1875 he compiled the vital statistics of Philadelphia. He was the author of "Statistics of Births, Marriages and Deaths in the City of Philadelphia," published in 1874. He was, for several years, one of the associate editors of the Philadelphia Medical Times.

It is known that at the commencement of the eighteenth century notice was made of provisions for a public slaughter-house, for draining hollows, for regulating the keeping of cows, for grubbing and cleaning land between Broad street and the River Delaware, and for the purpose of sowing grass. In 1748, on account of the danger of malarial disease, the swamp land on Dock Creek, near Spruce street, was filled in as a sanitary measure, advocated by Dr. Rush and others. In the primitive city, pumps were rarely seen. Such wells as existed were generally in the streets for general use. In 1784 it is said there was a well to every house, and the water was good and clear. The yellow fever epidemic in 1793 brought about a change of opinion with regard to pump water, which had hitherto been regarded with favor, and led to the construction of waterworks. The city waterworks were introduced in 1799 by building a power-house on the Schuylkill River, south of Market street, and a marble edifice at Centre Square as a "receiving fountain." In 1818 steam pumping was installed at Fairmount. The Schuylkill water was always unquestionably excellent and would be to-day but for constant extraneous pollution.

Watson, in his Annals, speaks of dyspepsia as a disease scarcely known among the primitive inhabitants, and of apoplexy as less frequent than it has now become. These he esteems as diseases of increased civilization and produced by the cares and anxieties of modern existence. The City Hospital was at first united with the Poor House. "At and before 1740 it was the practice when sick emigrants arrived to place them in empty houses about the city. Sometimes diseases were imported to the neighborhood as once occurred, particularly at Willing's alley. On such occasions physicians were provided for them at the public expense." "The Governor was induced, in 1741, to suggest the procuring of a pest house or hospital; and in 1742 a pest house was erected on Fisher's Island, called afterward 'Province Island,' because purchased and owned by the Province for the use of sick persons arriving from sea." This was, in reality, the first quarantine station ever organized on the Delaware.

Yellow fever was the great scourge that afflicted Philadelphia in its early history. Extensive commercial relations with the West Indies opened a channel for the introduction of the pestilence. Smallpox occasionally broke out among the early settlers; it was, in fact, introduced by them. Malarial fevers were prevalent, in some years proving very malignant. It has been only within the last two or three decades that these fevers have been rare in Philadelphia. Typhus fever was occasionally imported from Europe.

In the autumn of 1669, yellow fever was imported from the West Indies and proved very fatal, two hundred and twenty dying of the disease. The summer of 1717 was remarkable for the "great prevalence of fever and ague in the country parts adjacent to Philadelphia." In 1741, and then again in 1743, yellow fever prevailed. In 1747 the city was visited by what was called the "Bilious plague preceded by influenza." "Epidemic pleurisy" was very fatal in the spring of 1748. In 1754 and in 1755 there were many deaths from "Malignant Fever," which was called the "Dutch Distemper," supposed to have been communicated by immigrants from Germany and Holland. It is spoken of as "Jail fever" and was probably true typhus. Smallpox, which was introduced at the beginning of the settlement, has ever since prevailed to some extent. Before the discovery of vaccination great hope was placed in inoculation as a protection against the disease. It was first practiced in Philadelphia in 1731. It had been practiced in New England much earlier, as far back as 1721. Although there were cases of smallpox on Penn's ship in 1682, the first mention of the disease as prevalent in Philadelphia was in 1701. In the year 1726 a vessel infected with smallpox arrived at Philadelphia, and the passengers were taken to the Swedes' Church, below town, and conducted through the woods to the Blue House Tavern, at South street. All recovered without communicating the disease to the inhabitants of the city. Again, in 1730, there was "great mortality from smallpox." Inoculation was practiced until March 29, 1824, when a law was enacted making it a misdemeanor, except by special permission of the Board of Health. Thomas Jefferson was successfully inoculated in 1760. This practice was succeeded by vaccination, which was introduced into the country by Waterhouse in 1801. The mortuary records of smallpox in Philadelphia are very complete from 1807 to the present date. Since 1807, in only fourteen years has the city been entirely free from the disease. The years of the greatest mortality were 1808, 1811, 1823, 1824, 1834, 1841, 1852, 1861, 1871, 1872 and 1881. The death-rate from the disease was greatest in 1871 and 1872, the years of the great epidemic. Since 1881 the deaths have been very few; in six years none at all.

The lamentable experience of 1793 led to the adoption of general health laws. The hospital upon State Island, formerly Province Island, was ordered to be repaired for the admission of patients, and a resident physician appointed. Vessels coming up the river were ordered to anchor for inspection. By this act, a Board of Health was established in the city. It consisted of twenty-four inspectors appointed by the Mayor and corporation of the city and the six justices of Northern Liberties and Southwark. The Act was passed on the 22d of April, 1794, and the Board organized in the following May.

The Board of Health was abolished in 1797 and a new corporation created, entitled "The Managers of the Marine and City Hospital." The Board consisted of twelve persons and was invested with all the powers of the old Board of Health and with more extensive authority. In 1798 the new Board entered upon its duties. The presence of yellow fever was announced by the Board of Health on the 7th of August, 1798. The population of the city at this time was said to be 55,000. It is estimated that 40,000 people fled from the city on account of the pestilence.

On August 9, 1798, the City Hospital was opened at the Wigwam, on the banks of the Schuylkill, at Race street, and four cases of yellow fever were admitted. The disease was very malignant. It is said that in private practice three out of four died, while in the City Hospital only two out of four died. The number of deaths due to this epidemic was 3,645, occurring mostly during the summer. In 1793 the percentage of deaths was 22. In 1798 it is said to have reached 24, of the population remaining in the city. The old lazaretto property was sold to the United States Government and added to the Fort Mifflin property. The year 1803 began by the reappointment of the entire Board of Health. The quarantine season of 1803 opened April 1st. A building was constructed in 1805 at the lazaretto, for the detention of seamen and passengers from infected vessels.

Nothing very special occurred in quarantine legislation until the year 1818, when a code of laws, including quarantine, was passed by the Legislature, many of which are in existence at the present day. By this act the Board of Health was reorganized by changing the system of appointment to that of election, each ward electing one member annually. In January, 1831, the Board of Health memorialized Congress to appoint a commission to inquire into the nature of cholera and the prevention of its introduction into this country. The Board adopted stringent regulations. Thorough cleanliness was insisted upon. A Committee on Sickness was organized, and physicians appointed. Cholera hospitals were organized in different sections of the city. The first case of sporadic cholera was reported on July 9, 1832. By July 18th five hospitals were in readiness for the sick, and others were in preparation. By the middle of September the epidemic of cholera had largely subsided.

Yellow fever and smallpox occasionally prevailed, but not to any great extent up to the year 1847. This was a year of large immigration by sailing vessels from England and Ireland, and much typhus fever existed among the passengers. In the year 1848 Asiatic cholera appeared in the city. Cholera hospitals were established for the reception of patients. By July 4th forty-seven cases a day and twenty deaths were reported. It is said that this disease came by way of New York City and not by the river. The same year vessels were detained at the Lazaretto station on account of smallpox and typhus fever. The sick from typhus fever were removed to the Dutch House. Immigration this year was also considerable and the lazaretto was kept in active operation. Almost every arrival brought with it cases of typhus fever. The Board of Health was very active that year in making preparations for an epidemic of cholera, which did occur in the summer.

As early as 1768 there were Street Commissioners appointed, for we observe that in that year a contract was awarded to remove "all such dirt as shall arise from, and is incident to, common housekeeping within the paved streets of the city." In 1793, when the yellow fever raged, nearly five thousand persons died. On October 11th, the height of the epidemic, 119 burials took place, which, with the present population of Philadelphia, would correspond to over twenty-five hundred burials. On October 31st a hospital was established on "Bush Hill," in the mansion vacated by Vice-President Adams. The experience of this year led to improvements in the sanitary system and quarantine, the appointment of a Board of Health, a Lazaretto Physician and a Health Officer. In 1797, when yellow fever again appeared, hundreds of tents were placed along the Schuylkill and proved of great advantage. From August to October of that year there were 3,573 deaths.

Philadelphia has not suffered excessively from outbreaks of yellow fever since 1805. In 1855 the disease appeared on July 19th. Between that date and October there were 128 deaths. In June, 1870, it appeared again, at the Lazaretto, causing a number of deaths there and later several in the city, in all eighteen. Since that time, although yellow fever has been brought to the station, it has, in no case, been transmitted to the city. In all epidemics the fever has broken out and prevailed in some portion of the city fronting the Delaware River, from Vine to Christian street, and hardly ever beyond Second street. The epidemic years specially noted were as follows: 1699, 1747, 1762, 1793, 1794, 1798, 1799, 1802, 1805, 1819, 1820, 1855 and 1870. With the painstaking enforcement of the best devised system of quarantine regulations, primarily, and the rigid observance of municipal cleanliness, this disease is no longer feared in Northern cities, and under the maintenance of similar conditions will probably never again become epidemic in the North.

The quarantine station at the Lazaretto, on Little Tinicum Island, about 11 miles down the Delaware, is of historic interest. It was located there in 1799 and has been maintained continuously by the city, under the supervision of the Board of Health, until 1895, a period of nearly one hundred years. In 1895 a State Quarantine Board was created and soon after the station was removed to Marcus Hook, Pa., near the boundary between the State and Delaware. There are now practically three stations: One at Cape Henlopen, one at Reedy Island, both maintained by the National Government, and the State Station, at Marcus Hook, all acting in harmony. In recent years the quarantine station at the Lazaretto has been greatly modernized and improved and well equipped for its work. In anticipation of cholera in 1893 still further improvements were made, such as the erection of a large steam disinfecting oven and chambers for disinfection by chemical fumes. A floating quarantine detention vessel, capable of accommodating one thousand persons, and completely fitted up with every necessary appliance for disinfection, sterilizing water, bathing, steam disinfection of vessels, etc., was in constant use. This vessel, perhaps the most complete of its kind ever put into service, was kept in active operation during the entire season; in fact, until late in the fall of that year. Not a case of cholera reached the city in that or any succeeding years.

Since the year 1860, complete and accurate records have been kept of marriages, births and deaths, under the Registration Law, and the statistics have been published annually. Previous to that date, the deaths were published annually in tabular form on one large sheet of paper, from the year 1808 to 1860, by the Health Officer, by order of the Board of Health; with this there was also a monthly statement of deaths of adults and children, from 1837, inclusive. The weekly deaths were tabulated in the annual statement, together with the births, so far as they could be ascertained. Accounts of births and burials previous to the year 1807 have been preserved on printed sheets, from 1787, under the title of "An Account of the Births and Burials in the Associated Churches of Christ Church and St. Peter's in Philadelphia," but the series is broken. Previous to 1787 similar accounts of births and burials in Christ Church Parish, in Philadelphia, running up to 1774, have been preserved, with a number of intervening years left out. From 1774 to 1787 an eventful period in the history of Philadelphia, the records, if they were published, have not been kept. The valuable records which have been preserved are in the Health Office, having been collected years ago by an antiquarian and purchased by the city. It is observed that in the early account of births and deaths, for example, in the year 1740, the terms under which causes of deaths were reported are twenty-four, such, for example, as "Apoplex," "Dropsie," "Flux," "Imposthume in the Side," "Distempers." Consumption is mentioned in 1849. The list somewhat increases as the years pass on and we have mention made of bilious fever, cholera, convulsions, dysentery, whooping-cough, influenza, measles, rheumatism, typhus fever, etc. In 1808, as has been said, the Board of Health first published a statement of deaths, including the number for the months, and the total for the year 1807. This statement was further enlarged and improved, and is not very unlike, in nomenclature, the tabular statement made to-day. A weekly bulletin of deaths, variously classified, with meteorological tables, has been published since January, 1873. After vaccination was introduced in 1801, by Waterhouse, inoculation still continued to be practiced, for we observe in this first official statement of the Board of Health that in 1807 there were 30 deaths from natural smallpox and 2 deaths from inoculated smallpox. The total number of deaths for the year was 2,045. Mortality from inoculation is observed in the tables for several years. In 1811 there were 113 deaths from natural smallpox and 4 from inoculated smallpox. Typhus fever, otherwise called putrid fever, seems to have been very prevalent in the early part of the century. In 1808 there were 35 deaths ascribed to this cause; in 1809, there were 62; in 1810, there were 12; in 1811, there were 43; in 1812, there were 36; in 1813, there were 102; in 1814, there were 94; in 1815, there were 84, etc. In 1824 there were 307 deaths from typhus fever and 10 deaths from nervous fever. Whether or not typhus fever included what we denominate as typhoid fever or typhus mitior, it is impossible to say. In 1754 yellow fever caused 7 deaths. In 1750 smallpox caused 6 deaths; in 1756, 112 deaths; in 1757, 8 deaths; in 1759, 160 deaths; in 1763, 30 deaths; and yellow fever, 16 deaths. In 1764, smallpox caused 6 deaths, and yellow fever, 1 death; in 1765, smallpox caused 57 deaths; in 1766, 20 deaths; in 1768, 4 deaths; in 1770, 8 deaths; in 1772, 9 deaths; in 1774, 11 deaths. In 1798 yellow fever caused 95 deaths. In 1756 the deaths from all causes were 1,058; in 1768, 806 deaths; in 1769, 1,160 deaths; in 1772, 1,070 deaths; in 1795, 2,275 deaths; in 1798, 4,080 deaths; in 1806, 1,672 deaths; in 1807, 1,250 deaths. In 1832 there were 73 deaths from cholera morbus, 948 from cholera malignant, and 366 from cholera infantum. In the same year there were 681 deaths from consumption, 307 from scarlet fever, 196 from typhus fever, 39 from bilious fever and 25 from nervous fever. Inflammation of the lungs caused 225 deaths and influenza 41 deaths. The total deaths in this year were 6,699. The succeeding year, 1833, the deaths fell to 4,440, cholera having entirely disappeared. In 1837 the first mention is made of typhoid fever, in which year there were 28 deaths, and also 71 deaths from typhus fever. In 1853 there were 26 deaths from yellow fever. In 1854 there were 12 deaths from yellow fever, 186 deaths from typhoid fever, 162 deaths from scarlet fever, 77 deaths from typhus fever. The total number of deaths in that year was 11,814. The greatest mortality was in July and August. In 1855 there were 4 deaths from yellow fever, and in the same year 163 deaths from scarlet fever, 231 from typhoid and 58 from typhus. The same year there were 275 deaths from smallpox. The total number of deaths in 1855 was 10,505. In 1858 yellow fever caused 16 deaths, and in this year there were 9,741 deaths in all. In the old mortuary records the term diphtheria does not appear, this disease having been recorded under various names, particularly as croup and sore throat. Since the new registration act was passed, in 1860, diphtheria figures prominently as a cause of death. This is owing to a better knowledge of the disease, and, particularly within the last five years, to the valuable aid to diagnosis afforded by bacteriological examination, which all large cities and towns have provided at public expense. Early in the decade, 1860-1870, spotted fever became prominently mentioned in the statistical records, and was a subject of wide investigation. In 1863 and 1864 many deaths were attributed to it. In 1865 the term cerebro-spinal meningitis was substituted for spotted fever, and has been used ever since. Of late years it has not been very frequent. Typhus fever was present in epidemic form in 1863, 1864 and 1865, and to a less extent in the next five years, although it has figured in the records to a moderate extent until 1887, when not a single death took place. Since this year typhus has only occasionally been a cause of death. Until comparatively recent years this disease, like scarlet fever, measles, diphtheria, yellow fever, was treated in general hospitals, particularly in the Philadelphia hospital. Within the past ten years the Board of Health has exercised a rigid supervision over these diseases and treated the cases, demanding hospital care, in the Municipal Hospital of Contagious Diseases. In 1866 cholera caused 910 deaths. The disease was brought into the port of New York among immigrants and thence to Philadelphia. The first epidemic of relapsing fever occurred in 1807, following in the wake of typhus fever, with which disease it frequently coëxists in Russia. There were 162 deaths in 1870, 7 in 1871 and 1 in 1872, after which year the disease disappeared, and has not since returned. There were as many as 200 patients treated in the Municipal Hospital at one time. The mortality was not excessive. Scarlet fever, measles and whooping-cough are more or less prevalent annually, but in certain years these diseases have appeared in epidemic form. Provision is now made in the Municipal Hospital for scarlet fever and diphtheria, but whooping-cough and measles, except where they coëxist with the above mentioned diseases, are not treated in the hospital. There is a probability that, in time, these diseases, so contagious and fatal in early life, will receive the same care and restriction in hospitals as the other contagious diseases of early life.

Years ago Philadelphia was noted for the cleanliness of its streets. Citizens insisted on this hygienic measure and assisted in its maintenance. With the growth of the city, the deterioration of cobble-stone paving, and the difficulty of keeping so uneven a surface clean, a gradual neglect of civic cleanliness crept in. The contract system became a disgrace to the city, and reform movements were instituted, but with little success. The Board of Health frequently condemned the condition of the streets as a contributing cause of disease, and demanded improvements, especially improved paving of the streets. Finally, in 1869, after successive failures to retrieve the good fame of the city, the Legislature placed street cleaning in the hands of the Board of Health, but under the contract system, and also with the grave mistake of limiting the contracts to one year. For more than ten years the Board of Health struggled with this work and wrought a great improvement, but the fact was apparent that the city could never be kept in clean condition so long as the cobble-stone pavement and brick gutters for surface drainage were retained. The City Councils assumed the control of street cleaning under the agency of the Highway Department, but with no better results. Some improvement, however, was observed on streets newly paved with granite blocks. In 1875 and 1876, in view of the Centennial Celebration, an impetus was given to the construction of improved pavements, and this good work has continued ever since. Finally, cobble-stone pavements were prohibited, and from that time an improved condition in the cleanliness of the streets has been observed. Upon the establishment of the Department of Public Works, street cleaning and garbage removal (first established by the Board of Health in 1872), were placed under a separate bureau, organized anew, and excellent results have been obtained ever since. With new and improved pavements, mostly asphalt and granite blocks, the abandonment of surface drainage, and the systematic disposal of garbage by incineration and utilization, the city is maintained in a clean and satisfactory condition, which must necessarily have a beneficial influence on the public health. The original sewers were constructed to receive storm water and surface drainage, and when in the course of time it was proposed to empty water-closets and cesspools into them, the Board of Health strongly protested; contending that sewers should be specially constructed for this object and that it was important to have adequate flushing. The Board of Health was right in its view of the requirement of properly constructed sewers. But the water-carriage system is the only suitable system for large places, and it was better to utilize the old system with proper safeguards, and improve the construction of new sewers, than to continue the old system of accumulated filth. To-day privies or cesspools are not permitted where a sewer is accessible, and cesspools must be constructed strictly according to rule. The consequence is that cesspools and deep wells are diminishing in number yearly, while sewerage is increasing. The immense volume of water in the Delaware makes the pollution unappreciable, but the day may come when some plan of sewerage purification will be required, for which purpose there are ample facilities on the low lands below the built-up portions of the city. Early in 1876, the old bucket-and-cart system for removal of excreta was abolished, and for it was substituted the odorless method of air-tight apparatus, pumps and hose. The work is done in daylight instead of at night, and is therefore under possible strict supervision. No satisfactory method of disposal of excreta has yet been devised, although laborious efforts have been made to secure such a reform.

The regulation of the slaughtering of cattle has been attempted with only partial success. The first advance in this line was the establishment of immense cattle yards and abattoirs on the plateau west of the Schuylkill, between Market and Callowhill streets, in 1896, which, at the time, were among the most complete in the country. Later, a meat inspection service was organized with excellent results.

Under the new city charter, approved June 1, 1885, and effective April 1, 1887, important changes were made in the organization of the Board of Health. It provided that the members of the Board of Health "shall be five in number, to be nominated by the Mayor and confirmed by the Select Council for a period of three years." Before this change, the Board was constituted by the Act of April 7, 1859, and consisted of twelve members, three of whom were elected by City Councils and the remaining nine appointed by the courts, the term of service being three years. The new charter does not change the authority and duties of the Board, but places the executive control in the hands of the Director of Public Safety subject to the orders and resolutions of the Board. For system sake, the Board of Health is attached to the Department of Public Safety. The decade, 1887-1896, is probably the most important in the history of sanitary organization in Philadelphia. During this period the growth of the city has been rapid, and municipal improvements extensive and important, there has also been rapid advancement in preventive medicine and in the perfection of measures of sanitary administration. Greater efforts have been made to preserve public health. Less than twenty years ago the working force of the Board of Health consisted of a corps of unprofessional nuisance inspectors and one medical inspector, assisted by the Port Physician. To-day a large body of trained and expert officers are busily engaged in the performance of the various duties connected with the whole field of sanitary inspection and investigation, so that for emergencies and for ordinary routine work the preparations are comprehensive, precise, methodical, up-to-date and adequate, the results being satisfactory; the confidence of the community established and coöperation secured.

A system of house-to-house inspection established in 1888, on account of vessels arriving in port with yellow fever on board, has since been continued with beneficial results. This work is performed in the spring, summer and autumn and results in abating nuisances which would otherwise be unobserved. The expenditure of half a million of dollars in asphalting and paving, with smooth impervious surfaces, small streets and alleys in the crowded sections of the city, has returned markedly good results. This work has been continued and has changed whole districts from the dirtiest to the cleanest sections of the city. In 1888, an appropriation for a milk inspector was secured for 1889, under an obsolete law passed in 1878. A new law was proposed, but defeated in the Legislature of 1888 and 1889. Subsequently, Councils were induced to pass milk ordinances, and later on, the Legislature passed a law, the so-called "Pure Food Act," which gives ample authority for conducting this important service. There is now a complete inspection service and chemical and biological laboratories, where every necessary test can be made for use in enforcing the law. A law regulating house drainage and ventilation was passed in 1888, under which a most complete inspection service was organized. This division is self-sustaining. It is absolutely essential now that all house drainage in Philadelphia shall be controlled and approved by the Board of Health, the penalty for violation of the law being severe and prohibitory. An important improvement, much needed, was the construction of the intercepting sewer along the east bank of the Schuylkill River above Fairmount dam, and extending to all sections of the city, which naturally would drain into the city's water supply. The public schools are now subject to inspection; at first there was one medical officer detailed for this duty; at present there are sixteen. A plan is on foot to extend the inspection to the school children, employing from fifty to one hundred physicians for the purpose. The advantages of such service are at once apparent.

The last days of 1889 witnessed the commencement of an epidemic of influenza, which subsequently became widespread and very destructive to life, through its sequels and complications. The epidemic was remarkable from the fact that it swept over two continents almost simultaneously, affecting a very large proportion of the population, embarrassing trade and causing an amount of sickness and suffering that cannot be computed. It is also remarkable that in the face of so widespread and death-dealing a malady, recounted day by day with minuteness in the newspapers, the people maintained an indifference which can only be explained by a misconception of the seriousness of the evil. Had cholera, or yellow fever, or smallpox as suddenly appeared, a panic would have spread throughout the land. Since the above date this disease has frequently appeared, but in less fatal form. The microbic origin of the disease seems to have been established, although it is still difficult to explain the simultaneous appearance of the disease in widely separated countries. No special official restrictive measures have yet been attempted.

Public disinfection, established at first under the direction of a single officer, has since been organized on a large scale, with a chief and a number of assistants. This division is able to do all public disinfection required, and essays to keep abreast of all modern advances in disinfection. The latest advance is the use of formaldehyde gas, generated at the time of use, although the sprayed formaline has been in use by the Board of Health since 1892, probably the earliest application of this disinfectant on a large scale in the United States. Bacteriological tests show the spray to be effective, but probably less so than the fresh gas. The extensive steel disinfecting chamber constructed in 1892, answers every purpose for the city, thus far, for disinfecting, by steam, large articles, such as beds, mattresses, etc. Many public baths have been established in the city, and are frequented every season by great multitudes of people. Only a few of the smaller bathing establishments, and these private enterprises, are maintained all the year round. Auxiliary organizations have done much to reduce infantile mortality by providing excursions and days' outings in the country and on the river. In this line of relief, the Sanitarium Association and the Children's Country Week have been faithfully working for years. In one season as many as 178,000 children and caretakers have been provided a day's excursion seven miles down the river. The Country Week's operations are more limited, but proportionally effective.

In 1860, public vaccination, hitherto performed indifferently, was transferred to the Board of Health. Since that year the average annual vaccination has been 12,917, though in years of smallpox prevalence the operations have been far above this figure, as many as 30,000 in one year. The Act of Assembly of 1895, prohibiting the attendance at school of all unvaccinated children, has had a very salutary effect, and has been rigidly enforced. A child who has had smallpox is admitted without vaccination. An illustration of the vagaries of opinion is seen in the declaration of the Board of Health in 1860 that the maintenance of a hospital for contagious and infectious diseases beyond what is provided at the Lazaretto, is no longer essential, and as a result of this declaration notice was given of the intended vacation of the hospital early in 1861. A decided change in opinion, however, took place in the succeeding year, when smallpox broke out and measles, typhoid fever and other zymotic diseases appeared among the army recruits. The Board of Health, by request of Councils, promptly resolved to continue the existing hospitals, and furthermore declared "that a permanent and commodious hospital for the care and treatment of contagious diseases was demanded, and absolutely necessary, in so large and populous a city as Philadelphia." "The Managers of the Almshouse" rented the hospital at Bush Hill in the latter part of 1823 for the reception of smallpox cases, so that it would appear that the Board of Health was not always in direction of hospitals for contagious diseases. It is said that, up to the year 1743, there had not been an organized hospital in the city of Philadelphia. In 1826, smallpox broke out in the city, and a house located near where Ninth and South streets intersect one another was used as an isolation house. The victims of this disease, it is stated, were in those days taken to farmhouses. In the year 1743 a movement was started by the merchants of the city to provide for the sick, on account of the increase of smallpox, brought by immigrants from Germany. The Colonial Assembly built a small hospital on State Island, at a later period called Fisher's Island, near the mouth of the Schuylkill River. This remained in use for sick immigrants until the year 1800, when the Lazaretto, on Little Tinicum Island, in Delaware County, was organized. The calamitous visitation in 1793 had so alarmed the inhabitants that it was then considered absolutely necessary to establish some measure to insure the public safety. The Guardians of the Poor had already refused to receive smallpox patients into the Almshouse, at that time located on Spruce street, between Tenth and Eleventh streets. The Pennsylvania Hospital was closed at that time. The Guardians of the Poor took possession of the old circus at Sixth and Chestnut streets, but the residents of the neighborhood threatened to burn the place down unless the sick were removed. Application was then made to the magistracy of the city, and finally a place was selected on Bush Hill.

The Board of Health was organized in 1794, and purchased Fish Tavern on the west side of the bridge, subsequently occupied for years by the Pennsylvania Railroad Company. This was used for a time for hospital purposes. The first hospital established by the city was in 1796 or '97, at the foot of Race street, on the Schuylkill River, and known as the "Wigwam" Hospital. At this time it was a somewhat celebrated tavern, similar to those of the present day, along the banks of the Schuylkill. The hospital retained the name of the "Wigwam" Hospital for several years; the sign that used to swing there was removed to Germantown, where it became defaced by the ravages of time and use, and was afterward painted over. In 1805, the citizens in the vicinity of the "Wigwam" Hospital entered complaints against the institution. It was finally removed to a spot on the Wissahickon road, near where Ridge avenue and Wallace street now intersect each other. Here it remained for two seasons only, when the citizens demanded its removal. For a time the city was again without a hospital. The people seemed to be of the opinion that if another epidemic should visit the city buildings should be erected at some distant place to meet the emergency. In the year 1810 (s), a hospital for infectious diseases was erected on Bush Hill, where it remained until 1855, when it was removed. From that time until 1865 the city was without a hospital for infectious diseases. This was very inconvenient. The Board of Health was obliged to open the Lazaretto Hospital, and patients had to be removed twelve miles from the city. No one can form an idea of the amount of suffering they were subjected to. In 1865 the Municipal Hospital for Contagious Diseases, at Twenty-second and Lehigh avenue, was completed and handed over to the Board of Health. The plot of ground contains over ten acres. Part of the plot is unavailable for use on account of its location on the other side of the street. The buildings consisted of a main building containing a central administration building and two wings, the entire length of the structure being 280 feet, and the width 50 feet. There are now five separate buildings: A main building, one wing of which is used for scarlet fever, the other for occasional cases—it may be mixed cases or it may be typhus fever, etc.; a building for leprosy, accommodating four cases; a group of four buildings, each pair connected by a corridor, for mixed cases or for smallpox, and two pavilions, separated by an administration building and dormitory for nurses, which are used for diphtheria patients. There are no special private rooms for pay patients in any of the divisions of the hospital, except in the diphtheria pavilion. The nearest approach to private accommodations is by screening off a portion of a large ward in which there are but few other patients. The diphtheria pavilion, which is a modern structure with every useful appointment, accommodates one

---

(s) The old plate of the hospital says: "City Hospital, 1808."

hundred and ten patients. Besides the six wards, there are thirteen comfortable, well ventilated, well lighted, well furnished private rooms, each of which can accommodate a patient and a nurse. The disinfecting apparatus and ambulance service are ample and complete. The Municipal Hospital for Contagious and Infectious Diseases is located about three miles from the City Hall, but quite in the center of population. The site is preëminently well adapted for the work. But, as would be supposed, there is constantly an agitation of the question of its removal, not from public advantage or necessity, but rather for the benefit of property owners in its vicinity. Nevertheless, additions have been constantly made to the hospital buildings, and when, finally, public opinion has settled the question of retaining the present site, many needed improvements will be accomplished and the hospital made complete and efficient in all respects.

The threatened invasion of cholera in 1892 was a blessing in disguise. By it, the coöperation of the local legislative authority and favorable public sentiment were secured, which resulted in the introduction of many sanitary measures of lasting benefit to the city. The Lazaretto was completely equipped and quarantine surveillance almost perfectly maintained. Every necessary appliance for the treatment of suspects, and the sick, besides the disinfection of vessels and cargo, and personal effects of passengers, was secured. The Quarantine Commission of the International Conference of State Boards of Health concluded their report with the statement "that to Philadelphia at least the continent may confidently look for protection against the importation of cholera, so far as she can control its entry by way of the Delaware basin, and for limiting its spread within her own borders, should it unfortunately find its way into the city through other channels." The force of sanitary officers was largely increased and thereafter maintained. Nuisances in abeyance for years were removed because of availability of funds for the purpose. Domiciliary inspections over an extensive territory were rigidly performed. Stations for storing disinfectants, and for telegraphic communication with health officials, were established in all parts of the city. Inspection stations were established on various railroads entering the city, the ambulance corps enlarged, a new hospital pavilion constructed, and in brief, a condition of preparation attained which inspired confidence in the community.

On January 1, 1893, the Board prohibited the keeping of hogs in the city and county of Philadelphia, and also, necessarily, the feeding of garbage to swine, thus getting rid of two nuisances. The Chemical Laboratory, fitted up in 1891, in the City Hall, and supplied with all necessary apparatus and material for making chemical analyses of water, milk and food supplies generally, has been of great service to the health administration. The organization of a bacteriological laboratory, early in 1895, was another advance in the application of exact methods of scientific investigation to the protection of the public health. It was not until the International Congress was held at Budapest, in 1894, that a very widespread public interest became manifested in the flattering prospects which the treatment of diphtheria by the so-called antitoxin of diphtheria seemed to hold out. Very little experience in the use of this remedy had been gained in the United States. There was, however, sufficient to stimulate efforts to found a laboratory for cultivating and supplying the antitoxin, as well as for furnishing diagnostic tests and for cultivating the toxin diphtheria. Since its establishment, the laboratory has been extended in its scope, so that under the Chief of the Division of Pathology, Bacteriology and Disinfectants, it includes the investigation of the etiology of certain communicable diseases, their prevention and possibly their cure, the investigation of disinfectants and their uses, and the study and investigation of all subjects related to preventive and curative medicine, so far as they appropriately come within the scope of such an institution. In 1894, the Board of Health required of farmers or producers of milk supplying the city of Philadelphia, a certificate of clean bill of health of their cattle, based upon the tuberculin test; otherwise the milk was liable to be rejected as being "suspicious." This action excited very free discussion, especially in Farmers' Institutes, resulting in the dissemination of exact information and useful knowledge, and, in fact, prepared the way for the introduction of legislation authorizing the establishment of a "State Live Stock Commission," chiefly concerned in the eradication of transmissible diseases among cattle, and among these, tuberculosis. The introduction of the electric passenger railways, in 1893, caused a praiseworthy improvement in the substitution of smooth, impervious pavements for the less cleanly and unsanitary cobble-stones. As a preliminary to repaving, improved sewers, drainage and sidewalks were required. The effect of this change is apparent, not only in the increased comfort of citizens, the cleanliness of the thoroughfares, but also in the improved condition of the health of the city. Philadelphia to-day has not only the best system of electric passenger railways in the country, but the best paved and best lighted streets as well.

Perhaps the most important sanitary legislation adopted in recent years was the Act of June 18, 1895, to provide for the more effectual protection of the public health in the several municipalities of the commonweatlh. It is aimed chiefly against the spread of contagious and infectious diseases. It requires all cases of such diseases to be reported immediately to the health authorities; authorizes the placarding of houses where such diseases exist; holds the head of the family responsible for the preservation of the placard where placed; provides for the proper burial of the dead from infectious diseases; prohibits public funerals in such cases; directs the isolation of infected persons; requires disinfection; regulates the attendance of children upon schools; prohibits unvaccinated children from attending school and prohibits the use of infected articles until certified as disinfected. By supplementing the general health laws this Act has added greatly to the efficiency of sanitary administration.

The Division of Contagious Diseases, consisting of a chief and fifteen assistant medical officers, is charged with the execution of this and the other laws for restricting or preventing the spread of contagious and infectious diseases. Whenever, in the opinion of the Medical Inspector or of his assistants, a person suffering from any of the diseases required to be reported to the Board of Health cannot be properly cared for at home, full authority exists for having such person taken to the Municipal Hospital, even by the employment of force. The hospital has accommodation for about 350 patients, and the excellence of its administration is so generally recognized that objection is seldom made to removal there by patients whose cases require it. Quarantine guards are taken from 100 sub-policemen, specially selected for the purpose, and put under the control of the Medical Inspector. An Act of July, 1895, placed public lodging houses and tenement houses conjointly under several bureaus of the Department of Public Safety, including the Board of Health. Still another important law, passed in the same year, was the Act entitled, "An act for the prevention of blindness, imposing a duty on all midwives, nurses or other persons having the care of infants, and upon health officers, and fixing a penalty for neglect thereof." A law giving authority to the Board of Health to license lying-in establishments and to have supervision over the same, was passed by the preceding Legislature. The preparation of the antitoxin of diphtheria by the Board of Health, in quantity more than could be used at the Municipal Hospital, made it possible to supply this material to physicians for use in the treatment of the indigent sick. In addition to this aid to the poor, a special officer was appointed to inject antitoxin gratuitously and to practice intubation. The bacteriological laboratory has also been serviceable in applying a rapid and satisfactory method for the diagnosis of typhoid fever, which will compare not unfavorably in point of efficiency with the methods now employed for the diagnosis of tuberculosis and of diphtheria.

For several years past typhoid fever, owing to improved methods of treatment, has gradually become less fatal. The death-rate per 100,000 of population in the seventeen years, 1860-1896, has varied from 77.2 to 32.4, the last five years showing the lowest figures. The death-rate from consumption has also been steadily declining for many years past. Philadelphia has always enjoyed the distinction of being one of the healthiest large cities in the world. The death-rate has not varied greatly from year to year. The record of deaths is complete and accurate, while the estimated population between the census years is equally reliable, being approximately verified by the census figures; hence the death-rate can be depended on as giving a faithful representation of the state of the city's health. The death-rate of Philadelphia for the past ten years, 1887-1896, was as follows: 1887, 21.85; 1888, 20.04; 1889, 19.74; 1890, 20.76; 1891, 21.85; 1892, 22.25; 1893, 21.20; 1894, 19.90; 1895, 20.44; 1896, 20.17. The territory of Philadelphia, since the act of consolidation of 1854, is 129.4 square miles. The estimated population in 1896 was 1,188,793.

A prominent characteristic of Philadelphia is the very large number of houses, particularly for the accommodation of the laboring classes. Hence the city is known as the "City of Homes." Only a little over twelve per cent. of the population live in houses that contain ten persons; or, in other words, over ninety-five per cent. of the dwellings contain less than ten persons. This condition of domicile prevents crowding, and the absence of crowding has a very beneficial effect upon the health and morals of the people. Acres of small dwelling houses are the pride of the city. Building associations, which are very numerous, have been instrumental in fostering ownership of small houses by the laboring classes. The number of dwellings in Philadelphia in 1896 was 247,668; all other buildings, stores, etc., 23,499; total number, 271,167. Within recent years a great improvement has taken place in the paving of the city. Cobble-stones have been discarded, and there have been substituted Belgian block, vitrified brick and sheet asphalt, so that to-day Philadelphia is one of the best paved cities in the world. The introduction of impervious pavements, not only upon the main thoroughfares, but in the courts and alleys, which has been accomplished within the last few years, has been a factor in the improvement of the public health, as it prevents the accumulation of filth and the pollution of the soil. There are 1,400 miles of streets, of which 980 miles are paved: with sheet asphalt, 180 miles; with Belgian block, 345 miles; with vitrified brick, 85 miles; macadam, 170; cobble and rubble, 170; other kinds, 30. Number of miles of electric passenger railways, 450. The system of electric passenger railways is most complete, making every part of the city accessible at a moderate fare. The sewerage system has also been vastly improved, the modern sewers having been constructed water-tight and self-scouring and provided with vents. Up to January 1, 1897, 130.miles of main sewers have been constructed, 662 miles of branch sewers; total, 792 miles. The largest sewer is 20 feet in diameter, and the smallest 8 inches and composed of terra cotta pipe. There are in the city at the present time 7,036 electric lights, 21,981 gas lamps, 11,604 gasoline lamps; so that the city has the reputation of being the best lighted city on the continent. Fairmount Park, one of the most beautiful of parks, contains 2,791 acres, extending on both sides of the Schuylkill River and the Wissahickon. In addition, there are numerous small parks. These breathing places for the people are very attractive and deservedly popular. The water supply of the city is derived mainly from the Schuylkill; that is, ninety-four per cent. from the Schuylkill River and the remainder from the Delaware. The average daily pumpage (1896) is 239,600,116 gallons. The storage capacity of the reservoirs is 1,417,860,000 gallons. Average number of gallons of water used daily per capita, 175. The water is lavishly used. In Europe it is estimated that about thirty-five gallons per capita for all purposes are used. Here at Philadelphia the use has amounted to 250 gallons per capita per diem. The Schuylkill water is naturally excellent, but the increase of population along its banks has, by degrees, contributed to its pollution, so that the quality of the water is not all that could be desired. There are projects on foot to improve it, particularly by the introduction of natural sand filtration, and it is only a question of time when some such plan will be introduced, the result of which, with scarcely any doubt, will add to the improvement of the public health. The altitude of the city above mean sea level, at Broad and Market streets, is 48.73. The highest altitude is 446 feet; the lowest, 2 feet. The average is 110 feet. There are 183 cemeteries pertaining to the city, of which 20 are within the thickly populated parts and are still considerably used. The streets of the city are maintained in a clean condition. They are required to be cleaned, that is, the principal ones, once a day, and those streets upon which there is less traffic three times a week. The work is done largely by machinery, supplemented by hand labor. The material collected is transported beyond the city limits. Some of it is used for filling up low lands, etc. Ashes are removed from all dwellings once a week. The garbage is removed daily and is disposed of in a very satisfactory manner by incineration, and very largely by the reduction process, by which much valuable material is economized.

There are many conditions that contribute to Philadelphia's salubrity. There are the natural advantages of location, the moderate climate, the very large number of dwellings, permitting, as a rule, of most families being domiciled in separate houses, thus preventing overcrowding and the growth of the tenement-house system; the cheapness of living and the almost unsurpassed variety and excellent quality of food supplies; the thriftiness of the people, on account of the almost certain employment of the masses depending on the extensive industrial advantages of the city; the absence of that keen competition and struggle for wealth that characterize such cities as New York, which are so liable, if continued, to end in premature death; the unstinted liberality that provides for all conditions of men, the sick, the helpless and the unfortunate, from whatever cause, and the excellent sanitary and general administrative government that provides for the comfort and guards the health of the community The progress of the city from 1682 until the present day has been steady and surprising, and shows how well its founder planned for the great future, in which he had the most uncompromising faith.

Physicians, Presidents of the Board of Health of Philadelphia, from the year 1800 to 1897, inclusive, are as follow: 1806-1809, Thomas C. James, M. D.; 1820-1822, Samuel Jackson, M. D.; 1833-1835, Robert E. Griffith, M. D.; 1836-1838, Henry Bond, M. D.; 1845-1846, Nathan L. Hatfield, M. D.; 1854-1855, Wilson Jewell, M. D.; 1856-1857, Thomas F. Betton, M. D.; 1857-1858, Joseph R. Coad, M. D.; 1860-1861, Paul B. Goddard, M. D.; 1862-1867, James A. McCrea, M. D.; 1867-1871, Eliab Ward, M. D.; 1878-1880, William H. Ford, M. D.; 1886 to the present, William H. Ford, M. D.

Physicians, members of the Board of Health, from the year

1800 to 1897, inclusive, are as follows: 1803-1804, Charles Caldwell, M. D., and Felix Pascalis, M. D.; 1804-1806, William Currie, M. D., and James Reynolds, M. D.; 1806-1809, William Currie, M. D., and Thomas C. James, M. D.; 1809-1816, Elijah Griffiths, M. D.; 1816-1817, George T. Lehman, M. D.; 1817-1818, Thomas C. James, M. D., and Samuel Emlen, Jr., M. D.; 1818-1820, Samuel Emlen, Jr., M. D., and Nathan Shoemaker, M. D.; 1820-1821, Samuel Jackson, M. D.; 1821-1822, Samuel Jackson, M. D., Samuel Emlen, Jr., M. D., and Gilbert Flagler, M. D.; 1822-1823, Jno. Barnes, M. D., Jno. Eberle, M. D., Harvey Klapp, M. D., and Jesse R. Burden, M. D.; 1823-1824, Jno. Barnes, M.D., and Gouverneur Emerson, M.D.; 1824-1825, Gouverneur Emerson, M. D., and Joseph G. Nancrede, M. D.; 1825-1826, Governeur Emerson, M. D., Joseph G. Nancrede, M. D., and Thomas H. Ritchie, M. D.; 1826-1827, Gouverneur Emerson, M. D., Robert E. Griffith, M. D., Charles Lukens, M. D., and Thomas H. Ritchie, M. D.; 1827-1828, Robert E. Griffith, M. D., and Charles Lukens, M. D.; 1828-1829, Robert E. Griffith, M. D., Charles Lukens, M. D., and Jesse R. Binder, M. D.; 1829-1830, E. Cooper Cook, M. D., and Jesse R. Binder, M. D.; 1830-1831, John T. Sharpless, M. D.; 1832-1833, Jno. T. Sharpless, M. D., and William D. Brincklé, M. D.; 1833-1834, Henry Bond, M. D., Robert E. Griffith, M. D., Jno. T. Sharpless, M. D., and William D. Brincklé, M. D.; 1834-1835, Henry Bond, M. D., Robert E. Griffith, M. D., and D. Francis Condie, M. D.; 1835-1836, D. Francis Condie, M. D., and Henry Bond, M. D.; 1836-1837, D. Francis Condie, M. D., Henry Bond, M. D., and William W. Gerhard, M. D.; 1837-1838, Henry Bond, M. D., D. Francis Condie, M. D., and William W. Gerhard, M. D.; 1838-1839, William W. Gerhard, M. D., and Thomas Stewardson, Jr., M. D.; 1839-1840, William W. Gerhard, M. D., and Thomas Stewardson, Jr., M. D.; 1840-1841, William W. Gerhard, M. D., Nathan L. Hatfield, M. D., and Abraham Helfenstein, M. D.; 1841-1842, Jesse W. Griffith, M. D., Abraham Helfenstein, M. D., and Mark M. Reeves, M. D.; 1842-1843, Mark M. Reeves, M. D., D. Francis Condie, M. D., and Nathan L. Hatfield, M. D.; 1843-1844, Mark M. Reeves, M. D., and Nathan L. Hatfield, M. D.; 1844-1845, Mark M. Reeves, M. D., Nathan L. Hatfield, M. D., and John A. Elkinton, M. D.; 1845-1846, John A. Elkinton, M. D., and Nathan L. Hatfield, M. D.; 1846-1847, John A. Elkinton, M. D.; 1847-1848, D. Francis Condie, M. D., and John A. Elkinton, M. D.; 1848-1849, Jno. A. Elkinton, M. D., Wilson Jewell, M. D., and William Henry, M. D.; 1849-1851, Jno. A. Elkinton, M. D., Wilson Jewell, M. D., J. D. Logan, M. D., and Henry Pleasants, M. D.; 1851-1852, Jno. A. Elkinton, M. D., Henry Pleasants, M. D., Richard Gardiner, M. D., and J. D. Logan, M. D.; 1852-1853, Henry Pleasants M. D., and Richard Gardiner, M. D.; 1853-1854, John A. Elkinton, M. D., Richard Gardiner, M. D., Wilson Jewell, M. D., and Henry Pleasants, M. D.; 1854-1855, Eliab Ward, M. D., Thomas Harper, M. D., Wilson Jewell, M. D., Daniel Hershey, M. D., James Ash, M. D., Ephraim F. Leake, M. D., and William Gallagher, M. D.; 1855-1856, Eliab Ward, M. D., Joseph R. Coad, M. D., Wilson Jewell, M. D., Daniel Hershey, M. D., William H. Geyer, M. D., Benjamin Housekeeper, M. D., and William Gallagher, M. D.; 1856-1857, Joseph R. Coad, M. D., Thomas J. P. Stokes, M. D., Philip De Young, M. D., Wilson Jewell, M. D., James McClintock, M. D., Benjamin Housekeeper, M. D., Thomas F. Betton, M. D., William D. Woodward, M. D., and William Gallagher, M. D.; 1857-1858, Joseph R. Coad, M. D., William Gallagher, M. D., Philip De Young, M. D., Benjamin Housekeeeper, M. D., and Jno. A. Weir, M. D.; 1858-1859, William A. Piper, M. D., H. W. Siddall, M. D., William Young, M. D., and S. S. K. Christine, M. D.; 1859-1860, Paul B. Goddard, M. D., James McCrea, M. D., René La Roche, M. D., James Bond, M. D., and Wilson Jewell, M. D.; 1860-1861, Paul B. Goddard, M. D., James A. McCrea, M. D., James Bond, M. D., Wilson Jewell, M. D., and René La Roche, M. D.; 1861-1862, Paul B. Goddard, M. D., James A. McCrea, M. D., Wilson Jewell, M. D., René La Roche, M. D., and T. Stewardson, M. D.; 1862-1864, James A. McCrea, M. D., Wilson Jewell, M. D., René La Roche, M. D., and T. Stewardson, M. D.; 1864-1867, James A. McCrea, M. D., Eliab Ward, M. D., Wilson Jewell, M. D., René La Roche, M. D., and R. E. Rogers, M. D.; 1867-1871, Eliab Ward, M. D., René La Roche, M. D., James A. McCrea, M. D., and Thomas Stewardson, M. D.; 1871-1873, **James A.** McCrea, M. D., René La Roche, M. D., Thos. Stewardson, M. D., and William H. Ford, M. D.; 1873-1874, James A. McCrea, M. D., William H. Ford, M. D., C. P. La Roche, M. D., and Samuel Ashhurst, M. D.; 1874-1879, James A. McCrea, M. D., William H. Ford, M. D., and Samuel Ashhurst, M. D.; 1879-1880, William H. Ford, M. D., James A. McCrea, M. D., Richard A. Cleemann, M. D., and Samuel Ashhurst, M. D.; 1880-1881, William H. Ford, M. D., Richard A. Cleemann, M. D., and Samuel Ashhurst, M. D.; 1881-1882, Samuel Ashhurst, M. D., Jos. G. Richardson, M. D., and Richard A. Cleemann, M. D.; 1882-1887, William H. Ford, M. D., Richard A. Cleemann, M. D., and Jos. G. Richardson, M. D.; 1887-1889, William H. Ford, M. D.; 1889-1897, William H. Ford, M. D., and Peter D. Keyser, M. D.; and the present members, William H. Ford, M. D., and James W. Walk, M. D.

The event which may be said to have closed this period, and opened another, had its rise in a meeting of the County Medical Society in October, 1872, when Dr. J. G. Stetler introduced a resolution, proposing a meeting of the various medical societies and colleges in the city to consider what part should be taken by the Medical Profession of Philadelphia in the approaching celebration of the national centennial anniversary of 1876. "The form which the proposed celebration should assume," writes Dr. James H. Hutchinson, "had not, however, been fully agreed upon, and the time at which it was to take place was still far off in the future. Moreover, its advocates had not yet succeeded in convincing our people that it was destined to be one of the great events in our history." In consequence, it was not until January, 1874, that the County Society was persuaded to consider the matter by the appointment of a committee for that purpose, composed of Drs. L. Turnbull, J. G. Stetler and M. O'Hara. The result was a report, proposing a congress, to begin its sessions on National Day in 1876. This committee at once took measures to enlarge itself so as to make it completely representative, and with such success that it was organized on March 29, 1875, with Samuel D. Gross, M. D., LL. D., D. C. L. Oxon., as president; Alfred Stillé, M. D., LL. D., and W. S. W. Ruschenberger, M. D., U. S. N., as vice-presidents; Caspar Wistar, M. D., as treasurer; William B. Atkinson, M. D., as recording secretary; Richard J. Dunglison, M. D., as foreign secretary, and Daniel G.

Brinton, M. D., as home secretary. This body bore the title, the "Centennial Medical Commission of Philadelphia," and after securing the aid of every medical body in the city, it proceeded to make plans for a thoroughly representative International Medical Congress, independent, however, of the body generally known under that name. It proposed to make it commemorative of American medicine by having the mornings devoted to the following addresses: 1. Medicine and Medical Progress, by Dr. Austin Flint of New York; 2. Surgery, by Dr. Paul F. Eve of Tennessee; 3. Obstetrics, by Dr. Theophilus Parvin of Indiana; 4. Therapeutics, by Dr. Alfred Stillé of Pennsylvania (declined); 5. Medical Jurisprudence, by Dr. Stanford E. Chaillé of Louisiana; 6. Medical Biography, by Dr. J. M. Toner of the District of Columbia; 7. Medical Institutions and Education, by Dr. N. S. Davis of Illinois; 8. Medical Literature, by Dr. L. P. Yandell of Kentucky; 9. Hygiene and Social Science, by Dr. H. I. Bowditch, of Massachusetts; 10. Medical Hygiene, by Dr. John P. Gray of New York; and Medical Chemistry, by Dr. Theo. G. Wormley of Ohio. For the afternoons there were to be scientific discussions, distributed among nine sections: 1. Medicine; 2. Biology; 3. Surgery; 4. Dermatology and Syphilography; 5. Obstetrics; 6. Ophthalmology; 7. Otology; 8. Sanitary Science, and 9. Mental Diseases.

The committee was still further enlarged, and its work executed by a smaller representative conference of delegates from all societies in the city; and two more secretaries were chosen, Drs. William Goodell and Robert M. Bertolet. The plans having been so fully made, it was decided to put their execution into the hands of four committees: 1. On Arrangements were Drs. D. S. Gross, chairman, Edward Hartshorne, Washington L. Atlee, Albert Frické, Lawrence Turnbull, W. W. Keen, I. Minis Hays, J. Solis Cohen, N. L. Hatfield, A. K. Minich, Thomas G. Morton, George Strawbridge, William Goodell, John S. Parry, R. G. Curtin, John H. Packard, James H. Hutchinson, Louis A. Duhring, Alfred Stillé, William Thompson and Daniel G. Brinton, W. B. Atkinson acting as secretary; 2. On Finance, Drs. Caspar Wistar, H. Lenox Hodge, Levi Curtis, Thomas G. Morton, T. Hewson Bache, Albert H. Smith,

James Tyson and Charles Burnett; 3. An International Executive Committee, and 4. A Committee on Invitation. An effort was then made to induce the International Medical Congress proper, which met in Brussels in 1875, to meet in Philadelphia the next year. While not accepting this proposition, the Congress did adjourn for two years in order to allow its members to join the movement already begun. It was proposed, too, that the committee should convene the Congress and then that that body should conduct its own business.

The Congress assembled on Monday, September 4, 1876, at noon, in the chapel of the University of Pennsylvania. Dr. Gross, after prayer by Bishop Stevens, called Dr. Ruschenberger to the chair, and read an address of welcome. "In its wide range," said he, "the present Congress is without a parallel. Similar bodies have repeatedly met, but none on so grand a scale, or with such a cosmopolitan outlook. . . . The science of medicine has been completely revolutionized, and within our day. . . . The microscope, chemical analysis, clinical observation and experiment upon inferior animals are leading the medical mind with wondrous velocity in the pursuit of knowledge, and are daily adding new facts to our stock of information far beyond what the wildest fancy could have conceived, even a third of a century ago. . . . Hippocratic medicine is the order of the day. Everything bows before its divine behests." Dr. Gross then appointed a committee on nominations, and Dr. Flint delivered his address on Medicine and Medical Progress in the United States. "At the time," says he, "to which our survey of the history of medicine has extended, Philadelphia was the acknowledged seat of medical education. This preëminence she has held from that time to the present. In the number of medical men who have been educated at her schools, in the great preponderance of her medical literature, and in her large proportion of the distinguished representatives of the different departments of medicine, she has had no compeer in the new world. To the influence of her example is to be attributed much of the activity of progress in other cities of the Union. If, in future, she should cease to preserve the relative position which she now deservedly holds, it will be, in no small measure, from the spirit of honorable emulation awakened and sustained by her admirable example. In saying what I have said, I feel that I may assume to speak in behalf of the medical profession of the United Sates. It was most fitting that an International Medical Congress, in celebration of our centennial anniversary, should assemble in the City of Philadelphia." The report on nominations was unanimously adopted and Dr. Gross was made president. The other Philadelphians chosen as officers were: Dr. Caspar Wistar, as treasurer; Dr. I. Minis Hays, as secretary-general, with Drs. W. B. Atkinson, Richard J. Dunglison, Richard A. Cleemann, W. W. Keen and R. M. Bertolet as secretaries of the meeting. Philadelphians, as officers of sections, were: 1. Medicine, Dr. Alfred Stillé, president, and J. Ewing Mears as secretary; 2. Biology, Dr. James Tyson, secretary; 3. Surgery, Drs. John Ashhurst, Jr., as a vice-president, and John H. Packard, as secretary; 4. Dermatology and Syphilography, Drs. Edward Shippen, U. S. N., as a vice-president, and Arthur Van Harlingen, as secretary; 5. On Obstetrics, Dr. William Goodell, as secretary; 6. On Ophthalmology, Dr. William Thompson, as a vice-president; 7. On Mental Diseases, Dr. Isaac Ray, as a vice-president. On the second day, the Committee on Publication was chosen—all Philadelphians: Dr. John Ashhurst, Jr., chairman, Dr. R. J. Dunglison, Dr. William Goodell, Dr. James H. Hutchinson and Dr. Caspar Wistar. Dr. Bowditch also delivered his address on Hygiene and Preventive Medicine, in which he divided the century into periods:— 1776-1832, the era of dogmatism, giving prominence to Benjamin Rush; 1832 to '69, of observation, led by Gerhard and others; 1869, and subsequently the era of preventive medicine, Massachusetts leading with the first state board of health—an address that was really a powerful plea for state boards of health, and no doubt had great influence in bringing other states into line on that subject. He also referred to the national quarantine conventions, the first of which was held in Philadelphia in 1857. After his address, came that of Dr. Wormley on Medical Chemistry and Toxicology, in which he mentioned Priestly, at one time a Pennsylvanian, as the father of Chemistry, in his discovery of oxygen; and Benjamin Rush as the first American professor of that subject in the oldest medical school; Dr. John Redman Coxe, too, was mentioned, as contributing, "perhaps, more than any other, to the progress of medical chemistry in the United States," especially in measures that led to the first College of Pharmacy, that of Philadelphia; he referred to Drs. Jackson, Wood, Bache, the Mitchells, notably Dr. S. Weir Mitchell, and others who have made the city so great a center of chemistry. The sections also began their work, which is, of course, too voluminous for notice.

On the third day, three hundred and eighty-two had registered. Dr. Eve gave his address on Surgery, speaking of Physick as the "Father of American Surgery;" and of others who had followed him. Dr. Toner's address on Medical Biography was given also, in which nine names out of eighteen, chosen for special mention, were Philadelphians. Dr. Parvin's address on Obstetrics came on the fourth day. He spoke of Shippen as one of the first two American leaders in this subject, and of their instruction in London; he referred as well to Dr. T. C. James, the first professor of Obstetrics, and to Dewees, whom he would call "the father of Obstetrics in America," and whose name "should live forever in the memory of the American profession." Dr. C. D. Meigs was also given due honor, as well as Dr. Hodge. Dr. Chaillé's address on Medical Jurisprudence also came on the fourth day. On the fifth day were given those of Dr. Gray and Dr. Yandell, the latter being on Medical Literature, and devoted chiefly to the contributions of Philadelphians. "In the century," said he, "that has passed away since Rush appeared as an author, no one of all the medical writers of America has attained to the popularity which he enjoyed, nor exerted so wide and lasting an influence on the professional mind of his country," and but a glance at the names he mentions in his pages shows the vast preponderance of those of Philadelphia, the greatest medical center in the first century of American medical history. On the sixth day the session was closed with an address by the founder of the American Medical Association, Dr. N. S. Davis of Chicago, who surveyed the progress of American medical education, in which Philadelphia had displayed even more activity than in other lines of medical work, from the organization of the first medical school to the days of the greatest number of medical students. He referred also to the higher standards of the present day, the longer and graded courses and the increased clinical advantages. In detailing the foundation of the Medical School of the University, he said: "We have thus sketched briefly the progress of medical instruction from its incipient beginning in Philadelphia to the complete establishment of the University of Pennsylvania, by the formal election of the faculty above named, in January, 1792, not merely because it is the pioneer school, and one which still continues to exercise an important influence over the educational interests of our profession, but because it has served as the type or pattern for nearly all the medical schools subsequently organized in this country." The day and the Congress closed. "The International Medical Congress of 1876," said President Gross, "is about to pass into history as a thing of the past; but, although its exercises are at an end, its work will live and form an interesting era in our profession as marking the reunion of a great body of men in the centennial year of American independence."

CHAPTER V.

THE RECENT PERIOD.—1876 TO 1897.

The current period in history is, as a whole, too near to ever give assurance that its perspective has been adequately appreciated. Its personages of influence are always, or at least with rare exceptions, still living; and the movements that characterize it are, for the most part, in process of making. In the history of medicine in Philadelphia the situation is all the more difficult to depict, inasmuch as the development since 1876, and particularly in the last decade, has been so rapid and many-sided that even outlines are uncertain and exact detail impossible. Before an attempt at either is made a glance at some comparisons may enable us to make the rapidity of this development more manifest.

At the end of two hundred and thirty years after the first notice of a medical man in this territory, there were 606 physicians in Philadelphia. This was in 1868, when the population of the city was close to 674,000, the figures given by the census of two years later, making something less than one physician to a thousand inhabitants, a very considerable increase over the proportion of a half century before. Since that date the population has scarcely doubled, but the number of physicians has more than quadrupled, and even the regular practitioners alone more than treble the numbers of 1868. The number of the latter is given in the current directories at 2,061, while adherents of other medical schools are distributed as follows: 405 Homeopaths, 17 Eclectics and 30 irregular practitioners. The manager of a prominent directory estimates conservatively that Philadelphia, in 1897, contained 2,600 practicing physicians of all classes. The number had reached 1,215 in

1884-85 (a), and 2,484 in 1895, so that the two decades after the Centennial are seen to be remarkable for the increase of the medical population. It is notable, too, that the students of regular medicine are more than five to one in proportion to the adherents of homeopathy, while other schools have no following worth mentioning. These numbers show Philadelphia overwhelmingly conservative in the character of its medical constituents, as compared with other great cities. This is even more true of the students found in its medical schools, for while the regulars have five great medical institutions, the University, Jefferson, the Medico-Chirurgical, the Polyclinic and the Woman's Medical College (the first-mentioned alone having 926 students), the only non-regular school is that of homeopathy—Hahnemann Medical College, with an attendance of 258, less than one-third of the number at the University alone, not to speak of the grand total in this comparison. Thus the great development of the period is primarily that of *regular* medicine.

As to societies, in 1868, there were in existence the College of Physicians, which came down from the period of the Revolution; the County Medical Society, Northern Medical Association, and the Pathological Society from the third period; and the Union Medical Association, the Microscopical Society, the Southern Medical Society and the Obstetrical Society, organized within the previous three years. The rest have been organized since (b).

As to hospitals, in 1868, there were thirteen, not including those for the insane, or private hospitals and sanitaria. These were the the Pennsylvania and Philadelphia, from the period of the Revolution; the Protestant Episcopal, the Wills, St. Joseph, the Municipal, the Children's and the Preston Retreat, from the third period (although the Municipal, in other forms, dates back farther); and the Charity, the German, the Jewish, St. Mary's and the Ortho-

---

(a) In one directory of 1884, after the regular and homeopathist names, 87 others are given, with the note that they are from the schools of that date which were attacked in the bogus diploma war; and that 50 more were without diplomas, practicing under a sanction of the law.

(b) The Medico-Chirurgical College had an uncertain existence as a society for many years also, before it became a college proper.

pædic in the civil war period; the rest of the hospitals having since been established.

There were only six dispensaries in 1868; the Philadelphia of 1786, the Northern and Southern, both of 1817; the Lying-in Charity of 1828; one at the Howard Hospital, and the Society for Employment of the Poor, both of 1853.

These facts serve to show what a large part of the marvelous growth of the present day has come in the last thirty years; far the greater bulk of it since 1876, the year of the International Medical Congress, the period now under consideration. The chief developments of the present period naturally group themselves about the colleges, the societies, and the hospitals of the city, and may be considered in that order.

Philadelphia again became as great a student center as it was before the war, and Jefferson reached her old-time number of 1854 when she enrolled 630 in 1881-82. Southern students no longer constituted the majority in the classes of either Jefferson or the University. The former made gains from the West and the latter still greater gains from Pennsylvania, while in recent years the University has gained marvelously from the entire land. By 1876 the most radical changes had been made in the University. The old site on Ninth street was deserted for the splendid grounds now so well known, in West Philadelphia. The Arts Department was moved in 1872-73; the Medical Department in 1873-74; and the New University Hospital was ready in 1874-75, which, with the Philadelphia Hospital near at hand, gave the long desired clinical advantages within easy access. In 1865 the auxiliary summer faculty had been established and in 1871-72 daily clinical lectures had been begun with a list of clinical lecturers embracing Drs. Agnew, Pepper, Tyson, Goodell, Allen, Strawbridge, Norris and Garretson. These vigorous measures began to tell effectively on the attendance, the number of students in 1876 being 476, as against 310 in '70-'71, the lowest number recorded since 1861. In 1876 the faculty consisted of Drs. Wood and the two Smiths on the Emeritus list; Drs. Leidy, Penrose, Stillé and Agnew, and the newly elected professors, Dr. Horatio C. Wood to succeed Dr. Carson; Dr. John

Neill in Clinical Surgery; Dr. William Pepper, the younger, in Clinical Medicine, and Theory and Practice; Dr. William Goodell in Clinical Obstetrics; and Dr. James Tyson in General Pathology and Anatomy. The auxiliary faculty was also increased, Dr. S. B. Howell having been added the year before, and Drs. J. T. Rothrock and H. B. Hare, in the year 1876-77. The entire University, and notably the medical department, was entering upon modern scientific University methods and the latter announced the inauguration of a three years' course for the ensuing year. In 1877-78 the chair of Chemistry was filled by Dr. Theodore G. Wormley. Dr. Neill the same year was made professor emeritus, Dr. John Ashhurst, Jr., succeeding to his chair. Dr. J. G. Richardson was added to the auxiliary faculty and there began to be formed the long list of lecturers, instructors, demonstrators, and assistants necessitated by the new clinical and laboratory methods which were instituted from time to time. Post-graduate work was begun, and many of the features established that characterize the present work of the University. Indeed these years were a period of revolution in the methods of the medical school, in which foundations were laid for the remarkable development of recent years.

Of the new members of the regular faculty not now living, were Drs. Neill and Wormley, one from Philadelphia and the other from Ohio. Dr. John Neill was of an old Philadelphia family of Ulster Irish ancestry. His father, Dr. Henry Neill, married Martha Duffield, a daughter of Dr. Benjamin Duffield and a relative of Dr. Jonathan Potts, both familiar names of the period of the Revolution; so it will be seen that he came of a distinctively medical line. Born in this city in 1819, he entered the University by special permission because he was a year under the regulation age. He graduated in 1837 and at once entered the medical department, from which he received his degree in 1840 at the age of twenty-one. He then spent two years in Wills Hospital and was resident in the Philadelphia Hospital for a time. After a professional voyage to the West Indies, he began practice in Philadelphia in 1842. He began giving private medical instruction at once and was made assistant to Professors Horner and Gibson, and in 1845 became demonstrator of anatomy. In this position he was remarkably successful, and a few years later he joined Drs. Reese, Benedict and Frazier in reviving the old Medical Institute. Dr. Neill became a prominent member of the College of Physicians and did distinguished service in the cholera epidemic of 1849, in both a practical and scientific way. In 1854 he was called to the chair of Surgery in the Medical Department of Pennsylvania College, then on Ninth near Spruce street, and also served on the staffs of the leading hospitals. At the fall of Fort Sumter he was the first to make efforts to secure a military hospital by converting Moyamensing Hall on Christian street into one, and telegraphed to the Surgeon-General of the army for authority to establish it as a branch of the United States army. This was so timely for service after Bull Run that he was given charge of the establishment of hospitals and hospital arrangements for some time to come and was finally placed at the head of Broad Street Central Hospital. All of his work previous to 1862 was that of a contract surgeon, but in the latter year he was made Surgeon of Volunteers. In 1863, on the invasion of the state by Lee, he was made medical director of the state forces, and performed such able service that he received the brevet of Lieutenant-Colonel. He became Post-Surgeon after the war, and was associated with the founding of the Presbyterian Hospital. It was in 1874 that he was called to the new chair of Clinical Surgery in the University, where he was distinguishing himself as a lecturer, when, after one course, disease compelled his transfer to the Emeritus list, and his death followed a few years later, in 1880, at the age of nearly sixty-one years. "He was," says Dr. Edward Shippen, "a man of catholic mind—ever interested in literature, art, politics and the social topics of the day. He was a ready and pleasing writer, his style being remarkable for its curt, incisive sentences, divested of all redundancy or verbiage. With great power of concentration upon the subject of inquiry or interest at the moment before him, he was always true to his profession, giving it the first place. Although a conscientious and successful general practitioner, he was especially a surgeon, of surpassing skill in diagnosis and ability in operation. He loved his profession for itself, and found high compensation in the consciousness that he had devoted to its pursuit all the energy and ability which he possessed. . . . . Dr. Neill's most striking characteristics were quickness of apprehension, intensity of application and perseverance in execution. Of these, perhaps, the most prominent was his intensity; whatever he found to do he did with all his might."

Dr. Theodore G. Wormley, who came to the chair of Chemistry in 1877, was a native of Cumberland County, Pennsylvania, but had made his reputation in Ohio. He was born in 1826, of an old German-American family, and was educated in Dickinson College, at Carlisle. Here he came under the influence of President Allen of Girard College, then a Professor of Chemistry in Dickinson, and also accompanied Spencer Baird, afterward of the Smithsonian Institution, on scientific tours. He began the study of medicine in Carlisle, and finally graduated from the Philadelphia College of Medicine in 1849. After a year in Carlisle, he settled in practice in Columbus, Ohio, in 1850, and two years later became Professor of Chemistry in the University there. From 1854, he also held the chair of Chemistry in Starling Medical College, and it was while occupying that position that he delivered his address on the History of Chemistry in America before the Centennial Medical Congress of 1876. The following year, in June, he was called to succeed Dr. Rogers in the University of Pennsylvania, as Professor of Chemistry and Toxicology. He had then just passed his fiftieth year. He had made an eminent name in his chosen science and received many honorary degrees, among them being that of Doctor of Laws from Marietta College. He was a member of many societies, and was an acknowledged expert of national and international reputation in toxicology. His greatest work, "Micro-Chemistry of Poisons," is a standard throughout the world, and owes its excellent illustrations to his wife, who learned the art of engraving on steel especially for the purpose of illustrating her husband's book. "He was eminent in toxicology," said a colleague at the time of his decease, "which science he made his special department of study. He was a most capable teacher, and possessed, to a wonderful degree, the faculty of imparting knowledge to students. Personally, he was a modest, unassuming man, very much liked by all who knew him. He possessed, to a remarkable degree, that regard for truth and that humility of mind which are the basis of the true scientific mind. Dr. Wormley's knowledge of poisons naturally made him a leading witness in many famous cases of medical jurisprudence, and in all such cases his minute and deep knowledge was displayed to full advantage, and his devotion to truth for truth's sake shown in every way." Dr. Wormley died in 1897, at the age of seventy-one, having, with the aid of an assistant, fulfilled the duties of his chair for twenty years after his first introduction to it in 1877. The faculty, then, in 1877-8, consisted of Drs. Leidy, Penrose, Stillé, Agnew, Wood, Pepper, Goodell, Tyson, Wormley and Ashhurst, not to mention those who were emeritus professors, or those of the subordinate auxiliary faculties. To these, in 1878-9, were added Dr. Harrison Allen, for Physiology, and the men having charge of the summer course: Drs. Allen, Reese, Howell, Rothrock and Richardson. Dr. A. J. Parker was added to the summer faculty in 1882-3. No other additions were made until 1883-4, when Drs. W. F. Norris, George Strawbridge and Louis A. Duhring were made clinical professors, Dr. Wood also adding clinical teaching to his didactic work. The next year Dr. Louis Starr became a clinical professor, and Dr. William Osler was made Professor of Clinical Medicine. Dr. Allen was made Emeritus Professor in 1885-6, andABbr. Edward T. Reichert succeeded him, though not formally until a year later, when Dr. J. William White became a Clinical Professor in Surgery. In 1887-8, Dr. Norris became Honorary Professor of Ophthalmology, and the next year Drs. Barton C. Hirst and Howard A. Kelly became associates in the chair of Obstetrics. In 1889-90, Dr. Tyson succeeded Dr. Osler, and Dr. John Guitéras followed Dr. Tyson. Dr. J. William White became full Professor of Clinical Surgery, and Dr. Ashhurst succeeded Dr. Agnew, who was made Professor Emeritus. Dr. George A. Piersol became Professor of Histology and Embryology, Dr. S. G. Dixon of Hygiene, Dr. John Marshall assistant to Dr. Wormley, and Dr. De Forest Willard was made a clinical professor, as were Dr. Hobart A. Hare and Dr. B. A. Randall, the following year. By this time the developments in the University began to show marked results in the attendance, there being 582 students for the year 1890-91. This was increased to 693 and 847 for the next two years, and the current year enrolls the astonishing number of 926 matriculates. In 1891-2, Dr. Duhring was given the chair of Diseases of the Skin, and Dr. John S. Billings took the place vacated by Dr. Dixon. Drs. J. P. C. Griffith and Edward Martin were made clinical professors, and Dr. John H. Musser and John B. Deaver associates to Clinical Medicine and Applied Anatomy, respectively. In 1893-4, Dr. William Goodell was made honorary professor, and Dr. Charles B. Penrose succeeded to his duties. Dr. Charles K. Mills was elected Professor of Mental Diseases. In 1893 the course was extended to four years. Dr. William Pepper, then Provost of the University, had been intimately identified with all the advances in medical teaching since the founding of the University Hospital in 1874. The Dental Department was established in 1878, the Department of Veterinary Medicine in 1884, the Veterinary Hospital in 1885, and the Laboratory of Hygiene and the Wistar Institute of Anatomy and Biology in 1892.

The present faculty of the Medical Department of the University embraces the following: Alfred Stillé, M. D., LL. D., Emeritus Professor of the Theory and Practice of Medicine and Clinical Medicine; Richard A. F. Penrose, M. D., LL. D., Emeritus Professor of Obstetrics and the Diseases of Women and Children; William Pepper, M. D., LL. D., Professor of the Theory and Practice of Medicine and Clinical Medicine; James Tyson, M. D., Professor of Clinical Medicine; Horatio C. Wood, M. D., LL. D., Professor of Materia Medica, Pharmacy and General Therapeutics; John Marshall, M. D., Professor of Chemistry and Toxicology; John Ashhurst, Jr., M. D., LL. D., *John Rhea Barton* Professor of Surgery and Professor of Clinical Surgery; Edward T. Reichert, M. D., Professor of Physiology; William F. Norris, M. D., Professor of Ophthalmology; Barton Cooke Hirst, M. D., Professor of Obstetrics; J. William White, M. D., Professor of Clinical Surgery; John Guitéras, M. D., Professor of General Pathology and Morbid Anatomy; George A. Piersol, M. D., Professor of Anatomy; John Marshall, M. D., Nat. Sc. D., Assistant Professor of Chemistry and Dean of the Faculty; Louis

A. Duhring, M. D., Professor of Skin Diseases; Charles B. Penrose, M. D., Ph. D., Professor of Gynecology; and Alexander C. Abbott, M. D., *Pepper* Professor of Hygiene. The clinical professors are: William F. Norris, M. D., Clinical Professor of Diseases of the Eye; Horatio C. Wood, M. D., LL. D., Clinical Professor of Nervous Diseases; Louis A. Duhring, M. D., Clinical Professor of Skin Diseases; De Forest Willard, M. D., Clinical Professor of Orthopædic Surgery; B. Alexander Randall, M. D., Clinical Professor of Diseases of the Ear; J. P. Crozer Griffith, M. D., Clinical Professor of Diseases of Children; and Edward Martin, M. D., Clinical Professor of Genito-Urinary Diseases. John H. Musser, M. D., is Assistant Professor of Clinical Medicine; John B. Deaver, M. D., Assistant Professor of Applied Anatomy, and Charles K. Mills, M. D., Professor of Mental Diseases and Medical Jurisprudence. The lecturers, demonstrators and instructors are: Adolph W. Miller, M. D., Lecturer on Materia Medica; Henry R. Wharton, M. D., Demonstrator of Osteology; Thomas R. Neilson, M. D., Assistant Demonstrator of Surgery; Edmund W. Holmes, M. D., Demonstrator of Anatomy; Judson Daland, M. D., Instructor in Clinical Medicine and Lecturer on Physical Diagnosis; G. G. Davis, M. D., M. R. C. S. Eng., Assistant Demonstrator of Surgery; John K. Mitchell, M. D., Lecturer on General Symptomatology and Diagnosis; George H. Chambers, M. D., Assistant Demonstrator of Normal Histology; James K. Young, M. D., Instructor in Orthopædic Surgery; Henry W. Cattell, M. D., Demonstrator of Morbid Anatomy; Robert Formad, M. D., V. M. D., Demonstrator of Normal Histology; Arthur A. Stevens, M. D., Lecturer on Medical Terminology and Instructor in Physical Diagnosis; Benjamin F. Stahl, M. D., Instructor in Physical Diagnosis; John C. Heisler, M. D., Assistant Demonstrator of Anatomy and Prosector to the Professor of Anatomy; Frederick A. Packard, M. D., Instructor in Physical Diagnosis; Richard C. Norris, M. D., Instructor in Obstetrics and Lecturer on Clinical and Operative Obstetrics; Milton B. Hartzell, M., D., Instructor in Dermatology; Charles S. Potts, M. D., Instructor in Electro Therapeutics and Nervous Diseases; Walter I. Pennock, M. D., Assistant Demonstrator of Anatomy; Herman B. Allyn,

M. D., Instructor in Diagnosis; William Schleif, Ph. G., M. D., Instructor in Practical Pharmacy; James M. Brown, M. D., Instructor in Otology; W. Constantine Goodell, M. D., Instructor in Clinical Gynecology; M. Howard Fussell, M. D., and Samuel W. Morton, M. D., Instructors in Clinical Medicine; Alfred C. Wood, M. D., Instructor in Clinical Surgery; Elwood R. Kirby, M. D., and Charles L. Leonard, M. D., Assistant Instructors in Clinical Surgery; George C. Stout, M. D., Assistant Demonstrator of Histology; Robert S. J. Mitcheson, M. D., Assistant Demonstrator of Anatomy; David B. Birney, M. D., Assistant Demonstrator of Surgery; Joseph T. Tunis, M. D., Assistant Demonstrator of Surgery and Anatomy; Alfred Stengel, M. D., and T. Mellor Tyson, M. D., Instructors in Clinical Medicine; Charles W. Dulles, Lecturer on the History of Medicine; Daniel W. Fetterolf, M. D., Assistant Demonstrator of Chemistry; Harry Toulmin, M. D., Instructor in Physical Diagnosis; David Riesman, M. D., Demonstrator of Pathological Histology; Charles P. Grayson, M. D., Lecturer and Instructor in Laryngology; Henry D. Beyea, M. D., Instructor in Clinical Gynecology and Assistant Demonstrator of Obstetrics; William A. N. Dorland, M. D., Assistant Demonstrator of Obstetrics; William S. Wadsworth, Assistant in Physiology; Clarence W. Lincoln, M. D., Assistant Demonstrator of Pathological Histology; John H. Girvin, M. D., Instructor in Clinical Gynecology and Assistant Demonstrator of Obstetrics; Ward F. Spenkel, M. D., Assistant Demonstrator of Obstetrics; Lawrence S. Smith, M. D., Instructor in Clinical Gynecology; John M. Swan, M. D., Assistant Demonstrator of Anatomy; Charles H. Frazier, M. D., Assistant in Clinical Surgery; William R. Hoch, M. D., Instructor in Laryngology; James P. Hutchinson, M. D., Assistant Demonstrator of Surgery; J. Dutton Steele, M.D., Assistant Demonstrator of Morbid Anatomy; William S. Carter, M. D., Demonstrator of Physiology; Howard Mellor, M. D., Instructor in Ophthalmology; J. Rex Hobensack, M. D., Prosector to the Assistant Professor of Applied Anatomy; William H. Price, M. D., Instructor in Children's Diseases; Frederick G. Hertel, Ph. G., Assistant Instructor in Practical Pharmacy; Aloysius O. J. Kelly, M. D., Instructor in Physical Diagnosis; Frank

S. Pearce, M. D., Instructor in Physical Diagnosis; Alfred Hand, Jr., M. D., Assistant Demonstrator of Pathological Histology; James H. McKee, M. D., Assistant Demonstrator of Physiology; and Thompson S. Westcott, M. D., Instructor in Children's Diseases.

The work of this large faculty requires commodious buildings. These are the Medical Hall, which, beside lecture-rooms and the like, contains also the laboratories of Histology, Osteosyndesmology, Physiology, Pathology, Pharmacy and Experimental Therapeutics; the Laboratory Building, used for the Dental Department, the chemical laboratories and the dissecting-room; the Hospital, which treats about 12,000 cases annually, with its Gibson wing for chronic diseases, the D. Hayes Agnew Memorial Pavilion for clinical instruction, the William Pepper Laboratory of Clinical Medicine and the amphitheaters; the Maternity Hospital, begun in 1889 and completed in 1894, with a capacity of fifty beds; the Wistar Institute of Anatomy and Biology, containing the Wistar and Horner Museum, and other collections of Drs. Wood, Hodge, Smith, Neill and Agnew. Ample clinical facilities are also afforded by the neighboring Philadelphia Hospital. The Stillé Medical Library, presented in 1879, contains over six thousand volumes. About fifty graduates are appointed annually to the hospitals in this and other cities. The entire plant of the Medical Department is grouped with the other numerous structures of the University at Woodland avenue and Thirty-fourth street, near the Philadelphia Hospital, in West Philadelphia, and has been largely the product of this period. Indeed, the University's work has been so typical of the splendid advancement of medicine in the last quarter of a century—its elevation of medical educational standards, its highly developed scientific methods, its specialization, and a multitude of other no less important features—that, so far as Philadelphia is concerned, the era thus ushered in might be called the New University period. Happily, too, has it carried out the spirit of Franklin, Morgan, Shippen and Rush; the dominance of the scientific spirit of Franklin; the far-seeing, philosophic spirit of Rush; the high educational standards of Morgan, and the practical application and skill of

Shippen. It has preserved them all to an admirable degree, and thus the last period has attained the high aims of its founders. The chair of Theory and Practice has ever been most fortunately occupied in the University by men of brilliant attainments. In the early days of the University its occupant was the founder of the Medical School; in the present period the chair is filled by one whose name must ever be associated with many of the measures that have marked the development of the University Medical School—Dr. William Pepper.

The material equipment of the Medical School has this year (1897), under Provost Harrison, been greatly increased, by the fact that the large Dental Building, contiguous to Medical Hall, has been wholly given up to the uses of the Medical Department, the Dental School being commodiously lodged in a handsome structure, just completed. The resources of the University Hospital have also this year been largely increased by the opening of the D. Hayes Agnew pavilion—a fine memorial to the late distinguished surgeon, Dr. Agnew, so many years of whose life were devoted to surgical work at the University.

Another indication of the progressive spirit of the University is found in the marked rise in the requirements for admission to the Medical School—a further gradual rise being announced until the year 1899. This will insure hereafter a thorough general education on the part of all who hold the University's medical degree.

Jefferson Medical College, at the beginning of the present period, was located on Tenth street, near the Pennsylvania Hospital. To this institution belonged the enviable honor of having furnished from its chair of Surgery one of the two most highly honored men in the entire history of American medicine, to preside over the deliberations of the first International Medical Congress held in the United States. Its faculty in 1876 included Drs. Joseph Pancoast, Samuel D. Gross and Ellerslie Wallace, on the emeritus list, and Drs. B. Howard Rand, John B. Biddle, J. Aitken Meigs, J. M. Da Costa and W. H. Pancoast, as active professors. The final change in this faculty was that already mentioned, the accession of Dr. Rogers to the chair of Chemistry in 1877-8, in place of Dr. Rand,

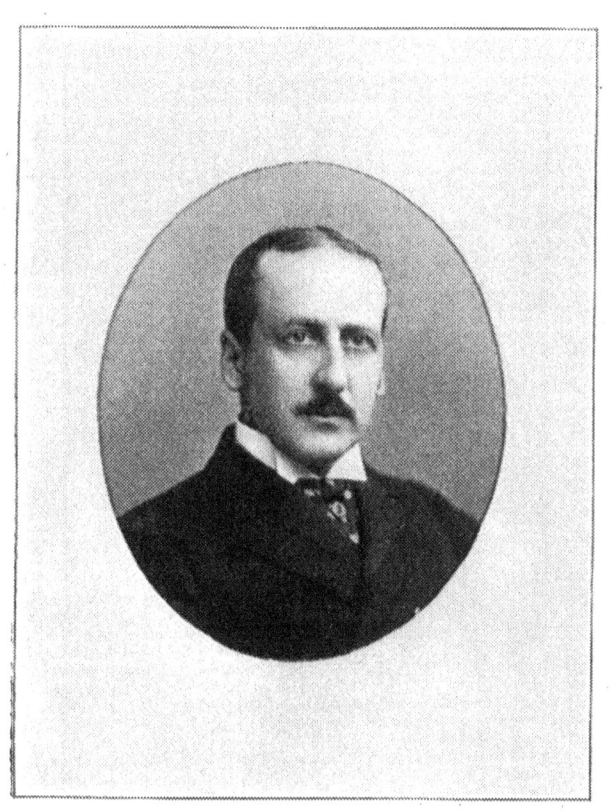

when Dr. Rogers left the University. Two years later Dr. Roberts Bartholow succeeded Dr. Biddle, and the year following that, 1880-81, Dr. Henry C. Chapman took the place of Dr. Meigs. The faculty had been more and more impressing itself upon the profession at large. The work of Dr. Gross as a teacher of Surgery, and of Dr. Da Costa, equally strong in the chair of Medicine, as well as the general strength of the faculty and the progressive spirit of the institution, all succeeded in bringing up the attendance in 1881-2 to 630 matriculates, the famous record of ante-bellum days. The year 1882-3 witnessed a change in the chair of Surgery; Dr. Gross, the elder, was made emeritus professor, and his chair was divided between his son, Dr. Samuel W. Gross, who was elected Professor of the Principles of Surgery, and Dr. John H. Brinton, who was assigned the chair of the Practice of Surgery.

Samuel W. Gross, M. D., LL. D., was the eldest son of the eminent surgeon whom he succeeded. "He was a learned surgeon," said a writer in the Medical News, "deeply versed not only in the medical literature of his own language, but also in that of Germany and France. He was a constant reader of periodicals, reports and transactions of societies. His memory was retentive, and the precise information thus stored up was always at his instant command. His professional judgment was unusually correct, and his surgical treatment was based upon an accurate knowledge of the pathological anatomy of diseased or injured parts. As an operator, he was bold and self-reliant. He was systematic in the highest degree. Every step in the operation was thoughtfully planned and boldly, judiciously and promptly carried out. He was fertile of resources, undaunted and well able to meet and deal with the contingencies of operative surgery. He was a thorough and careful operator, seeing to the final steps and dressing of an operation with an unremitting attention. His operations were well done to the end. As a lecturer, Dr. Gross was eloquent, earnest and enthusiastic. He was loved and respected by his class, who fully appreciated his rare power of imparting knowledge and his unflagging efforts for their instruction. He was indeed a model teacher. His style was clear, logical and terse. He taught, in an eminent degree, principles, and seeing clearly he sought to make others see. He succeeded, and his lectures, didactic and clinical, were thronged with listeners of maturer years, who came to profit by his lessons." Dr. Gross was about forty-five years old when he came to this chair. He was born in 1837, in Cincinnati, O., and was educated at Shelby College, Kentucky. His medical studies were, of course, begun under his father and continued in the Medical Department of the University of Louisville, although he finished in Jefferson Medical College, from which he was graduated in 1857. He spent some time in Europe before he settled in practice in Philadelphia, and soon after locating, he was made coëditor of the North American Medico-Chirurgical Review, founded by his father. In 1861 he entered the United States service as brigade surgeon of the United States Volunteers, acting with the Army of the Ohio, where he was medical director of the Fifth Division until the summer of 1862. He then served in De Camp General Hospital, New York harbor, until the summer of 1863, when he was sent to South Carolina, in charge of hospitals there and in Florida, and rose to be the chief medical officer of the Northern District of that department. In 1864 he was in charge of Haddington Hospital in this city, and for his services brevetted lieutenant-colonel. The transfer to other hospitals and the lectureship on Genito-Urinary Diseases in the summer course in Jefferson Medical College, were natural and easy steps after the war, and were followed in due time by the succession to his father's chair, which he filled for the seven years previous to his death in 1889. He was a prolific writer and was associated with his father in much of it. His own chief works are those on *Tumors of the Mammary Gland* and *Diseases of the Male Sexual Organs*, appearing respectively in 1880 and 1881, and showing him to be an authority on genito-urinary diseases, to which he had given especial attention for many years. He was active in professional organizations, especially in the College of Physicians and in the two societies which were founded by his father: the Pathological Society and the American Surgical Association, the first of the last two mentioned conferring upon him its highest honor, that of the office

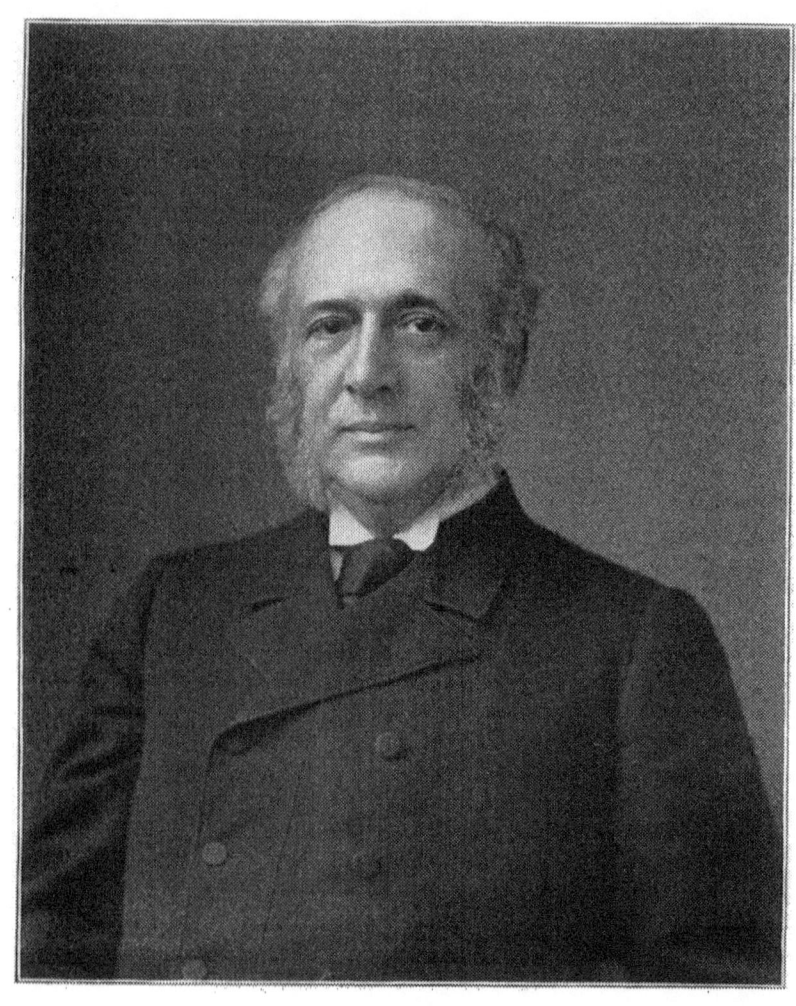

J. M. DA COSTA.

of president. Such was the man who, with Dr. Brinton, assumed the duties of Jefferson's greatest professor in 1882.

It was in 1883-4 that the next change occurred, when Dr. Wallace was made emeritus professor, and Dr. Theophilus Parvin of Indiana was called to succeed him. Chairs of Ophthalmology and Laryngology were created about this time, and Drs. William Thomson and J. Solis Cohen appointed to them, though they were ranked as honorary chairs for a time. These enlargements were due in some measure to the post-graduate courses that were begun the following year, and to the successful work of the summer courses. Dr. J. W. Holland succeeded Dr. Rogers in 1885-6, and the next year Dr. Pancoast, the younger, having withdrawn, his chair was occupied by Dr. William S. Forbes. In 1888-9, a large staff of clinical and other lecturers were added: Drs. Morris Longstreth, O. H. Allis, Charles E. Sajous, Oliver P. Rex, A. Van Harlingen and James C. Wilson (c); and the following year, on the death of Dr. Gross, his successor, Dr. W. W. Keen, the present incumbent of the chair of Surgery. A chair of General Pathology and Pathological Anatomy was created in 1891-2, and Dr. Longstreth elected to it, while Dr. Hobart A. Hare succeeded Dr. Bartholow, who became Professor Emeritus, and Dr. James C. Wilson came to the chair so long made famous throughout the professional world by Dr. Da Costa's ability as a teacher. Dr. Da Costa, now emeritus professor, is at present the honored president of the College of Physicians. In 1892-3, when preparations were making for enlarging the course to three years of study, Dr. E. E. Montgomery was made Professor of Clinical Gynecology, and a large staff of honorary and clinical professors was created. These were Drs. Thomson, Cohen, Stelwagon, H. A. Wilson, E. E. Graham, F. X. Dercum; in after years, Dr. W. L. Coplin, in 1893-4; Drs. E. de Schweinitz and Orville Horwitz, in 1894-5; Drs. W. J. Hearn, Edward P. Davis, S. MacCuen Smith and Howard F. Hansell, in 1895-6, and Dr. A. P. Brubaker, in 1896-7. Dr. Thomson was made full professor in 1895-6, and Dr. Coplin in 1896-7, when the establishment of a four years' course still father advanced the standards of

---

(c) Dr. H. W. Stelwagon was added to this list in 1890-91.

Jefferson, and numerous clinical and laboratory advantages were provided for.

The present faculty of Jefferson is as follows: J. M. Da Costa, M. D., LL. D., Emeritus Professor of Practice of Medicine and Clinical Medicine; Roberts Bartholow, M. D., LL. D., Emeritus Professor of Materia Medica, General Therapeutics and Hygiene; Henry C. Chapman, M. D., Professor of Institutes of Medicine and Medical Jurisprudence; John H. Brinton, M. D., Professor of the Practice of Surgery and of Clinical Surgery; Theophilus Parvin, M. D., LL. D., Professor of Obstetrics and Diseases of Women and Children; James W. Holland, M. D., Professor of Medical Chemistry and Toxicology and Dean of the College; William S. Forbes, M. D., Professor of General Descriptive and Surgical Anatomy; William W. Keen, M. D., LL. D., Professor of the Principles of Surgery and of Clinical Surgery; H. A. Hare, M. D., Professor of Materia Medica and Therapeutics; James C. Wilson, M. D., Professor of Practice of Medicine and Clinical Medicine; E. E. Montgomery, M. D., Professor of Clinical Gynecology; W. M. L. Coplin, M. D., Professor of Pathology and Bacteriology; and G. E. de Schweinitz, M. D., Professor of Ophthalmology. The honorary and clinical professors are: J. Solis-Cohen, M. D., Honorary Professor of Laryngology; Henry W. Stelwagon, M. D., Clinical Professor of Dermatology; H. Augustus Wilson, M. D., Clinical Professor of Orthopædic Surgery; Edwin E. Graham, M. D., Clinical Professor of Diseases of Children; F. X. Dercum, M. D., Clinical Professor of Diseases of the Nervous System; Orville Horwitz, M. D., Clinical Professor of Genito-Urinary Diseases; Edward P. Davis, M. D., Clinical Professor of Obstetrics; S. MacCuen Smith, M. D., Clinical Professor of Otology; W. Joseph Hearn, M. D., Clinical Professor of Surgery; Howard F. Hansell, M. D., Clinical Professor of Ophthalmology; D. Braden Kyle, M. D., Clinical Professor of Laryngology; J. Chalmers Da Costa, M. D., Clinical Professor of Surgery; and Albert P. Brubaker, M. D., Adjunct Professor of Hygiene, and H. E. Harris, M. D., Associate in Pathology. S. Solis-Cohen is Lecturer on Clinical Medicine, and the demonstrators are: A. Hewson, M. D., for Anatomy; E. Q. Thornton, M. D., for Therapeutics, Pharmacy and

Materia Medica; Thomas G. Ashton, M. D., for Clinical Medicine; Julius L. Salinger, M. D., for Clinical Medicine; Albert N. Jacob, M. D., for Chemistry; C. H. Reckefus, Jr., M. D., for Obstetrics; J. M. Fisher, M. D., for Clinical Gynecology; L. Bevan, M. D., for Morbid Anatomy and Bacteriology; C. A. Veasey, M. D., for Ophthalmology; J. Torrance Rugh, M. D., for Orthopædics; and George W. Spencer, M. D., for Surgery. The instructors and assistant demonstrators are: Max Bochroch, M. D., Instructor in Electro Therapeutics; Emanuel J. Stout, M. D., Instructor in Dermatology; F. K. Brown, M. D., Instructor in Diseases of Children; E. L. Klopp, M. D., Instructor in Otology; C. W. Hoopes, M. D., Instructor in Otology; W. M. Sweet, M. D., Instructor in Ophthalmology; John Lindsay, M. D., Assistant Demonstrator of Anatomy; W. H. Wells, M. D., Assistant Demonstrator of Clinical Obstetrics; J. P. Bolton, M. D., Assistant Demonstrator of Chemistry; H. R. Loux, M. D., Assistant Demonstrator of Surgery; C. H. Reckefus, Jr., M. D., Assistant Demonstrator of Anatomy; C. D. S. Fruh, M. D., Assistant Demonstrator of Anatomy; Howard Dehoney, M. D., Assistant Demonstrator of Anatomy; J. R. Crawford, M. D., Assistant Demonstrator of Anatomy; Randle C. Rosenberger, M. D., Assistant Demonstrator of Histology; E. H. Irvine, Assistant Demonstrator of Chemistry; E. H. Green, M. D., Assistant Demonstrator of Surgery; Henry L. Dexter, M. D., Assistant Demonstrator of Surgery; Lynford L. Moore, M. D., Assistant Demonstrator of Surgery; W. Krusen, M. D.., Assistant Demonstrator of Clinical Gynecology; W. N. Sedgwick, M. D., Assistant Demonstrator of Clinical Medicine; J. C. Da Costa, Jr., M. D., Assistant Demonstrator of Clinical Medicine; F. Hurst Maier, M. D., Assistant Demonstrator of Clinical Gynecology; John Gibbon, M. D., Assistant Demonstrator of Anatomy; Henry Tucker, M. D., Assistant Demonstrator of Clinical Medicine; W. J. Gillespie, M. D., Assistant Demonstrator of Morbid Histology; Nathan G. Ward, M. D., Assistant Demonstrator of Morbid Histology; A. F. Targette, M. D., Assistant Demonstrator of Morbid Histology; J. Coles Brick, M. D., Assistant Demonstrator of Anatomy; D. Gregg Matheny, M. D., Assistant Demonstrator of Surgery; C. R. Adams, M. D., Assistant Demonstrator of Morbid

Anatomy; T. L. Rhoads, M. D., Assistant Demonstrator of Morbid Histology, and Charles Braddock, M. D., Assistant Demonstrator of Surgery.

The four fine buildings that constitute the plant of the Jefferson Medical College are situated on Tenth and Sansom streets. The Medical Hall has its two large lecture-rooms, each with a capacity of 750; a museum, containing the collections of Drs. Gross and Da Costa; the dissecting-room, with its forty tables; the laboratories of Pharmacy, Therapeutics, Chemistry and Obstetrics, and the reading-room and private rooms for various professors. The Laboratory Building proper contains laboratories of Chemistry, Physiology, Morbid Anatomy, Major and Minor Surgery and the faculty-room. The Hospital Laboratory Building has three floors, with especial desk arrangements for 110 students, with 100 microscopes and other appliances for bacteriological and other study. The hospital has long been the pride of Jefferson, and its 140 beds are constantly filled, while its out-patient department averages 300 cases daily. It has a large amphitheater, even larger than the lecture-rooms, and smaller rooms for the use of classes. During the past year, 1,587 cases were cared for in the wards alone, and 16,487 in the out-patient department. Besides these, there is a Maternity Department at 224 South Seventh street, a Training School for Nurses at the hospital, a Nurses' Home at 228 South Seventh street, and a Students' Reading-Room at Tenth and Walnut streets. The Pennsylvania Hospital is near at hand, and twenty other hospitals of the city are easily accessible, many of them having Jefferson teachers on their staffs. About fifty students from the college are appointed as residents to hospitals every year in this and other cities, and about twenty-five prizes are awarded. Such is Jefferson's development after seventy-three years. It is interesting to observe that while the University was founded by a *physician*, and produced, perhaps, as her most eminent figure, a physician, (although she also produced the "Father of American Surgery"), Jefferson was founded by a *surgeon*, and has produced in the present period, in the incumbent of the chair of surgery, one of the most eminent of American surgeons. She has not, however, lacked a representative in medicine, having during this period also furnished one of the foremost teachers of medicine in the land—Dr. J. M. Da Costa. For Jefferson, this has been a period dominated by the fame of Gross, its first year ushered in by his presidency of the first International Medical Congress, and its last distinguished by the erection of his statue in the grounds of the National Capitol, an event due largely to the impetus given the movement by the Jefferson Alumni Association.

Besides the University and Jefferson, there was but one other of the present medical schools of Philadelphia in existence in 1876, the beginning of this period. This was the "Woman's Medical College of Pennsylvania." It has already been observed that, although it was founded by men, and suffered for no short period the misfortune of having among its friends some who were not believed to be free from medical heresies, it bravely overcame these disabilities. During the present period the school has won recognition equal to that accorded to the first institutions in the land, from the last stronghold of opposition—the County Medical Society. It will be recalled that this college won the battle for the recognition of women by the National Medical Society in 1871. "Ten years passed by," says Dr. Clara Marshall, in her outline history of the college, "and still women practitioners of medicine in Philadelphia were excluded from the County Society, and were, therefore, ineligible to membership in the State Society and in the American Medical Association, both made up of delegates from the county societies; and it seemed to them and their friends in Philadelphia rather an anomaly, when, in 1876, Dr. Sarah Hackett-Stevenson was sent as a delegate from Chicago to the meeting of the American Association in Philadelphia, and received, without question, to membership in an association from which women, long well-known to the profession and to the public as professors in the college, and as successful practitioners in the city, were excluded. Alumnæ of the college, resident in Montgomery County, the home of Dr. Corson, were also at this time members of the County Society, and, therefore, eligible to membership in both the State Society and the American Medical Association, while some members of the faculty of the college whose names gave validity to their diplomas were ineligible." In 1877 the college sent Dr. Frances E. White, as the woman member of its delegation, to the Association of American Medical Colleges, of which Dr. Gross was president, and she was admitted, although the great surgeon had been one of the opponents of recognition in the County Medical Society, all of which shows the curious situation brought about by the conflict between conservative Philadelphia and other more radical sections of the constituency of the National Association. In the spring of 1881, however, some members of the County Society presented the names of five women physicians for membership. The question of their admission had been a chronic one for so long, and, like the slavery question in national politics, was composed of such irritating and inflammable materials, that the members strove to avoid it. The by-laws of the society provided only for male membership, and, although that was the case, in October of that year it was resolved, "That female medical practitioners in good standing in the profession are eligible to membership in this society under the same laws and regulations now governing the admission of men." The by-laws, however, were held to stand in the way, and in April, 1882, when these candidates were again presented, they were defeated, and women continued to be defeated for five succeeding elections thereafter. Efforts to change the by-laws at last secured the necessary two-thirds vote, and in 1884 an heroic canvass was made for the election of women.

Even the medical journals, as well as the daily papers, made efforts to speed the day for their recognition. A writer in the Philadelphia Medical Times, 1883, says: "It must be acknowledged that the strictly regular instruction imparted in the principal medical schools for women has excited respect and greatly tended to overcome former prejudices. The admission of women is now a fixed fact." It was not, however, until 1888, that the Philadelphia County Medical Society elected its first woman member—Dr. Mary Willets.

The Neurological and the Medical Jurisprudence Societies admitted women the same year, and in 1890 Dr. Frances Emily

White represented the College and the County Society in the International Medical Congress at Berlin. The women organized their Alumnæ Medical Society that same year (1890), and two years later they were admitted to the Obstetrical Society of the city. The Northern Medical Association was the first society in Philadelphia to admit women, but only for temporary reasons, and returned to their original custom after their entrance into the County Medical Society. This struggle for recognition was in one sense a society, rather than a college question, but as it was far more vital to, and more characteristic of, the progress of this college than of the societies, it has been considered solely in connection with the Woman's College, whose growth toward excellence made its success possible.

It has already been noted that Dr. Ann Preston was the first woman to enter the faculty of the Woman's Medical College, taking the chair of Physiology, and that Dr. Emeline H. Cleveland was the second. The latter occupied the chair of Anatomy. In 1857, besides these two women professors, there were five men professors, the dean being a man—Dr. Edwin Fussell. This was when the college was at 229 Arch street (d). Ten years later, after its removal to North College avenue and Twenty-second street, these proportions were reversed, there being but two men on the regular faculty, and Dr. Ann Preston was dean. The women were Drs. Ann Preston in Physiology, Emeline H. Cleveland in Obstetrics, Mary J. Scarlett in Anatomy and Rachel L. Bodley in Chemistry. There were then forty-two students from all parts of the country. In 1869-70, two able men, Drs. Charles H. Thomas and Henry Hartshorne, joined the faculty, and were the most successful of any up to that time in winning respect for the college among the profession at large—at least the respect that brings professional recognition. This year was one of great prosperity for the college in the legacies left it, and in the opening up of the clinical facilities afforded by the Philadelphia and Wills Hospitals to its students. The term of study required was three years. In 1872-3 its faculty was increased to nine members, the four seniors being women, although Dr. Pres-

---
(d) The present number of the same building is 627.

ton's death during 1872 removed one of them. A staff of four auxiliary instructors was introduced in 1874-5, which, with Dr. Frances E. White as demonstrator, in 1872, added four women to the faculty. These were Dr. Hannah T. Croasdale in Surgery, Dr. Elizabeth C. Keller in Practice and Obstetrics, Dr. Clara Marshall in Materia Medica and Pharmacy, and Dr. White in Anatomy and Physiology. A spring course had been established with success, and the following year one more woman was added, Dr. Anna E. Broomall, as instructor in Obstetrics, making a faculty of fourteen, eight of whom were women. These changes, together with the fine new college building on Twenty-first street, gave great impetus to progress, and in the year that opens the present period, three more women were added—Drs. Mary Branson, Anna M. McAllister and Mary E. Allen—as instructors, making nine women. Dr. Alice Bennet became Demonstrator of Anatomy in 1877-8 and among the men occupying professorships in the institution was the present Professor of Surgery at Jefferson, Dr. W. W. Keen. In 1878 Dr. Amy S. Barton was made Instructor in Medicine, and the following year the whole teaching corps numbered nineteen members, ten of whom were women. It was now evident that the college included in its faculty some of the best men in the profession. Dr. Horatio C. Wood of the University was among the additions that year. Among other new names in the list of instructors were those of Drs. Sophia Presley, Frances N. Baker and Ida E. Richardson. In 1883 the faculty recommended a four years' course, and Dr. Anna M. Fullerton, Dr. Lena V. Ingraham and Grace L. Babb were added to the corps of teachers. Later, Drs. Elizabeth R. Bundy, Emma V. Boone, Susan P. Stackhouse and Emma E. Musson were added, so that by the time the first woman was admitted to the County Medical Society the list of teachers included twenty-six members, twelve of whom were women. Among the men on the staff were the well-known practitioners, Keen, Wood, Reese, Mills and others of like reputation. Drs. M. Helen Thompson, Mary Willits and Emma Putnam were later elected to positions. Dr. Marie K. Formad, Dr. Caroline M. Purnell, Dr. Lucy N. Tappan, Dr. Elizabeth E. Peck, Dr. Eleanor C. Jones, Dr. Eleanor M. Hiestand, Dr. Mary B. McCollin and Dr.

Louise M. Harvey were added by 1892, and by the following year the complete staff numbered forty-nine, including many of the brightest professional lights of Philadelphia. Thus it will be seen that the splendid struggle of the Woman's College for recognition terminated in victory in consequence of the evidence afforded by its aims and its attainments, of its worthiness to rank with its sister institutions, as a center for medical instruction.

The present faculty includes the following professors: Clara Marshall, M. D., Professor of Materia Medica and General Therapeutics; Frances Emily White, M. D., Professor of Physiology and Hygiene; Anna E. Broomall, M. D., Professor of Obstetrics; Hannah T. Croasdale, M. D., Professor of Gynecology; William H. Parish, M. D., Professor of Anatomy; Henry Leffman, M. D., Professor of Chemistry and Toxicology; John B. Roberts, M. D., Professor of the Principles and Practice of Surgery; Frederick P. Henry, M. D., Professor of the Principles and Practice of Medicine and Clinical Medicine; Arthur A. Stevens, M. D., Professor of Pathology. The following are Auxiliary Instructors: Elizabeth R. Bundy, M. D., Adjunct Professor of Anatomy and Demonstrator of Anatomy; Amy S. Barton, M. D., Clinical Professor of Ophthalmology; Charles K. Mills, M. D., Clinical Professor of Neurology; Henry W. Stelwagon, M. D., Clinical Professor of Dermatology; Charles H. Burnett, M. D., Clinical Professor of Otology; Emma E. Musson, M. D., Clinical Professor of Laryngology and Rhinology; Lawrence Wolff, M. D., Clinical Professor of Medicine; Edward P. Davis, M. D., Clinical Professor of Pediatrics; James K. Young, M. D., Clinical Professor of Orthopedic Surgery; Anna M. Fullerton, M. D., Clinical Professor of Gynecology; Alfred Stengel, M. D., Clinical Professor of Medicine; Edward Martin, M. D., Clinical Professor of Surgery; Charles K. Mills, M. D., Lecturer on Medical Jurisprudence; F. G. Ryan, Ph. G., Lecturer on Pharmacy; Eleanor C. Jones, M. D., Lecturer on Symptomatology, and Demonstrator and Clinical Instructor in Practice of Medicine; Lydia Rabinowitsch, Ph. D., Director of the Bacteriological Laboratory; Caroline M. Purnell, M. D., Demonstrator and Clinical Instructor in Gynecology; Kate W. Baldwin, M. D., Demonstrator and Clinical Instructor in Surgery; Emma L. Billstein, M. D., Demonstrator of Histology and Embryology; Mary W. Griscom, M. D., Demonstrator of Obstetrics; Helen Kirshbaum, M. D., Instructor in Chemistry; Annie Bartram Hall, M. D., and Ruth Webster Lathrop, M. D., Assistant Demonstrators of Physiology; Ruth W. Lathrop, M. D., Agnes B. Robinson, M. D., and Georgine I. Hochman, M. D., Assistant Demonstrators of Anatomy; Mary Thornton Wilson, M. D., Assistant Demonstrator of Obstetrics; Mary Getty, M. D., and Ada Howard-Audenried, M. D., Assistant Demonstrators of Pathology; Florence Mayo, M. D., Assistant Demonstrator of Histology and Embryology; Katherine A. Williamson, M. D., and Mary Getty, M. D., Assistant Demonstrators of Surgery; Alice M. Hackley, M. D., Assistant Demonstrator of Gynecology; Amelia A. Dranga, M. D., Assistant Demonstrator of Chemistry; Frances C. Van Gasken, M. D., Assistant in Hygiene and Instructor in Medical Diagnosis; Clara T. Dercum, M. D., Instructor in Therapeutics; Helen Murphy, M. D., Instructor in Materia Medica; Ruth Webster Lathrop, M. D., Prosector; A. A. Stevens, M. D., Curator of Museum; and seven student assistants.

The work of this Medical School is carried on in the following buildings: The College, the Laboratory, Brinton Hall, and the adjoining Clinic Hall, and in the wards of the Woman's Hospital of Philadelphia. It possesses excellent laboratories of Chemistry, Histology and Embryology, also Physiological, Pharmaceutical, Pathological, and Bacteriological laboratories. The Maternity of the Woman's Hospital, and the hospital proper, in which over seven thousand cases annually are treated, and which has a clinical amphitheater, with a seating capacity of about three hundred; the hospital and dispensary of the Alumnæ Association, at 1212 South Third street; the Maternity Hospital of the Woman's Medical College, at 335 Washington avenue, and the West Philadelphia Hospital for Women, furnish the best of hospital advantages, not to speak of the clinical lectures at the Pennsylvania, Philadelphia, German, Children's, Lying-in Charity, Wills, and other hospitals now open to the students. The students, also, have a good reading-room, library and museum, and the advantages of Brinton Hall, a

Young Women's Christian Association home. A large number of internes are appointed each year to hospitals in this and other cities, and as the required course has been, since 1893, four years, the students are able to enter into competition with those of the best schools of the country. The matriculates for the current year number 164, and the last graduating class enrolled twenty-eight, nine of whom were from Pennsylvania. Forty-eight years have passed since its establishment, but, undoubtedly, the greatest achievements of this, the oldest woman's medical college in the world, have been wrought within the present period. Beginning with the appointment of Dr. Cleveland in 1878, as gynecologist to the Department of the Insane in the Pennsylvania Hospital, one after another of the public institutions has added its representatives to their staffs, until the number has already grown very large, and is constantly increasing. The Woman's Medical College of Pennsylvania has won an enviable place in the history of medicine as the leader in a country that leads in the professional advancement of women.

Besides the wonderful development of the University in West Philadelphia, Jefferson in the old central part of the city, and the Woman's College in the northern part, facing Girard College grounds, this period has had enough vitality to produce, in locations midway between these three, a third college for men, and an advanced school for graduates in medicine, giving Philadelphia five strong schools devoted distinctively to the regular medical profession, not to speak of numerous other semi-medical institutions devoted to dentistry, pharmacy, and the like. These are the Medico-Chirurgical College of Philadelphia, with its beautiful clinical Amphitheater, Hospital, Lecture Hall and Laboratories, at the corner of North Eighteenth and Cherry streets, and the Philadelphia Polyclinic and College for Graduates in Medicine, with its great four-story combined clinic and hospital building on Lombard street, above Eighteenth.

The Medico-Chirurgical College had its origin, according to the earliest records, on the 13th of May, 1848, as a society whose plans and purposes were intended to be somewhat similar to those of the College of Physicians, which, as is well known, is in no sense a college, as the term is commonly used, but a permanent association of physicians. It will be recalled that just the year before this the American Medical Association was formed and its first annual meeting appointed to be held on May 2, 1848, at Baltimore, with delegates from all medical schools, societies, hospitals, dispensaries and other institutions. It was held as arranged, and the Philadelphia institutions that sent representatives were the old Philadelphia Medical Society, the College of Physicians, the University, the Medical Institute, Jefferson, Pennsylvania Medical College, the "Summer Association," as it was called, the Franklin Medical College, the Philadelphia College of Medicine, the Pennsylvania Hospital, the Philadelphia Dispensary, the Northern Dispensary, and the Northern Medical Association. Of these, the old Philadelphia Medical Society, which afterward converted itself into the County Society, sent as its representatives Drs. B. H. Coates, W. Ashmead, John Bell, Gouverneur Emerson, Isaac Parrish, Francis West, John D. Griscom, Lewis Rodman, Samuel Jackson (professor), John B. Biddle, and James Bryan. Of these, the last mentioned, Dr. James Bryan, it will be recalled, had a private school in Arch street for a time. The Baltimore meeting closed on the 5th, and on the 13th there met at the house of Dr. Bryan, at the northeast corner Arch and Tenth streets, Drs. James Bryan, Levi Curtis, Thomas N. Flint, Zebedee R. Jones, John T. Nicholas, Henry Y. Smith, William P. White, and Allen Ward, the first members of a new society. Other members were added during the succeeding months of 1848, so that by the close of the year there were fifty-three members. In February, 1849, they adopted a permanent constitution, and the title, Medico-Chirurgical College, the constitution declaring that "Its object shall be the dissemination of medical knowledge, the defense of the rights and the preservation of the repute and dignity of the medical profession." In form it was somewhat suggestive of the College of Physicians, with senior, junior and honorary members, the only condition of senior membership being a degree from some reputable school and a reputable standing.

Its professional exercises were to be directed by twelve sections: Anatomy, Surgery, Obstetrics, Practice, Materia Medica, Chemistry, Physiology, Medical Jurisprudence, Public Hygiene, Diseases of Women and Children, Pharmacy and Pathology, and all members were to join some section or sections, while its regular meetings were to be on Saturday evenings throughout the year, excepting in midsummer. The first officers elected were as follows: Dr. James Bryan, president; Drs. Charles M. Griffith and John Dawson, vice-presidents; Dr. H. S. Porter, senior recording secretary; Dr. L. Gebhard, junior recording secretary; Dr. Henry Y. Smith, corresponding secretary; Dr. William Gardiner, treasurer; Drs. A. H. Todd and William Bryan, curators; Dr. James Bryan, orator; Dr. R. Foster, alternate; counselor, T. Dunn English, Esq. A year later, on February 12, 1850, the society was incorporated, with ninety-four members, with power to "grant diplomas of fellowship, honorary membership, senior membership, and junior membership, but this grant shall not be construed into the grant of any power to confer the degree of Bachelor of Medicine or Doctor of Medicine." It is interesting to note that among these incorporators was Dr. George P. Oliver, who became a member September 23, 1848, and was therefore one of the latest additions of that year. This was more than four months after the formation of the organization. The society does not appear among those represented in the American Medical Association, however, until its fifth annual meeting at Richmond in 1852, when Drs. Henry Wadsworth and Samuel Walsh (formerly of Virginia) were received as delegates. The next year Dr. James Bryan alone was its representative, while Dr. Samuel H. Meade and Dr. J. B. Bell were delegates in 1854. Dr. Henry Y. Smith was a delegate in 1855, but there was none the next year, nor thereafter until 1872, when Drs. S. B. W. Mitchell, H. W. Ozias, and Alfred G. Reed were sent. Dr. Bryan had once, soon after 1855, attended, as a permanent member, but the society did not have a very vigorous existence from that time until after the war closed.

During the revived activity of the renaissance in medicine, when new colleges were springing up, it occurred to Dr. George P.

Oliver and a few associates, members of the old society, that "Whereas, the members of the Medico-Chirurgical College, believing that the objects of their association would be greatly benefited by having additional privileges granted to them, of appointing or electing professors to lecture on the different branches of medicine, and to confer the degree of Doctor of Medicine," they could, by securing changes in their charter, completely transform the organization into a regular medical college. Consequently, on April 10, 1867, an amendatory act was secured, according to a previous resolution of the society, providing that "George P. Oliver, Charles M. Griffith, Edward Donnelly, H. St. Clair Ash and George H. Cooke, Doctors of Medicine, and members of the said college, with their associates, are hereby empowered to meet on the first Saturday in May, one thousand eight hundred and sixty-seven, at four o'clock in the afternoon, in the city of Philadelphia, and elect such officers and professors for said college as may be necessary for the proper dissemination of medical knowledge in all its various branches," and that "the said officers and professors, by this act, shall have conferred upon them all the rights, immunities and privileges, as to lecturing, granting diplomas, and conferring degrees in medicine, as are possessed by the officers and professors of the University of Pennsylvania at this time." The faculty so ordered was composed of Drs. George P. Oliver, J. A. Meigs, J. Solis Cohen, Edward Donnelly, D. D. Richardson, D. D. Clark and Samuel Walsh. For various reasons, this faculty gradually dissolved and nothing was done until about the time, in 1880, when there was considerable activity throughout the profession in correcting abuses of various kinds. Dr. Oliver still had the charter and he and others began the formation of a faculty, of which Dr. G. B. H. Swayze was dean. The reorganization took place at Dr. Stubbs' home, on the northeast corner of Seventeenth and Jefferson streets, in October. Drs. Oliver, Stubbs and Swayze were appointed a committee to secure a building, and they succeeded in obtaining the upper story of the bank building on the southwest corner of Broad and Market streets, opposite the Broad street station. On April 4, 1881, when arrangements had been made for an embryo hospital, dispensary, and college, Dr. Oliver delivered the opening address. The faculty for the spring session consisted of Drs. Oliver for Practice, H. E. Goodman for Surgery, G. B. H. Swayze for Obstetrics, G. E. Stubbs for Anatomy, W. F. Waugh for Materia Medica, A. S. Gerhard for Physiology and Medical Jurisprudence, and C. L. Mitchell for Chemistry. There was but a handful of students, and the faculty underwent some changes before the following autumn, when its first real work began.

Before turning to that subject, however, it will be of interest to glance at the real founder of this institution, an organizer of more than ordinary talent. Dr. George P. Oliver was a Philadelphian, born in 1824, the son of Major W. G. Oliver, of the 42d United States Infantry, who served in the War of 1812. Dr. Oliver, after receiving an education in the academies of the city, began the study of medicine with Dr. J. P. Bethell, in 1842. After one year at the medical department of Pennsylvania College (1847-8), he entered the Philadelphia College of Medicine in 1850, and graduated in 1851. In 1854 he became a resident at the Philadelphia Hospital and afterward became chairman of its clinical committee. In 1859, he attended a course of lectures in the Medical Department of the University, and received his degree from that institution, after which he spent the following year, 1860, in pursuing his studies in Europe. He had already, in 1851, begun practice, which was interrupted by a brief residence in Cincinnati, where he served as city physician. In 1861, he was made assistant surgeon of the 98th Volunteers, but the following year was made post-surgeon of the 111th Volunteers, and served for three years. He was twice wounded and once taken prisoner, and made an excellent record as an army surgeon. On his return he resumed practice, but in 1878 removed, first to New York and then to Brooklyn, returning in 1880 to his native city. It was at this time that the new college was begun. He only lived four years longer, his decease occurring on February 20, 1884, in his sixtieth year. Dr. Oliver was the life of this institution, and was active in many others, being one of the charter members of the Methodist Episcopal Hospital. In 1881 he received the degree of

Master of Arts from Westminster College. He also held honorary degrees from several other institutions. "As a teacher," says Dr. Stubbs, "he was impressive, clear, and particular, insisting upon the student's fixing the facts and principles advanced firmly in his mind. . . . . . Professor Oliver was a warm-hearted, sympathetic physician, to whom the poor patient could look ever for help and counsel in time of trouble." Dr. Oliver must always be regarded as having been to the Medico-Chirurgical College what Dr. McClellan was to Jefferson.

"The first teaching faculty," says Dr. J. M. Anders, in his history of the institution, "consisted of George P. Oliver, A. M., M. D., President of the College, and Professor of the Principles and Practice of Surgery and Clinical Surgery; George E. Stubbs, A. M., M. D., Professor of Anatomy and Clinical Surgery; Charles L. Mitchell, Ph. D., M. D., Professor of Chemistry, Sanitary Science and Medical Jurisprudence; William F. Waugh, M. D., Professor of the Principles and Practice of Medicine and Clinical Medicine; Abraham S. Gerhard, A. M., M. D., Professor of Physiology, Pathology and Clinical Medicine; William S. Stewart, M. D., Dean, and Professor of Obstetrics, Gynecology, and Clinical Gynecology; Frank O. Nagle, M. D., Professor of Materia Medica, Therapeutics and Clinical Medicine. The opening address of the first regular session of the College was delivered April 4, 1881 (beginning of the spring course), by Professor Oliver, who took occasion to define the policy of the school, announcing that it would adhere to the aims of its founders, and that it would adopt the methods of higher medical education, and the graded three-session course of study. Touching these points, I prefer to quote his own words: 'It is the intention of the faculty to use every means that can be made available to advance students and to render them proficient in the duties of their profession. We deprecate the system of cramming, now in use in many medical colleges, in various parts of the country, crowding into two winter sessions the entire medical tuition of the student. Owing to the shortness of time, sufficient instruction cannot be given, and the student fails to complete his medical education properly. With a view of elevating the standard of medical education, our college has adopted a curriculum embracing a full three-years graded course. By this action we believe we will assist in placing some safeguards around society that are being sadly neglected by many medical colleges in America.' His masterful address closed with these encouraging and inspiring sentiments: 'To both old and young, in our profession, who are resting satisfied with the laurels already gained in former days, we desire to say, fall in line and march to the front; assist your brethren to break down the formidable barricades that have been erected by unscrupulous men, who have almost run their course, but who are still attempting to control the destiny of our profession. To our friends who have honored us with their presence to-day, we tender the thanks of grateful hearts. We feel that our success will not depend upon ourselves alone; much will be due to the encouragement we receive from those who are in full sympathy with us. Give our college and our sister colleges, who are engaged in this noble work, your aid and counsel, and the great object will, in a short time, be effected. We know we will have a severe struggle at first, but we are determined to hold on, even though we have to fight the battle alone. Other colleges may falter, as one in New York already has, but with the full assurance that we are doing right, we intend, with the assistance of Divine Providence, to persevere manfully until victory shall crown our efforts.'

"The original faculty continued unbroken until the death of Dr. Nagle in 1884. During the first session, thirty-one students were in attendance, during the second twenty-seven, and during the third session (1883-84), only twenty-four students. The first class was graduated March 10, 1882, and consisted of three men. The valedictory address was delivered by Professor Charles K. Mitchell, Professor of Chemistry. It was determined to make a stand for higher medical education from the outset. This principle, be it remembered, was affirmed at a time when but two sessions, without regard to grading of the course of instruction, were required by the many medical institutions, a fact to which may be rightfully attributed the comparatively slow growth of the College during the first few years of its existence. From its inception, too, the Medico-Chirurgical College was in all other respects in the van of progress. Thus, candidates for admission were required to pass a preliminary examination; attendance of the students was required at the College six hours per day; and no student was admitted to advanced standing, until he had passed a satisfactory examination in the branches of the preceding grade. The autumn term began the first Monday in September, during which the instruction was elementary and preliminary to that of the winter term, which commenced on the first Monday in October, and was continued for six months. The policy of this school embraced, thus early, certain important and distinguishing characteristics, and, to render appreciable in some measure the *genius loci* of the institution, a few of the original and progressive features introduced from time to time may here be mentioned. Besides didactic and clinical lectures, laboratory work, and practical training at the bedside, forming an exceptionally advanced course of study, the old college year embraced from the outset a spring, or auxiliary, literary term of three months, beginning on the first Monday in April. This was especially designed for students whose qualifications were not sufficient to enable them to fully comprehend the didactic and the clinical lectures of the regular winter term. During this session instruction was given in Natural Philosophy, Botany, Physical Geography, Mental Philosophy, Principles of English Composition, Elements of the Greek and Latin Languages, Mathematics, Comparative Anatomy, and Zoölogy, Mineralogy and Geology. Another conception of the founders of this school related to the supreme importance of personal instruction of the students by the members of the faculty. The first faculty daily conducted personal examinations, or quizzes, of the classes, on the subjects of the preceding lectures, thus fixing permanently in the minds of the students the instruction previously given. This method of teaching also furnished opportunity for essential explanations by the professors themselves of any truths not clearly understood. So valuable an adjunct did this measure prove that it has been continued down to the present time. Moreover, the recognition of the superior advantages of personal instruction over the old method of didactic lectures early led the authorities of the Medico-Chirurgical College to abandon the traditional lectures for recitation and personal laboratory and dissection-room work. Indeed, it may be claimed that the phenomenal growth and development of this institution has been, in no small measure, due to the thorough execution of this primal conception, viz.: That personal instruction not only enables the teacher to impart facts, but, also, to furnish the reasons upon which those facts are founded. The trend of thought of the faculty of the Medico-Chirurgical College, at the present time, leans strongly in the direction of the seminar method of instruction—a method that enables the student to understand the facts imparted to him, and, what is of no small importance, enables the teacher to determine the amount of work actually performed by the student, and the quantity of practical knowledge acquired. This mode of teaching is about to be applied by the Medico-Chirurgical College to all of the branches embraced in the curriculum. Here should be mentioned the fact that, at the time of the reorganization, there was established a system of quizzes, free of charge, and this has been continued until the present time. They are conducted by the professors, assisted by competent tutors; their object is twofold, first to remove the expense of private quizzes, and, secondly, to prepare the students thoroughly for their life's work on all of the branches.

"To show the confidence of the pioneers of this institution in the practical value of laboratory training in the basal sciences, and of practical work in surgery, as a means of qualifying the student for exact work, courses in the following branches were given: Practical Pharmacy, Analytic Chemistry, Practical Anatomy, Histology, Pathologic Histology, and Operative Surgery and Bandaging."

In prominent connection with the dental and hospital departments was Dr. James E. Garretson, A. M., M. D., D. D. S., who was long associated with Agnew in the School of Anatomy. A native of Wilmington, Delaware, he was born in October, 1828. During his youth he became interested in dentistry and graduated from the Philadelphia Dental College in 1857. Realizing the medical relations of dentistry, he also graduated in medicine from the University of Pennsylvania in 1859. It was then that Dr. Agnew secured him as an associate in the School of Anatomy, of which he took sole charge on Dr. Agnew's withdrawal to the University work a few years later. About this time he began to make a specialty of the surgery of the mouth and neighboring parts and soon became widely known as an "oral surgeon." In 1869 he took the chair of Oral Surgery in the University and had charge of its oral hospital service. Nine years later he was chosen Professor of Anatomy and Surgery in the Philadelphia Dental College, of which he became dean in 1881. In this position and as a founder of the hospital of the Medico-Chirurgical College, he rendered great service to the institution. He died October 26, 1895, best known, probably, by his work, "A System of Oral Surgery." Dr. Garretson achieved distinction in other than the scientific fields of literature, and is perhaps as well known to the general public by his "Odd Hours of a Physician" and other books, as he is to the profession by his surgical treatises.

Previous to the changes above mentioned, there came to the faculty men who infused into it such a spirit of energy as to institute the beginning of a new period in its development. One of these was the late Dr. William H. Pancoast, A. M., M. D., who came from Jefferson Medical College, where he had been Professor of Anatomy for the eleven years since his father's resignation. Dr. Pancoast was fifty years of age when he joined the Medico-Chirurgical College in 1885. He was a native of Philadelphia, born in 1835, and was educated in Haverford College, from which he received his diploma in 1853. He had studied medicine under his distinguished father, Joseph Pancoast, and was graduated from Jefferson Medical College in 1856. Going abroad, he spent three years in the hospitals and other medical institutions of London, Paris, Vienna and Berlin, and pursued special work under Civiale, who desired him to remain as his assistant. In 1862, however, he returned to Philadelphia and became Demonstrator of Anatomy in the school, in which he succeeded his father in 1874. In 1885, on his resignation from Jefferson, he was contemplating an extended visit abroad, when he was induced to join the Medico-Chirurgical College. The chair he accepted was, as a matter of course, similar to that which he had occupied at Jefferson. He at once became one of the greatest powers in the new developments of the school, and soon became president of its board of trustees. "Dr. Pancoast," says one of his biographers, "was a man of striking personality, of courtly manners and greatly beloved by his students and friends. As a lecturer on anatomy he was pre-eminent, and as an operator he was equally successful." During the civil war he was surgeon-in-chief and second in command at one of the military hospitals. He was surgeon to the Philadelphia Hospital for many years and was prominent in nearly all the leading medical societies of Philadelphia. He was especially active in the county, state and national societies, and was vice-president of the American Medical Association in 1884, and delegate to various international congresses. Dr. Pancoast died in January, 1897, having lived long enough to witness the remarkable development of the school of which he was so great a promoter.

Just before Dr. Pancoast came to the institution, Dr. Henry Ernest Goodman was called to the chair made vacant by the death of Dr. Oliver. A glance at the career of this man, also one of the founders of the institution, will be of interest before attention is directed to the latter. Dr. Goodman was of German descent, grandson of an officer in our Revolutionary Army of '76. A native of Speedwell, near Philadelphia, he was born in 1836, so that he was almost the exact age of Dr. Pancoast. He graduated from the University Medical School in 1859, in the same class with Dr. Oliver, and also became a resident in the (Philadelphia) Blockley Hospital. On completing his term, he became a resident at Wills Hospital, where he became interested in the specialty to which he devoted the greater part of his time in after life. He was also one of the surgeons of the Orthopædic Hospital from its opening until his death. He held many public positions, as well. Thus for six years he served as port physician. "In 1885," says Dr. Anders in a memoir before the College of Physicians, "he was made Professor of Surgery at the Medico-Chirurgical College, a position he filled most worthily and acceptably for six years. His lectures were noteworthy for their perspicuity, as well as for the safety and soundness of their substance. As a teacher he was concise yet expressed fully enough the truths he wished to impart, while his sympathetic nature and warmth of manner quickly led to the establishment of pleasant personal relations between himself and his students." He was a member of various leading societies and did eminent service in the civil war, acting as surgeon to the 28th Pennsylvania Infantry from 1861 to 1864, and becoming Medical Director of the Army of Georgia, with the rank of colonel. Dr. Goodman lived to the age of sixty years, his death occurring on February 3, 1896, and he was in his fiftieth year when he joined the faculty of the Medico-Chirurgical College.

"In 1885," says Dr. Anders, "the late Dr. H. Ernest Goodman was chosen to succeed Dr. Oliver, as Professor of Surgery and Clinical Surgery. At this period, the Medico-Chirurgical College joined forces with the Philadelphia Dental College, and procured buildings more commodious and appropriate for the uses of both institutions. The site selected was the north side of Cherry street, below Eighteenth street, the same as that occupied by the Medico-Chirurgical College and Hospital at the present time. From the year 1886 up to 1895, the Medico-Chirurgical College and the Philadelphia Dental College constituted a firm, so to speak, with equal rights and privileges, so far as appertained to the direction and control of the buildings, while, at the same time, maintaining a separate existence, as institutions of medical and dental learning. In 1895 it was mutually agreed to dissolve the previous business relations that had existed between the two institutions, this action to take effect at the end of the session of 1896-97, and, since the latter date, the Medico-Chirurgical College has assumed the ownership of the entire property, consisting of a number of buildings, all devoted to hospital and college purposes.

"In 1885, such well-known teachers as the late Dr. William H. Pancoast, Profs. John V. Shoemaker and E. E. Montgomery entered the faculty, and the Board of Trustees of the College. Prof. Shoemaker, who for several years had lectured on diseases of the skin in the post-graduate course of the Jefferson Medical College, was elected Professor of Dermatology in the Medico-Chirurgical College, and, soon after, also to the chair of Materia Medica and Therapeutics. The Philadelphia Hospital for Skin Diseases, under his charge, with all its appurtenances, was transferred to the new location at Cherry street, and there continued with increased accommodations, as a department of the Medico-Chirurgical College and Hospital. Dr. E. E. Montgomery was elected Professor of Gynecology, a separate chair having been created for him, and this important department became a special feature of the course. At this time, the Hospital of Oral Surgery, under Professor Garretson, was also merged into the Medico-Chirurgical Hospital, and there continued to hold its unrivaled clinics in that specialty. These gentlemen, from the moment they became connected with the school, displayed much energy and financial courage, and, by their exertions, rendered it possible for the institution to consummate the removal to the present site. Professor Pancoast, who brought with him his extensive and valuable Anatomical and Pathological Museum, which was collected during many years by his father and himself, and subsequently freely used in illustration of his lectures, was at once elected to the presidency of the College, and many examples could be cited to show his great ardor, zeal, and genius, as the leader of the new combination, striving to wrest from a conservative public, professional and popular applause and favor. Resting confidently upon the wise and comprehensive basis upon which the school was reorganized by the founders, and under the impetus given to the institution by the gentlemen named above, the Medico-Chirurgical College moved forward with remarkable vigor in the face of many discouraging influences. Fresh additions to the faculty followed, consisting, for the greater part, of young, able and energetic men.

"The list of professors from the date of reorganization is, for the various chairs, as follows: The chair of the Principles and Practice of Medicine and Clinical Medicine, Hugo Engel, A. M., M. D., 1881-83; William F. Waugh, A. M., M. D., 1883-91; James M.

Anders, M. D., LL. D., 1891. The chair of Surgery and Clinical Surgery was first occupied by George P. Oliver, A. M., M. D., in 1881-84; H. Ernest Goodman, M. D., 1884-91; Ernest Laplace, M. D., LL. D., 1891. The chair of Materia Medica and Therapeutics, William F. Waugh, A. M., M. D., 1881-82; Frank O. Nagle, A. M., M. D., 1882-84; Frank Woodbury, M. D., 1884-89; John V. Shoemaker, M. D., LL. D., Professor of Materia Medica, Pharmacology and Therapeutics, 1889. The chair of Obstetrics, Gynecology and Clinical Gynecology, George B. H. Swayze, M. D., 1881 (during preliminary term); William S. Stewart, A. M., M. D., 1881-91; E. E. Montgomery, A. M., M. D., 1881-92; W. Frank Haehnlen, M. D., Ph. D., 1892. Gynecology, E. E. Montgomery, A. M., M. D., 1886-92; W. Easterly Ashton, M. D., 1892. The chair of Clinical Medicine, Frank Woodbury, A. M., M. D., 1891-94; William E. Hughes, M. D., Ph. D., 1894. Clinical Surgery, George E. Stubbs, A. M., M. D. (including surgical pathology), 1886-92. William H. Pancoast, A. M., M. D., Professor of Anatomy and Clinical Surgery, 1893-97; William L. Rodman, A. M., M. D., Professor of the Principles of Surgery and Clinical Surgery. Ophthalmology, P. D. Keyser, A. M., M. D., 1884-93; L. Webster Fox, A. M., M. D., 1893. Anatomy, George E. Stubbs, A. M., M. D., 1881-86; William H. Pancoast, A. M., M. D., Professor of General Descriptive and Surgical Anatomy, 1886-97; John C. Heisler, M. D., 1897. Physiology and Medical Jurisprudence, Abraham S. Gerhard, A. M., M. D., 1881-86; Thomas C. Stelwagen, A. M., M. D. (Physiology only), 1886-89; Samuel Wolfe, A. M., M. D. (lecturer), 1889-90; Samuel Wolfe, A. M., M. D. (professor), 1890-93; Henry T. Slifer, M. D., 1893-94; Isaac Ott, A. M., M. D., 1894. The chair of Chemistry, Charles L. Mitchell, M. D., Ph. D., 1881-86; S. B. Howell, A. M., M. D., 1886-93; H. H. Boom, M. D. (adjunct professor), 1893-97; J. H. Meeker, B. S., M. S., 1897. Pathology—This chair was held by different lecturers up to 1886, but as some of the records are missing, their names cannot be furnished. Abraham S. Gerhard, A. M., M. D., Professor of Pathology, Medical Jurisprudence and Clinical Medicine, 1886-90; Ernest Laplace, M. D., LL. D., Professor of Pathology and Bacteriology, 1890-96; Joseph MacFarland, M. D., 1896. Sanitary

Science and Pediatrics, William B. Atkinson, A. M., M. D., 1884-89; James M. Anders, M. D., LL. D., 1889-92; Charles M. Seltzer, M. D., Professor of Hygiene, 1892-93; Seneca Egbert, A. M., M. D., 1893. In 1893 the authorities made a progressive departure in the establishment of a Board of Censors, composed of well-known physicians. A certificate of successful examination, as directed by the faculty, before one of these gentlemen, is sufficient for admission to the study of medicine in the College.

"As I have already stated, the College occupied, during the first five years of its existence, the upper stories of the Third National Bank building, at the southwest corner of Broad and Market streets. Here the facilities and accommodations offered to the student were plainly inadequate. In 1886 the valuable property on the north side of Cherry street, east of Eighteenth street (a building earlier known as the Home for Aged and Indigent Women), was so altered as to meet the requirements of a modern hospital, and was under the joint control of the faculties of the two schools named above. Its inmates, then, as now, furnished the means of supplying the major clinics, and of imparting bedside instruction to the student. At this time the hospital staff was composed of members of the medical and dental faculties and with equal representation. Upon the severing of the relations of the two schools, the staff was made up of representatives from the major and minor faculties of the Medico-Chirurgical College alone. Sufficient adjacent property was purchased at the outset to erect thereon a college building, containing three spacious lecture halls or amphitheaters, including a magnificent clinical amphitheater. These were well lighted, ventilated, and furnished with comfortable chairs for the students. The upper floor of the south side of this structure was furnished as a dissecting-room, with every needed appliance. This was leased by the Philadelphia School of Anatomy, with the distinct proviso that the students of the Medico-Chirurgical College and of the Philadelphia Dental College be privileged to dissect therein, under certain express terms and regulations. It may be mentioned here that immediately after the separation of the Medico-Chirurgical and Philadelphia Dental Colleges, the dissecting-room reverted to the latter institution. Within the ample confines of the College and hospital adequate space was found for the histologic, pathological, bacteriologic and chemical laboratories, all of which were at once properly equipped. It was soon discovered, however, that by reason of a lack of accommodations it would be necessary to enlarge the hospital building, and to this end it was, in 1890, determined to reconstruct the same on a larger scale. As a result, the original hospital was replaced by an extensive six-story building, which doubled its former capacity—a proceeding 'that marked a second peculiarly eventful period in the history of the institution, the first being the purchase of the site now occupied, and the removal of it from Broad street.' The plans called for an extension of the hospital buildings, twenty feet to the front, and the addition of two new stories. The hospital was then thoroughly equipped with the most modern conveniences for lighting, heating, drainage and ventilation. After the completion of these alterations, the hospital afforded accommodation for not less than 126 beds for patients; the two upper floors have been devoted to private rooms (twenty in number) for the reception of patients. Although the Medico-Chirurgical Hospital is located to the west of the College building, it is connected with the latter by an L posteriorly, so that the two buildings are virtually one. And now, for a time, both the new College building and the newly-remodeled hospital seemed to afford ample facilities, and to possess great adaptability to the purposes of medical teaching and hospital work. With the steady growth of the medical school, and the constantly increasing demands for hospital accommodations, it was again found needful to provide increased building accommodations. In view of this fact, six properties, located at the northeast corner of Eighteenth and Cherry streets, were purchased singly, though in quick succession, and devoted to the maternity department of the College, the children's ward of the hospital and the laboratories. The capacity of the hospital buildings was thereby increased from 126 to 200 patients, the maternity department alone having forty beds. A little later, the property extending from the College to the corner of Seventeenth and Cherry streets was also purchased, and it has been determined to erect thereon, immediately, a large laboratory building, suitably arranged in its details for teaching purposes. In consequence of these repeated acquisitions of property, the plant grew until it covered an extensive superficial area, extending from Eighteenth street to Seventeenth street on Cherry street, 120 feet northward on the east side of Eighteenth street, and 60 feet northward on the west side of Seventeenth street. The rapid progress of scientific thought concerning asepsis having made it imperative to surround surgical operations with certain definite conditions, particularly if the latter be performed in the presence of large numbers of medical students, the Board of Trustees of the Medico-Chirurgical Hospital have recently erected a new clinical amphitheater and operating-rooms, designed to fulfill the most advanced surgical and educational requirements. It is believed to be the most perfect, as well as the largest, clinical amphitheater that has yet been erected, either in the United States or Europe. In 1892 there were admitted to, and treated in, the wards and rooms of the hospitals, 585 patients; in the receiving ward, 774 so-called 'accident' cases, and in the out-patient department, or dispensary service, 5,537 cases. In 1896, the number of patients admitted to the wards and private rooms was 1,242; the number of 'accident' cases treated was 2,036, while in the out-patient department, there were treated not less than 37,907 cases. During the session of 1891-2 the number of matriculates was 122, while during the term of 1896-97 the number was 363.

"The college has recently adopted a four-session, graded course of instruction, with special features, looking to the establishment of the 'seminar' method, so as to afford the greatest possible opportunity for individual investigation by the student, and for personal examination by the teacher in sections of classes. In 1897, the institution, having become independent of the Philadelphia Dental College, owing to the removal of the latter to its present site, has established its own dental department."

The present teaching force is composed as follows: John V. Shoemaker, M. D., LL. D., Professor of Materia Medica, Pharmacology and Therapeutics; James M. Anders, M. D., LL. D., Ph. D., Professor of Theory and Practice of Medicine and Clinical Medicine; Ernest Laplace, M. D., LL. D., Professor of Surgery and Clinical Surgery; W. Frank Haehnlen, M. D., Ph. D., Professor of Obstetrics; W. Easterly Ashton, M. D., Professor of Gynecology; L. Webster Fox, A. M., M. D., Professor of Ophthalmology; William E. Hughes, M. D., Ph. D., Professor of Clinical Medicine; William L. Rodman, A. M., M. D., Professor of the Principles of Surgery and Clinical Surgery; Isaac Ott, A. M., M. D., Professor of Physiology; Seneca Egbert, A. M., M. D., Professor of Hygiene; Joseph McFarland, M. D., Professor of Pathology and Bacteriology; Charles E. de M. Sajous, M. D., Dean, Professor of Laryngology; John C. Heisler, M. D., Professor of Anatomy; J. H. Meeker, B. S., M. S., Professor of Chemistry. Emeritus and honorary professors: George E. Stubbs, A. M., M. D.; William S. Stewart, A. M., M. D.; W. B. Atkinson, A. M., M. D. Clinical and assistant professors: John V. Shoemaker, M. D., LL. D., Clinical Professor of Skin and Venereal Diseases; Charles W. Burr, A. M., M. D., Clinical Professor of Nervous Diseases; W. C. Hollopeter, A. M., M. D., Clinical Professor of Children's Diseases; Arthur H. Cleveland, A. M., M. D., Clinical Professor of Laryngology; E. B. Gleason, M. D., Clinical Professor of Otology; James P. Mann, M. D., Clinical Professor of Orthopedic Surgery; Benjamin T. Shimwell, M. D., Assistant Professor of Surgery; Albert E. Roussel, A. M., M. D., Adjunct Professor of Practice and Clinical Medicine; Spencer Morris, Ph. D., M. D., Adjunct Professor of Medical Jurisprudence; Henry Fisher, Ph. G., M. D., Assistant Professor of Materia Medica and Pharmacy. Lecturers and Instructors: Spencer Morris, M. D., Lecturer on Differential Diagnosis; Emanuel S. Gans, M. D., Lecturer on Skin Diseases; Michael O'Hara, Jr., M. D., Lecturer on Minor Surgery and Bandaging; Howard S. Anders, A. M., M. D., Lecturer and Clinical Instructor on Physical Diagnosis; I. N. Snively, Lecturer on Physical Diagnosis; W. N. Watson, M. D., Lecturer on Genito-Urinary Diseases; George W. Pfromm, M. D., Lecturer on Therapeutics and Materia Medica and Clinical Diagnosis; Charles L. Furbush, M. D., Lecturer on Histology and Director of the Histologic Laboratory; C. H. Gubbins, Ph. D., M. D., Instructor in Materia Medica and Pharmacy; Henry Parrish, M. D., Instructor in Physiology; Philip R. Cleaver, M. D., Instructor in Surgery; Matthew Beardwood, Jr., A. M., M. D., Instructor in Chemistry; J. G. Herschelroth, M. D., Instructor in Medicine; N. Napoleon Boston, Instructor in Obstetrics; E. F. Kamerly, Jr., M. D., Instructor in Ophthalmology; F. K. Brown, M. D., Instructor in Ophthalmoscopy; Alexander Ramsay, M. D., Instructor in Children's Diseases; L. C. Peter, M. D., Instructor in Neurology; R. D. Newton, M. D., Instructor in Therapeutics and Materia Medica. Demonstrators: J. Thompson Schell, M. D., Demonstrator of Obstetrics; Walter V. Woods, M. D., Demonstrator in Gynecology; W. Wayne Babcock, Demonstrator of Pathology; Joseph D. Wallace, M. D., Demonstrator of Anatomy; Edwin H. Miller, M. D., Demonstrator of Hygiene, and E. F. Kamerly, Jr., M. D., Demonstrator of Ophthalmology. The Medico-Chirurgical College, as has been seen, is wholly a product of the present period, and in the rapidity and vigor of its growth is probably without a parallel in the history of medical schools.

The four medical schools in existence in 1881-2, after the opening of the Medico-Chirurgical College, were covering the conventional ground of medical instruction, but that instruction had recently made such strides in progress that many older practitioners found that post-graduate work was almost a necessity in order to keep abreast with medical progress. Furthermore, the growth of specialization had become so remarkable in its proportions, and the call for special knowledge so frequent, that interest in post-graduate work was widespread. It was in the summer of 1882 that Dr. John B. Roberts, finding himself free from his School of Anatomy, conceived the idea of a combined hospital and specialist school, where graduates in medicine might spend such time as they chose under the personal instruction of a specialist. Gathering friends about him in sympathy with the purpose, a meeting was held at the residence of Dr. R. J. Levis, at 1601 Walnut street, where it was decided to form such an institution. "The institution, of whose early history I have been asked to give a brief history," said Dr.

Roberts, at the ceremonies of laying the corner-stone of the new building, in November, 1889, "was born on a December morning, in 1882, when I suggested to the distinguished surgeon, now president of the Board of Trustees (e), the establishment of an institution for post-graduate medical instruction, to be called the Philadelphia Polyclinic. The idea, which had long occupied my mind, had been partially realized some years before, in the practical courses in anatomy, surgery, physical diagnosis, chemistry, diseases of the eye, diseases of the throat, etc., carried on at the Philadelphia School of Anatomy by Drs. Henry Leffmann, H. Augustus Wilson and myself, with a number of associates. Dr. Levis accepted my suggestion with favor, and within a few minutes called upon Dr. T. G. Morton, who, with his usual energy, cordially approved the project. Upon that day, or the next, Dr. J. Solis-Cohen was asked by Dr. Levis to add his distinguished name to the trio, and to aid in the founding of the new medical college. To this nucleus others were joined, and, on December 21, a meeting was held, which resolved to organize an institution for giving advanced instruction in medicine and surgery. The polysyllabic name, 'The Philadelphia Polyclinic and College for Graduates in Medicine,' was the result of a compromise. . . . . The dispensary was opened at the southeast corner of Thirteenth and Locust streets, on March 12, 1883; the first pupil matriculated March 26, 1883, while the charter incorporating the institution 'for the purpose of furnishing gratuitous medical services and advice to the sick poor, and affording physicians facilities for study in special branches of practice,' was granted March 19, 1883." The incorporators were Drs. Charles H. Burnett, J. Solis-Cohen, Edward L. Duer, George C. Harlan, Henry Leffmann, Richard J. Levis, Charles K. Mills, Thomas G. Morton, John B. Roberts, Edward O. Shakespeare, Arthur Van Harlingen and James C. Wilson. The building opposite the College of Physicians was fitted up for hospital and instruction purposes, and the faculty consisted of Dr. R. J. Levis, for Operative and Clinical Surgery; Dr. T. G. Morton, for General and Orthopædic Surgery; Dr. J. Solis-Cohen, for Diseases of the Nose and

---

(e) Dr. Richard J. Levis.

Throat; Dr. James C. Wilson, for Diseases of the Chest; Dr. John B. Roberts, for Applied Anatomy and Practical Surgery; Dr. Charles H. Burnett, for Diseases of the Ear; Dr. Charles K. Mills, for the Mind and Nervous System; Dr. Henry Leffmann for Clinical Chemistry and Hygiene; Dr. Arthur Van Harlingen, for Diseases of the Skin; Dr. Charles L. Duer, for Diseases of Women and Children; Dr. George C. Harlan, for Diseases of the Eye; Dr. J. Henry C. Simes, for Genito-Urinary and Venereal Diseases; and Dr. Frederick P. Henry, for Pathology and Microscopy. The year was divided into six-week sessions. The school was successful from the first, and has ever since enjoyed a prosperity which is largely due to the unremitting interest in its welfare displayed by Dr. John B. Roberts. All but one of the original faculty are still living: Dr. Richard J. Levis, the first president and senior professor, died in 1890, in Kennett, Pennsylvania, at his home, "Cedarcroft," famous as the former home of Bayard Taylor. He retired from practice in 1887 at the age of sixty. He was the son of a physician, and was born in Philadelphia in 1827. After his graduation from Jefferson Medical College in 1848, he settled in Philadelphia and at various periods was connected with several of the leading hospitals. He served as president of the trustees of Jefferson for ten years and was honored with the presidency of both the County and State medical societies.

There were but few changes in the faculty while the institution was at Thirteenth and Locust streets. Drs. Levis and Wilson resigned in 1883-4, and Dr. W. H. Parish joined the obstetrical department for a time; Dr. W. H. Baker also became an adjunct professor. The next year Dr. Charles B. Nancrede succeeded Dr. Morton and Dr. L. W. Steinbach became adjunct to Dr. Roberts. Dr. Louis Genois also was an accession for the chair of Pharmaceutical Chemistry. The growth had been so great in every way, and the staff of clinical assistants so very numerous, that larger quarters were obtained in a four-story building at the corner of Broad and Lombard streets, and opened on March 1, 1886. Dr. B. F. Baer succeeded Dr. Duer that year, Dr. W. Barton Hopkins took the chair of Clinical Surgery, and Dr. Baker became a full professor, as did Dr. Steinbach, who took the chair of Operative Surgery. In 1887-8 there were numerous additions as adjuncts, instructors and assistants, and in 1888-9 several important changes occurred: Drs. Henry and Solis-Cohen resigned, also Drs. Genois, Hopkins, and Baker. The additions were: Dr. Thomas J. Mays, for Diseases of the Chest; Dr. Alex. W. MacCoy, for those of the Throat and Nose; Dr. H. Augustus Wilson, for General and Orthopædic Surgery; Dr. Edward Jackson, for Diseases of the Eye; Dr. S. Solis-Cohen for Clinical Medicine and Applied Therapeutics. The years 1889 and 1890 were witnesses of still greater things for the Polyclinic, for it was in November, 1889, that the corner-stone was laid for "the finest hospital building devoted to post-graduate instruction in the world," situated farther west on Lombard street, on the South Side, but a few doors west of South Eighteenth street. Dr. S. Weir Mitchell was the most notable accession to the faculty that year, his professorship being that of the Mind and Nervous System, a department in which he first became famous for his work in the Turner's Lane Military Hospital of this city during the Civil War. Dr. B. Alex. Randall was also elected to the professorship of Diseases of the Ear. In 1890, Drs. Levis, J. Solis-Cohen, Bennett and Nancrede, and, in '91, Dr. Harlan, became the first professors of the emeritus list. Dr. E. P. Davis, in 1890, became professor of Obstetrics, Dr. Thomas S. K. Morton, of Clinical Surgery, and Dr. Mays, of Experimental Therapeutics, while the Auxiliary list was still further enlarged. In 1891-2 the accessions were: Dr. S. D. Risley for the Eye, Dr. John B. Deaver for Surgery, Dr. J. P. Crozer Griffith for Clinical Medicine, Dr. J. Montgomery Baldy for Gynecology, Dr. A. W. Watson for the Throat and Nose, and Dr. George E. de Schweinitz for Diseases of the Eye. Dr. J. Madison Taylor for Diseases of Children, Harris A. Slocum for Gynecology, and Benjamin Lee for Orthopædics— although Dr. Lee withdrew later—were the additions of 1892-3; and those of the following year were: Dr. Thomas Neilson for Genito-Urinary Diseases, Dr. Wharton Sinkler for Nervous Diseases, Dr. Ralph W. Seiss for the Ear, and Dr. W. J. Taylor for Orthopædic Surgery. In 1895, when Dr. Simes became emeritus professor, the faculty had been increased so as to number thirty-five professors and forty auxiliary instructors. Those added in that year were: Dr. Lewis H. Adler, Jr., for Diseases of the Rectum, Dr. Harrison Allen for the Throat and Nose, Dr. Max J. Stern for Operative and Clinical Surgery, Dr. J. Abbott Cantrell for Diseases of the Skin, Dr. Edward Martin for Genito-Urinary Surgery, and Dr. Orville Horwitz for the same subject. Dr. Horwitz, however, resigned the next year. In 1896-7 there were several accessions, and Dr. Van Harlingen was made emeritus professor; Dr. Charles W. Burr was made professor of Diseases of the Mind and Nervous System; Dr. Howard F. Hansell, of Diseases of the Eye; Dr. James K. Young, of Orthopædic Surgery; Dr. David D. Stewart, of Diseases of the Stomach and Intestines; Dr. A. A. Eshner, of Clinical Medicine; Drs. Walter J. Freeman and E. L. Vansant, of Diseases of the Throat and Nose, and Dr. Judson Daland, professor of Diseases of the Chest.

The present Faculty consists of the following: J. Solis-Cohen, M. D., Emeritus Professor of Diseases of the Throat; Charles H. Burnett, M. D., Emeritus Professor of Diseases of the Ear; Charles B. Nancrede, M. D., Emeritus Professor of General and Orthopædic Surgery; George C. Harlan, M. D., Emeritus Professor of Diseases of the Eye; J. Henry C. Simes, M. D., Emeritus Professor of Genito-Urinary and Venereal Diseases; Arthur Van Harlingen, M. D., Emeritus Professor of Diseases of the Skin; John B. Roberts, M. D., Professor of Anatomy and Surgery; Charles K. Mills, M. D., Professor of Diseases of the Mind and Nervous System; Henry Leffmann, M. D., Professor of Clinical Chemistry and Hygiene; B. F. Baer, M. D., Professor of Gynecology; Lewis W. Steinbach, M. D., Professor of Operative and Clinical Surgery; Thomas J. Mays, M. D., Professor of Diseases of the Chest and of Experimental Therapeutics; H. Augustus Wilson, M. D., Professor of General and Orthopædic Surgery; Edward Jackson, M. D., Professor of Diseases of the Eye; Solomon Solis-Cohen, M. D., Professor of Clinical Medicine and Therapeutics; B. Alexander Randall, M. D., Professor of Diseases of the Ear; Edward P. Davis, M. D., Professor of Obstetrics and Diseases of Infancy; Thomas G. Morton, M. D., Professor of Orthopædic Surgery; Thomas S. K. Morton, M. D., Professor of Clinical Surgery; Samuel D. Risley, M. D., Professor of Diseases of the Eye; Arthur W. Watson, M. D., Professor of Diseases of the Nose and Throat; J. P. Crozer Griffith, M. D., Professor of Clinical Medicine; J. Montgomery Baldy, M. D., Professor of Gynecology; George E. de Schweinitz, M. D., Professor of Diseases of the Eye; John Madison Taylor, M. D., Professor of Diseases of Children; Harris A. Slocum, M. D., Professor of Gynecology; Thomas R. Neilson, M. D., Professor of Genito-Urinary Surgery; Ralph W. Seiss, M. D., Professor of Diseases of the Ear; Lewis J. Adler, Jr., M. D., Professor of Diseases of the Rectum; Max J. Stern, M. D., Professor of Operative and Clinical Surgery; J. Abbott Cantrell, M. D., Professor of Diseases of the Skin; Edward Martin, M. D., Professor of Genito-Urinary Surgery; Howard F. Hansell, M. D., Professor of Diseases of the Eye; James K. Young, M. D., Professor of Orthopædic Surgery; David D. Stewart, M. D., Professor of Diseases of the Stomach and Intestines; Augustus A. Eshner, M. D., Professor of Clinical Medicine; Walter J. Freeman, M. D., Professor of Diseases of the Throat and Nose; Eugene L. Vansant, M. D., Professor of Diseases of the Throat and Nose; Judson Daland, M. D., Professor of Diseases of the Chest; Assinell Hewson, M. D., Professor of Anatomy; Joseph S. Gibbs, M. D., Professor of Diseases of the Throat and Nose; T. B. Schneideman, M. D., Professor of Diseases of the Eye; G. Hudson Makuen, M. D., Professor of Defects of Speech; Henry R. Wharton, M. D., Lecturer on the Surgical Diseases of Children; Charles P. Noble, M. D., Lecturer on Gynecology; Collier L. Bower, M. D., Adjunct Professor of Clinical and Operative Surgery; John T. Carpenter, Jr., M. D., Adjunct Professor of Diseases of the Eye; Frank W. Talley, M. D., Adjunct Professor of Gynecology; James Thorington, M. D., Adjunct Professor of Diseases of the Eye; William H. Wells, M. D., Adjunct Professor of Obstetrics and Diseases of Infancy; Clarence A. Veasey, M. D., Adjunct Professor of Diseases of the Eye; Herbert D. Pease, M. D., Adjunct Professor of Bacteriology; J. D. Moore, M. D., Adjunct Professor of Diseases of the Rectum; David Riesman, M. D., Adjunct Professor of Clinical Medicine and

Therapeutics; Hilary M. Christian, M. D., Adjunct Professor of Genito-Urinary Surgery; A. O. J. Kelly, M. D., Adjunct Professor of Pathology; J. Torrance Rugh, M. D., Adjunct Professor of Orthopædic Surgery, and Anna M. Fullerton, M. D., Associate in Surgery. The instructors are: J. William McConnell, M. D., Instructor in Nervous Diseases and Electro-Therapeutics; L. J. Hammond, M. D., Instructor in Diseases of the Throat and Nose; W. A. N. Dorland, M. D., Instructor in Gynecology; Edward W. Stevens, M. D., Instructor in Diseases of the Eye; Morris B. Miller, M. D., Instructor in Surgery; Elizabeth R. Bundy, M. D., Instructor in Nervous Diseases and Electro-Therapeutics; Theodore A. Erck, M. D., Instructor in Gynecology; George E. Stout, M. D., Instructor in Diseases of the Ear; Henrietta Dougherty, M. D., Instructor in Diseases of the Ear; Archibald G. Thomson, M. D., Instructor in Operative Ophthalmology; Florence Mayo, M. D., Instructor in Diseases of the Eye; James H. McKee, M. D., Instructor in Diseases of Children; John Lindsay, M. D., Instructor in Genito-Urinary Surgery; Bertha Lewis, M. D., Instructor in Orthopædic Surgery; Philip Fischelis, M. D., Instructor in Diseases of the Throat and Nose; John H. Gibbon, M. D., Instructor in Surgery; W. M. Sweet, M. D., Instructor in Diseases of the Eye; J. W. H. Rhein, M. D., Instructor in Neuropathology; Wilson Bowers, M. D., Instructor in Diseases of the Throat and Nose; Frank Woodbury, M. D., Instructor in Diseases of the Throat and Nose; Kate W. Baldwin, M. D., Instructor in Diseases of the Throat and Nose; Truman Augé, M. D., Instructor in Clinical Medicine; Jay F. Schamberg, M. D., Instructor in Dermatology; Helen Murphy, M. D., Instructor in Diseases of the Eye; Philip R. Cleaver, M. D., Instructor in Diseases of the Rectum; A. F. Witmer, M. D., Instructor in Diseases of the Mind and Nervous System; B. F. R. Clark, M. D., Instructor in Diseases of the Throat and Nose; W. S. Shimer, M. D., Instructor in Diseases of the Ear; Maurice A. Bunce, M. D., Instructor in Clinical Medicine; Howard Reed, M. D., Instructor in Orthopædic Surgery; Joseph I. Smith, M. D., Instructor in Clinical Medicine; William G. Spiller, M. D., Instructor in Diseases of the Mind and Nervous System; Mary A. Schively, M. D., Instructor in Neuropathology; George C. Küsel, M. D., Instructor in Diseases of the Throat and Nose; A. A. Stevens, M. D., Instructor in Clinical Medicine; Miss J. M. Ward, M. D., Instructor in Massage; and clinical assistants in all departments to the number of sixty, all but four of whom are graduates in medicine. The annual average attendance of physicians is now above one hundred, the exact number of 1896 being 117, about half of whom were from Pennsylvania. Its clinical service, in its own hospital, averages about 18,000 new cases annually. The Polyclinic is distinguished among Philadelphia schools for exceptional advantages. It is really a great hospital elaborately equipped for personal, clinical, specialist instruction in the midst of patients. As its services are designed for the poor, it also thus becomes one of the greatest of the city's medical charities. Its hospital service is supplemented by its dispensary, which had 77,000 visits in 1896, and its Training School for Nurses has already graduated nine students. The Polyclinic, significantly situated as it is, almost equidistant from the three great men's colleges—those of the University, Jefferson and the Medico-Chirurgical—is a complement to them and a bond of union between them, while its abundant facilities for women students make it a helpful coadjutor of the Woman's College, on North College avenue, in the northern part of the city. It thus occupies a keystone place in the medical education of Philadelphia. The Polyclinic is the crowning type of the present period—a specialist's school in a period characterized by the increasing subdivisions of the field once covered by the general practitioner, and yet a school by which the general practitioner is kept in touch with the various specialties.

These great schools are the centers of power in Philadelphia's vast ranks of conservative medicine. Through them the city has always exerted its greatest influence upon the medical profession, and some of their professorships are everywhere acknowledged to be among the first prizes and honors the medical world has to offer. Each has its own mission and character; and from them in a large degree the medical societies take their tone. With them the hospitals and dispensaries are largely colaborers, and to them are in many cases tributary. The colleges have undoubtedly been most largely instrumental, during the present period, in founding hospitals and dispensaries. This, it may be said, has been done from motives of self-interest, but the interest of the highest type of medical school is undoubtedly identical, from a sanitary standpoint, with that of the community at large.

It is not the purpose here to consider those semi-medical institutions—dental, pharmaceutical and the like—of which Philadelphia has such excellent examples, but, although this is a city of conservative and what is called regular medicine, and but one other system of medical tenets has gained any appreciable constituency, no history of medical development, in the present period especially, can overlook the growth of the homeopathic institution known as the Hahnemann Medical College. This, with its hospital and other fine buildings, facing both Broad and Fifteenth streets, above Race, has a faculty of thirty-six professors, instructors and demonstrators, annually instructing about 258 students. The institution embraces five large buildings. The college proper, fronting on Broad street, is one of the numerous attractive structures in the region just north of the City Hall. It contains "a large anatomical amphitheater and three lecture rooms, a well-lighted dissecting room, large laboratories for microscopic work in Biology, Histology, Pathology and Bacteriology; a large room for manual practice in Bandaging, Application of Surgical Dressings, and Surgical Operations on the Cadaver; a smaller room for manual practice in Obstetrics; a chemical laboratory; the College Museum, with its thousands of selected specimens, and the College Library of over 15,000 volumes, besides other apartments for the use of the students and teachers. The next building of the group is known as Clinical Hall. This structure is designed to accommodate the immense out-patient service of the institution, amounting to about one hundred new patients daily the year round. Besides the general reception and assignment rooms, there are waiting-rooms and examination and prescribing rooms for each and every department of the clinical service, each one being specially arranged and equipped for the particular work of the department it is intended to accommodate. Then there are six special clinic-rooms, in which as many clinics can be in progress at one time. Each room accommodates a small sub-class of the students engaged in examining and treating patients, under the instruction and supervision of the various clinical professors, while at the top of the building there is provided one of the most comfortable and best adapted clinical amphitheaters in America, with a seating capacity of nearly four hundred, and communicating with the anæsthetizing and recovery rooms and with the general wards of the hospital. The basement of the Clinical Hall contains the heat, light and motor plant of the entire institution. The remaining three buildings, the largest fronting on Fifteenth street, constitute the hospital proper, comprising the receiving wards, the administrative offices, resident physician's office, private operating rooms and chapel, small wards for special classes of patients, private rooms for pay patients, nurses' rooms, etc. The entire hospital contains two hundred beds," and averages about 28,000 cases of all kinds annually. This concise description shows that the adherents of homeopathy in Philadelphia have as excellent educational facilities, in proportion to their numbers, as have those of regular medicine; especially since clinical instruction in such hospitals as the Pennsylvania and Philadelphia are free to their students. Over 2,300 students have been graduated since 1849. The College requires a four years' course. Its faculty consists of: Pemberton Dudley, M. D., Professor of Institutes of Medicine and Hygiene; Charles M. Thomas, M. D., Professor of Ophthalmology and Otology; John E. James, M. D., Professor of Gynecology; Charles Mohr, M. D., Professor of Materia Medica and Therapeutics; William C. Goodno, M. D., Professor of the Practice of Medicine; William H. Bigler, M. D., Professor of Physiology and Pediatrics; William B. Van Lennep, M. D., Professor of Surgery; Herbert L. Northrop, M. D., Professor of Anatomy; Charles Platt, Ph. D., F. C. S., Professor of Chemistry and Toxicology; Edward Mercer, M. D., Professor of Obstetrics; Rufus B. Weaver, M. D., Professor of Regional and Applied Anatomy and Demonstrator; Erving Melville Howard, M. D., Associate Professor of Materia

Medica; Oliver S. Haines, M. D., Clinical Professor of Medicine; Edward R. Snader, M. D., Professor of Physical Diagnosis; Clarence Bartlett, M. D., Professor of Neurology and Medical Seminology; P. Sharples Hall, M. D., Professor of Pathology and Director of Histological Laboratories; William Shippen Roney, A. M., Attorney at Law, Lecturer on Medical Jurisprudence; Edward M. Gramm, M. D., Lecturer on Dermatology; Frederick W. Messerve, M. D., Lecturer and Demonstrator in Histology and Instructor in Ophthalmology; Landreth W. Thompson, M. D., Lecturer on Minor Surgery and Emergencies; Carl V. Vischer, M. D., Lecturer on Surgical Pathology; Isaac G. Shellcross, M. D., Lecturer on Rhinology and Laryngology and Clinical Instructor; Thomas Lindsley Bradford, M. D., Librarian and Lecturer on History of Medicine; Willett Enos Rotzell, M. D., Lecturer on Botany and Zoölogy; Duncan Campbell, M. D., Lecturer on Medical Terminology; Halton I. Jessup, M. D., Lecturer on Ophthalmology and Otology and Clinical Instructor; Isaac G. Smedley, M. D., Lecturer on Gynecology and Clinical Instructor; J. Percy Moore, Ph. D., Instructor in Biology; Weston D. Bayley, M. D., Lecturer on Insanity and Clinical Instructor in Neurology; William W. Speakman, M. D., Clinical Instructor in Otology; Leon P. Ashcraft, M. D., Lecturer on Venereal Diseases; Frank C. Benson, Jr., M. D., Demonstrator of Surgery; Thomas H. Carmichael, M. D., Lecturer on Pharmaceutics; Raymond J. Harris, M. D., Assistant in Chemistry; Walter W. Maires, M. D., Demonstrator of Histology; and Alfred Cookman, M. D., Demonstrator of Pathology. Its student constituency, like that of other colleges in Philadelphia, is about half from Pennsylvania, but it also has large numbers from New Jersey and New York, and the rest are well scattered over this and even other lands. Some post-graduate work is done and its last class of graduates numbered thirty-seven. It has now entered upon its fiftieth year.

Besides these institutions, there are one other Homeopathic school and several societies and hospitals, with the usual nurse and dispensary service. The Philadelphia Post-Graduate School of Homeopathics, at 613-15 Spring Garden street, was opened in

March, 1891, and now has a faculty of fourteen, of which Dr. J. T. Kent is dean. Besides the old Hahnemann Alumni Association, organized in 1857, there is the Germantown Society; the Philadelphia County Society, organized in 1886, and now having 266 members; the Twenty-third Ward Society; the Clinical Society, and several clubs. The Homeopathic Hospital, beside the Hahnemann, was opened in 1871; the Children's Hospital was opened in 1877, with 60 beds; the Woman's Hospital was opened in 1884, with 75 beds; and St. Luke's, with 11 beds, was opened in 1896. There are also four independent dispensaries, and five journals published. This is the result of sixty-six years of Homeopathy in Philadelphia, the first physician to locate here being Dr. George Butts, who came in 1831. Two years later Dr. Butts was joined by his friend, Dr. Constantine Hering, who, in 1848, with Dr. Jacob Jeans and Dr. Walter Williamson, started the first permanent Homeopathic Medical College in this country. This Homeopathic Medical College began its first course October 15, 1848, at the rear of 627 Arch street, with 15 students. A rupture occurred in the organization in 1867, and Dr. Hering, leading the seceders, founded Hahnemann Medical College on July 17 of that year. As Hahnemann survived, and was the successor of the first institution, it now claims to be the oldest medical college in the world teaching the system of treatment originated by Samuel Hahnemann. Its dean, Dr. Pemberton Dudley, was president of the National Homeopathic Society during the current year.

Next in importance to the colleges come the medical societies. This is true, not only locally, but also nationally, and even in worldwide relations. Indeed, it is probable that Philadelphia has influenced the medical world as much through her societies as through her institutions of learning, although their spheres of action are so different as hardly to be comparable. This has been done chiefly through the two great representative medical societies of the city. All the others are sectional, either in location, aim, constituency, or some other feature. These two societies have practically gone on side by side for over a hundred years (f), and during

---

(f) The old Philadelphia Medical Society must always be considered the County Society under another form.

all that time have served as a sort of senate and house of representatives to the profession of Philadelphia, except that the members of the senate, in this case, are almost invariably members of the house, and that between the two bodies there does not necessarily exist any community of action. The County Medical Society is the popular body, to which any reputable physician of the regular school, in its territory, may be elected, and, in a sense, it is also the greatest of the societies, because it is the sole representative of the physicians of the city in both the state and national bodies. The College of Physicians, on the other hand, has no connection with any other society, is sufficient unto itself in that respect, and is practically, though not formally, a limited and somewhat exclusive body, to which, with very rare exceptions, all the greatest names in the city's medical history have belonged. The County Society is purely a society; the College of Physicians is a great institution also, whose professional treasures, accumulating generation after generation within its ivy-grown walls at Thirteenth and Locust streets, invest it with an interest which, to the cultured physician, is almost sacred. In the hall of the College of Physicians the County Society holds its meetings, as well as the Academy of Surgery, the Pathological, Neurological, Obstetrical, and Pediatric societies. Both the College and the County Society, so far as national medicine is concerned, have always caused Philadelphia to be acknowledged as the leader of the conservatives, but, locally, the County Society leads the liberal wing and the College of Physicians is and always has been the conservative fortress. The County Society, since it became the sole representative of the profession in the national society, has been the more actively practical body, the College of Physicians the more purely scientific. The County Society, in recent years, has been the more usual leader of movements, while the College of Physicians, because of its principles and traditions, has been the main determiner of standards in most of the professional questions that have arisen within the last century. The relative positions of the two bodies and the course of events which determined them belong to the present period of the medical history of Philadelphia, and as they are chiefly concerned with the rise of the County Society they will be considered in that connection. A glance at the history of the College of Physicians will first be necessary to an understanding of these events, and of the entire course of medical history in Philadelphia since the Revolution.

The College of Physicians has had, since its formation in 1787, the following presidents: Dr. John Redman, elected in 1787; Dr. William Shippen, elected in 1805; Dr. Adam Kuhn, elected in 1809; Dr. Thomas Parke, in 1818; Dr. Thomas C. James, in 1835; Dr. Thomas T. Hewson, in 1835, also; Dr. George B. Wood, in 1848; Dr. W. S. W. Ruschenberger, in 1879; Dr. Alfred Stillé, in 1883; Dr. Samuel Lewis, in 1884; Dr. J. M. Da Costa, in 1884, also; Dr. S. Weir Mitchell, in 1886; Dr. D. Hayes Agnew, in 1889; Dr. Mitchell again, in 1892; and Dr. Da Costa, the present incumbent, again in 1895. Of these distinguished men some accounts have been given elsewhere in this volume, excepting those still living and Drs. Ruschenberger and Lewis, the former of whom has written the only history of the college, and the latter of whom, in the gift of the Lewis Library, has been one of the greatest benefactors of the institution. Dr. Ruschenberger was born in 1807 and died in 1895, after a valuable service of nearly sixty-nine years in the United States Navy, in which he bore the relative rank of commodore at his decease. He was a native of New Jersey and a graduate of the University of Pennsylvania. His most notable work was the organization of the Naval Laboratory. Dr. Lewis died in 1890 at the age of seventy-seven, desiring evidently that his library should be his only monument, as he requested that no memoir of his life should be written. He was born in Barbadoes, W. I., in 1813, and graduated in Edinburgh in 1840, returning to Philadelphia thereafter to engage in practice. He was well known and successful in his profession, but his love for books and his passion for their collection were his most striking characteristics, and resulted in the gift of the Lewis Library. The nucleus of this superb collection of books and journals, now numbering about 15,000 volumes, was formed on February 27, 1864, when Dr. Lewis presented to the College his library, consisting of more than 2,500

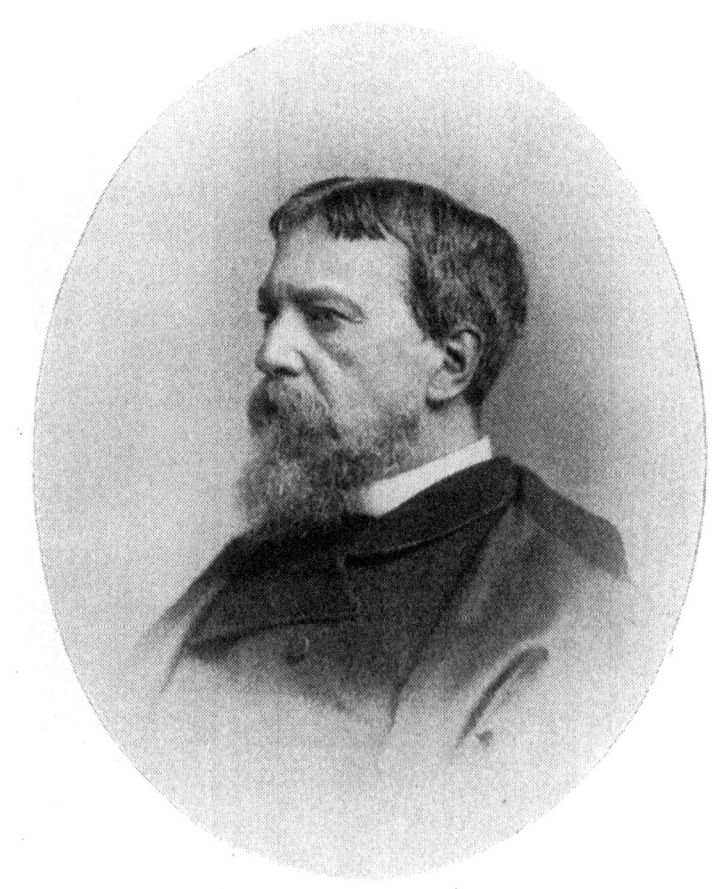

S. WIER MITCHELL.

volumes. Although the gift was without conditions, it was resolved, on motion of Dr. Alfred Stillé, then chairman of the Library Committee, that the books "shall be preserved as a separate collection, under the name of the Lewis Library." From that time until his death, nearly thirty years later, Dr. Lewis continued to add to his collection. As he was thoroughly versed in ancient and modern medical literature, and made his purchases with the most discriminating judgment, the library which bears his name is probably unequaled by any other medical library of similar size in the world. The last two presidents are still living and are too well and widely known to need more than mention. No one but must instantly admit that of all the names of the living physicians of Philadelphia, the fame of these two extends the most widely both within and without the profession; the one as a great physician and teacher; the other great in original scientific research, and so favorably known as poet and novelist as to have been described as succeeding to the mantle of the "Autocrat of the Breakfast Table."

These executives have presided in different places. The first meetings were held in the old "Academy"—the forerunner of the University—at Fourth and Arch streets, and in 1791 a room was secured in the hall of the American Philosophical Society, which was used for over fifty-three years. In 1845 the College found new quarters in a hall at the southeast corner of Fifth and Library streets, which was used until 1852, when "the picture house of the Pennsylvania Hospital," containing the celebrated painting of Benjamin West and located at 820 Spruce street, was rented. These experiences brought up the question of an independent permanent home, and in 1849 a building fund was begun. In 1860 the lot at Thirteenth and Locust streets was purchased, and in March, 1863, the present building, except the third story, which was built in 1886 chiefly for the Mütter Museum, was opened for meetings. It is now a three-story brick structure fronting on Thirteenth street, where the door opens into vestibules, on the left of which are the janitor's rooms and those of the Nurses' Directory, and on the right a stack-room for books and a room used for meetings of various societies. The accumulation of the library has grown so great that the entire building, except half of the first floor and all of the third, which contains the Mütter Museum, is given over to its books, and other collections. The second floor is the main one. The south side is divided into two large rooms, one known as the General Library and the other as the Lewis Library. The walls of both are banked with cases, portraits, curios and busts of medical celebrities. Leading from the General Library to the north end is a smaller room—the S. D. Gross Library. It is in the north room of the second floor that the meetings are held. The "Hall" contains an interesting collection of life-sized portraits of Rush, Redman, Shippen, Morgan and others, down to Agnew, Stillé, Da Costa and Mitchell of the present day, while in its vestibule are commemorative tablets, busts of Gross and Pancoast, portraits of Thomas Cadwalader, Oliver Wendell Holmes and others, and an excellent reproduction of Rembrandt's "The Lesson in Anatomy." This is the home of a medical library, second only, as to the quantity and quality of its books, to that of the Surgeon-General's office at Washington, and of an ancient society that stands unique among all the medical organizations of America.

The membership now includes 319 Fellows, of whom the following constitute the present officers: President, Dr. J. M. Da Costa; vice-president, Dr. John Ashhurst, Jr.; censors, Drs. Alfred Stillé, William F. Norris, Arthur V. Meigs and Richard A. Cleeman; secretary, Dr. Thomas R. Neilson; treasurer, Dr. Henry M. Fisher; honorary librarian, Dr. Frederick P. Henry; councillors, Drs. Henry R. Wharton, Frederick A. Packard, G. E. de Schweinitz, Thomas S. K. Morton, Charles W. Dulles and John K. Mitchell.

The nine committees are as follows, the first name mentioned being that of the chairman: Drs. G. G. Davis, Damaso T. Lainé and Thompson S. Westcott, on Publication; Drs. George C. Harlan, Charles A. Oliver, Charles B. Penrose, F. X. Dercum, William J. Taylor, and the honorary librarian, *ex officio*, on the Library; Drs. John H. Brinton, Harrison Allen, and George McClellan, on Mütter Museum; Drs. J. Ewing Mears, Morris J. Lewis, William Barton

Hopkins, J. K. Mitchell, and Caspar Morris, on the Hall; Drs. Wharton Sinkler, James E. Wilson, and James V. Ingham, on the Directory for Nurses; Drs. I. Minis Hays, Charles S. Wurts, William Thomson, and the president and treasurer, on Finance; Drs. Barton C. Hirst, E. E. Montgomery and John B. Shober, on the William F. Jenks Prize (g); Drs. J. Madison Taylor, Louis Starr, Robert G. Le Conte, Henry Morris, and the president, on Entertainments; Drs. H. C. Wood, Roland G. Curtin, John B. Roberts, Edward Jackson, and Henry W. Cattell, on the Alvarenga Prize. The chairmen and clerks of sections are: Drs. William F. Norris and H. F. Hansell, on Ophthalmology; Drs. Charles H. Burnett and Eugene L. Vansant, on Otology and Laryngology; Drs. W. W. Keen and Alfred C. Wood, on General Surgery; Drs. Barton C. Hirst and John B. Shober, on Gynecology; and Drs. James C. Wilson and S. M. Hamill, on General Medicine. In direct charge of the Library is Mr. Charles Perry Fisher, with an assistant librarian, Miss M. C. Rutherford. The public are admitted to the library through the introduction of members. This form of organization is the result of two important changes, since the adoption of the constitution. The first of these occurred in 1834, when the charter was made to supersede the constitution, and the second in 1893, when sections were introduced, one of the most important movements in the history of the institution, and due largely to the suggestion of the president, Dr. Mitchell. The work of the College and its general position as the chief representative of the profession of Philadelphia, up to the time that the County Medical Society was made exclusive representative in the national society, has been suggested in earlier chapters. One of the most important works in which it participated was the formation of a national Pharmacopœia. In this enterprise it persisted from 1788 until the publication of the volume in 1831. The work on the Pharmacopœia occupied many of its ablest members during that time, those most

---

(g) The W. F. Jenks Memorial Fund is in the hands of four trustees: Dr. James V. Ingham, Charles S. Wurts, Horace Y. Evans and the chairman of the Finance Committee.

closely connected with it being Drs. Hewson, Wood and Bache. "The founding and publishing of this very important work," says Dr. Ruschenberger, "is ascribed very largely, if not exclusively, to the enterprise of the College of Physicians." Out of this, as is well known, grew the Dispensatory of the United States, by Drs. Wood and Bache, and the College was equally prominent in later revisions. Its museum, one of the finest collections of physiological and pathological specimens in this country, was begun in 1849, and received its greatest accession in 1863 with Dr. Mütter's collection. This collection and the library and its accompaniments are to medicine in Philadelphia what the Academy of Natural Sciences, the Philosophical Society, and the Historical Society are to general scientific culture, and its present constant accumulation gives promise of a remarkable future. The Directory for Nurses was the result of a suggestion of Dr. Mitchell, who has been one of the most effective powers in the recent growth of the College. This was established in 1882, and at the end of four years the number of applications for nurses filed averaged considerably above a thousand annually. In 1883 Dr. Mitchell gave the College $5,000 as a permanent entertainment fund, and one of the first uses of it was the celebration of the centennial anniversary in January, 1887, the chief features of which were a "Commemorative Address" by Dr. Mitchell, "Reminiscences of the College", by Dr. Alfred Stillé, "An Account of the Institution of the College of Physicians" by Dr. Ruschenberger, and an elaborate program of addresses, toasts and responses. The presidency of Dr. Mitchell was the beginning of a new era in the life of the institution. Recently, under Dr. Da Costa's influence, the membership has been considerably increased, and the greatest growth of the past decade has been in the development of the sections. But these marks of progress in the career of the society are not sufficient, in any measure, to indicate the present power of the College as a framer of professional standards, or its general influence, here and elsewhere. It has been a quiet, unostentatious force in conservative medicine in this country for over a century. If it has been somewhat less active in popular movements in recent years, it has not been less influential in medical thought, and only needs the adjunct of a journal to make that fact more evident to the profession at large. If its library is the memory of the medical profession of Philadelphia, its journal would be its not less distinguished current thought.

The rise of the Philadelphia County Medical Society may be dated from June 3, 1874, when it became the sole representative of the profession of Philadelphia in the American Medical Association, by an amendment to the plan of organization of the latter, making its constituency thereafter composed of state, district and county societies. This action was merely a fulfillment of the original plan of the national body, which intended its representation to be territorial, rather than institutional, as compromise had compelled it to be ever since its organization. It will be remembered that this point was discussed in the very earliest meetings for the organization of the national society, and it will also be recalled that Philadelphia furnished the advocates for institutional representation; and Dr. N. S. Davis and his New York (State) constituency, those for the territorial, the latter aiming to have medical organization somewhat like that of our governmental structure. For more than twenty-seven years. Philadelphia was successful in upholding institutional representation, i. e., representation from societies, colleges, hospitals and dispensaries, rather than from counties and districts, but the sentiment of the country, stimulated by the perseverance of Dr. Davis in the original plan, made the adoption of the latter only a question of time. It was the object of democracy in medical organization, to secure an organ of expression of the American medical profession, but this did not imply that there was not a proper field for independent organization outside of it, although that idea, now fast disappearing, involved the situation for some time. The question has always been one of professional democracy and exclusiveness, and it has been so mingled with the allied questions of the cities versus the country, the East versus the West, and the specialist versus the general practitioner, that unless one keeps all these antitheses in mind the movement seems inexplicable. It required a long struggle to achieve the victory of democracy, and Philadelphia was the chief battlefield during twenty-seven years and over. Fortunately, the question seems practically settled by the recognition that the national body and its constituents have each a field of their own, in no way conflicting with those of the independent, specialist, scientific, social, or sectional societies, in medicine, that have been and will be found desirable; for there is a territory that only such bodies can cover. As memories of the struggle fade, the adjustments which have certainly been affected by them will undoubtedly be restored, and every branch of the profession receive its due consideration.

It will be of interest to trace the development of these questions, since they raised the County Medical Society to its present position, and caused within it one of the greatest struggles in the history of Philadelphia medicine, whose fading memories had at one time something of the sensitiveness of those of the late Civil War. It was a struggle, the effects of which were felt throughout the medical world. The Philadelphia County Medical Society is, virtually, though not actually, the oldest medical society in the city, for from the time Morgan organized the first Philadelphia medical society down to the present, there has been almost without cessation a popular society of which the great majority of the physicians, great and small, alike, were members. Up to 1847 these successive organizations were the popular discursive bodies of the profession, with hardly the dignity of the College of Physicians, although comprising most of the fellows of the College in their membership. In 1848 the County Society was founded. Its origin, to use the words of one of its former presidents, Dr. William Mayburry, can be traced "to the reflex influence which the institution of the American Medical Association exerted on the professional mind of the country." It was the purpose of some of the far-seeing founders of the latter organization, notably of Dr. N. S. Davis, that its delegates should be solely composed of members of the State and County societies, and this scheme was undoubtedly entertained by some of the founders of the Philadelphia Society. The prospect of such an alliance imparted new dignity and activity to the County Society, to which it was evident that all vital professional questions, such as those relating to ethics, the admission of women, and the like, must sooner or later be submitted, and through which all great movements of medical progress initiated by the national society would soon be represented in this territory. From that time until 1874, when the project was realized, was a long period of waiting, and during it all the most serious leader of opposition was the College of Physicians, supported by the other medical institutions of the city. The College of Physicians, by natural position, and at times by definitely adopted policy, performed those public offices of watchfulness over State medicine that are now more naturally undertaken by County and National bodies, so that the alliance of County, State, and Nation was suggestive of local rights giving way to federation. In 1874 the inevitable was accepted, and all Philadelphia institutions ceased to be represented in the national body as institutions, and their members, for the most part already members of the County Society, began to devote more attention to the work of that organization. They were not slow to appreciate the importance of a society through which alone a national representation could be secured. This change in the mode of representation in the national society was not secured without some compromises and conciliations to such leaders as required them. That they were wisely made is shown by the remarkable unity of the Congress of 1876, under the leadership of the elder Gross. For about ten years this close union of the profession in the movements of the national body, through the County Society, was productive of great mutual advantage to the profession of the city, and that of the nation. Philadelphia's influence upon the profession at large was, during this period, worthy of comparison with that of the brightest days of her history.

But the relations of the County Medical Society toward a certain portion of the profession were somewhat strained, on account of the various questions already mentioned, and it only needed the loss of the active and conciliatory influence of such a wise leader as Gross to precipitate a struggle. Nearly every question that has arisen in the present period—that of the code, the admission of women, and others—were in active discussion during the latter part of the decade mentioned. Trouble arose in connection with the first regular International Medical Congress held in the United States. It will be recalled that the Congress of 1876 in Philadelphia was not a meeting of the International Medical Congress proper, but the latter body did propose to hold its first meeting in the United States at Washington, in 1887, the same year, by the way, that the College of Physicians celebrated its centennial anniversary.

At the Washington meeting of the American Medical Association, in 1884, its president, suggested that an invitation be extended to the meeting in Copenhagen to hold the ninth International Medical Congress in the United States at Washington, in 1887. In accordance with this suggestion, it was decided that a committee be appointed by the president to give the invitation and, in case of its acceptance, that it should "proceed to act as an executive committee, with full power to fix the time and to make all necessary and suitable arrangements for the meeting of such congress, and to solicit funds for that purpose," and that it "have power to add to its membership, to perfect its organization," and all that was necessary thereto. President H. F. Campbell, of Georgia, appointed Dr. Austin Flint, Sr., of New York; Dr. I. Minis Hays, of Philadelphia; Dr. L. A. Sayre, of New York; Dr. C. Johnson, of Baltimore; Dr. George Englemann, of St. Louis; Dr. J. M. Brown, U. S. N.; and the president himself was added by vote, making eight members. The invitation was accepted; the committee added between fifteen and twenty prominent members of the profession to its list, and a meeting was held November 29, 1884, in Washington. A sub-committee of the original eight presented an outline plan of organization and rules similar to those governing previous congresses, the selection of names being based entirely on their reputation both at home and abroad, without regard to sectional or society representation. Membership depended upon invitation of the Executive Committee. This plan was, in some measure, modified so as to secure society and sectional representation, and a slightly wider representation of officers and readers of papers. The committee adjourned, after having chosen the following officers: Dr. Austin Flint, Sr., of New York, for president; Drs. Alfred Stillé of Philadelphia, Dr. Henry I. Bowditch of Boston, and Dr. R. P. Howard of Montreal, vice-presidents; Dr. John S. Billings, U. S. A., secretary-general; Dr. J. M. Brown, U. S. N., treasurer; and an executive committee, composed of the president, secretary-general, and treasurer; and Dr. I. Minis Hays of Philadelphia, Dr. A. Jacobi of New York, Dr. Christopher Johnson of Baltimore, and Dr. S. C. Busey of Washington. This executive committee was to proceed to complete the work of organization, and the General Committee was to meet some time before the New Orleans meeting of the national society. "The Executive Committee, however," says an editorial in the *Journal of the American Medical Association*, "regarded their work as so far advanced as to render a meeting of the General Committee in New Orleans unnecessary, and proceeded to the publication of their work as far as completed. This, we think, was an unwise step. We think the General Committee should have assembled at New Orleans and reported its action to the Association before its formal publication to the world. It would have afforded an opportunity for conference and adjustment of differences at once, and would have avoided the charge of having ignored the body from which its existence and all its powers had been derived. If an error, however, it was certainly one of judgment and not of design. Regarding the power conferred upon the committee by the resolutions we have quoted, as ample and unreserved, the members were simply intent on the early and efficient discharge of the duties imposed on them, without unnecessary expenditure of time and money. The idea that the members of the committee having charge of the work of organizing the International Congress had acted from any other than an honest desire to execute the trust committed to them to the best of their ability, is without the slightest foundation, and should be discarded by any honorable mind. But it is plainly evident, both from the expressions in a large part of the medical press, and from the sentiments freely expressed in private conversation, as well as publicly, that two important errors had been committed in the work of the committee. The first was committed by the original committee of eight members, appointed at Washington, in the selection of additional members of their own body. Actuated, perhaps, by an injudicious liberality, it is claimed that they included in their selection some who had placed themselves in antagonism to the National and State organizations of the profession, by openly repudiating the national code of ethics, which constitutes the common bond of union for all these organizations. By this step, they placed the American Medical Association, from which the committee had derived all its power, in an inconsistent position, and failed to sustain the large majority of the profession in the state of New York who had faithfully sustained the national code, and maintained their fraternal relations to the national and state organizations of the whole country. The second alleged error consisted simply in a failure on the part of the enlarged committee to appreciate the importance of so distributing the officers of sections as to represent and interest, as far as possible, the members of the profession in all the leading geographical divisions of our country."

Philadelphia was chiefly connected with the second "alleged error," the first one being of concern to New York. In fact, the struggle was primarily one of Philadelphia and New York, leading the great eastern cities, versus the West and the country at large. The editor of *The American Journal of the Medical Sciences*, Dr. I. Minis Hays, represented Philadelphia, or that part of Philadelphia which stood for the dominance of the great cities, in the Executive Committee. This committee claimed that, while they were appointed by the American Medical Association, they were to follow the precedent of the international body, which was a purely scientific one, unconcerned with codes or representation, and that there was a considerable and able minority who were not members of the national society, and could not be ignored. The position, character and ability of Dr. Hays, as well as the striking excellence of the committee's program, led the profession generally to ascribe it to his influence. A single glance at the names enrolled showed an array of the ablest scientific medical men in America, who would be recognized everywhere as eminently suitable delegates to such a congress. But, it is also evident at a glance that these men were largely from Philadelphia and New York and from distinguished circles in those cities. It might have been contended by some that these were the natural places in which to look for America's most distinguished medical men, but the democratic spirit of the American Medical Association manifested itself, demanding that the national body and those in sympathy with it should be the only representatives in the coming congress, and that all sections should be given recognition on the program. The leader in this movement in Philadelphia was Dr. John V. Shoemaker, a member of the faculty of the Medico-Chirurgical College, who had but recently been a participant in the International Congress. At the New Orleans meeting of the national society in 1885, after the program had been practically completed and published, the opposition to it became so formidable that a resolution was passed on April 29, to the effect that the General Committee "be enlarged by the addition of thirty-eight members, one from each State and Territory, the army, the navy, and marine hospital service," and a few days later the General Committee thus to be enlarged was defined as *"the original committee of seven!"* This of course removed all the previous additional members, and made it evident that the offending program should be thoroughly remodeled on the lines above indicated. The result was a wholesale resignation of nearly all those connected with the first program, and a general exodus of many of their sympathizers from any connection with the congress, while the whole affair was looked upon as an unfortunate scandal in the history of the international body. It was a struggle that resulted in the triumph of the principles of the American Medical Association and its claims to represent the profession in this country. The new committee met at once, while at New Orleans, and elected Dr. R. Beverly Cole of San Francisco temporary chairman, and Dr. John V. Shoemaker temporary secretary, and these, with a vice-president, were soon made permanent. Those Philadelphians who became presidents of sections—for there were none among the proposed officers of the Congress—were:

Dr. Henry H. Smith, formerly of the University Medical School; Dr. W. H. Pancoast of the Medico-Chirurgical College, and one other, who soon resigned. The new Executive Committee consisted of Drs. Austin Flint of New York, president; Dr. N. S. Davis of Chicago, secretary-general; Dr. Richard J. Dunglison of Philadelphia, Dr. Henry H. Smith of Philadelphia, Dr. W. H. Pancoast of Philadelphia, Dr. A. B. Arnold of Baltimore, Dr. E. S. F. Arnold of New York, Dr. A. R. Robinson of New York, Dr. J. Lewis Smith of New York, Dr. W. T. Briggs of Nashville, Dr. J. Taft of Cincinnati, Dr. J. P. Gray of Utica, and Dr. S. J. Jones of Chicago. Drs. Smith and Dunglison became respectively permanent chairman and secretary, and, later, Dr. William B. Atkinson of Philadelphia, who has so long served the national society as secretary, was made an associate secretary of the Executive Committee. Overtures were again made to a number of the eminent men, who had withdrawn their support, with a view to their taking part in the program, but these were not successful. The president, Dr. Flint, died before the time for the meeting at Washington arrived, and Dr. N. S. Davis became his successor as chief executive of the Ninth International Medical Congress, the first and only one so far held in the United States. The action of the American Medical Association was naturally resented by the leaders of the profession in Philadelphia, and this resentment was not long in manifesting itself. In October, 1885, nominations for delegates to the Association were made and a copy of the ticket was sent to every member of the society, with the notice of the January meeting. Shortly before this meeting a new ticket was issued, which, at the January meeting, was elected by the overwhelming majority of 169 to 36. The first, or regular, ticket was largely composed of indorsers of the action of the American Medical Association at New Orleans; the second, of those who were "opposed to this action and the dissensions it has engendered in the profession."

On May 4, 1886, when the American Medical Association met at St. Louis, under the presidency of Dr. William Brodie of Detroit, the delegates from the Philadelphia County Medical Society were not permitted to register as such, on the ground that a protest had been filed against their admission. On their inquiring concerning the nature of the protest, they were referred to the Judicial Council. On May 5th a committee of the Philadelphia delegation appeared before the Judicial Council, which allowed but one of its members to testify. No report of the Judicial Council was read at the general meeting of that day, although it was known to have been given to the permanent secretary of the Association. On the same day Dr. John B. Roberts, chairman of the committee of the Philadelphia delegation, was informed by a member of the Judicial Council that this body had decided in favor of the admission of the Philadelphia delegation and that this decision had been handed to President Brodie, to be read at the close of Dr. Senn's address. The Philadelphia delegation was then allowed to register as delegates to the American Medical Association, and did so. On the following day, on motion of Dr. Toner, the chairman of the Judicial Council, the report of that body was referred back for the hearing of further evidence, and "at length, within an hour of the closing of the last session of the annual meeting, a report from the Judicial Council, containing the following remarkable decision, was read:

" 'In the case of the protest again the registration of the delegates from the Philadelphia County Medical Society, which, upon petition, was reopened to admit new testimony, after a long and careful reëxamination, including evidence not before presented, the Judicial Council decide that, notwithstanding the fact that said delegates hold documents usually entitling to registration, it also appeared in evidence that the methods employed at their election were of such an irregular character as to compel their rejection as delegates by the council. The council would also suggest the return of any dues which may have been paid to the treasurer by said delegates. The council also refers the protest, and all the papers accompanying it, to the Philadelphia County Medical Society for adjudication.'"

Dr. John B. Roberts then offered a series of resolutions, containing eight questions concerning the action of the Judicial Council. They were seconded by Dr. Charles K. Mills, and were promptly laid on the table. Whereupon Dr. Roberts resigned the position of secretary of the Section on Anatomy and Surgery for 1887, to which he had recently been elected. Dr. Edward Jackson presented a protest against the action of the Judicial Council, which was signed by Drs. Roberts, Jackson, W. Joseph Hearn, Charles K. Mills, L. D. Judd and R. M. Girvin. The protest was laid on the table.

At a special meeting of the Philadelphia County Medical Society, held May 18, 1886, the delegates of the society to the thirty-seventh annual meeting of the American Medical Association submitted their report, which, being received, the following resolutions were offered by Dr. D. Hayes Agnew, and adopted:

"*Resolved*, That the Philadelphia County Medical Society has learned with surprise of the action of the American Medical Association, at St. Louis, in excluding the duly elected delegates from this society;

"*Resolved*, That, as the subject has been referred back to this society for final action, the legality of said election is hereby reaffirmed, and that, while it would be perfectly right for the delegates to vindicate the validity of their election by a resort to legal measures, yet, in the interest of peace, such action is not urged;

"*Resolved*, That in excluding the delegates from this society the Judicial Council has violated the plain rules of evidence and justice."

This, in brief, is the history of this unfortunate episode. Referring the reader to the admirable report of the delegates for full details of the transaction, it need only be added that the validity of the election of the Philadelphia delegation was affirmed by two eminent authorities on parliamentary law: Col. A. K. McClure and the late Hon. Samuel J. Randall.

This cleavage in the profession was thought, for a time, to be a serious menace to the success of the Congress, and it undoubtedly did interfere with it to some degree; but, on the whole, it was successful. Doubtless, at the time, all acted conscientiously; but few would now deny that the disagreement was a great misfortune, which a little more wisdom might easily have avoided. For a while its effects were very marked, but a decade has passed since then, and Time has shown his usual power in removing obstacles and in smoothing rough places; so that the day may soon come when all traces of the unfortunate difference will have disappeared from the practical life of the profession, if they have not done so already.

The County Society has thus naturally taken the lead in the two great international gatherings. These have been great events in its history, but it has also had a prominent place in all public professional movements by virtue of its connection with the National and State bodies. This connection, too, has been far more intimate than that of almost any other county society in the entire country, because Philadelphia has been so preëminently the home of the national body and of its permanent officers ever since its organization fifty years ago. This has been happily recognized in the celebration here of the semi-centennial jubilee of the national society during 1897. The latter is an event of such recent occurrence, and so identified with the entire profession of the city, that it will be noticed elsewhere in this volume.

The successive presidents of the County Society, since it took that form in 1849, have been as follows: Samuel Jackson, M. D., 1849-52; John F. Lamb, M. D., 1853; Thomas F. Betton, M. D., 1854; D. Francis Condie, M. D., 1855; Wilson Jewell, M. D., 1856; Gouverneur Emerson, M. D., 1857; John Bell, M. D., 1858; Benjamin H. Coates, M. D., 1859; Isaac Remington, M. D., 1860; Joseph Carson, M. D., 1861; Alfred Stillé, M. D., 1862; Samuel D. Gross, M. D., 1863; Lewis P. Gebhard, M. D., 1864; Nathan L. Hatfield, M. D., 1865; William Mayburry, M. D., 1866; Andrew Nebinger, M. D., 1867; George Hamilton, M. D., 1868; William L. Knight, M. D., 1869; William H. Pancoast, M. D., 1870; James Aitken Meigs, M. D., 1871; D. Hayes Agnew, M. D., 1872; William B. Atkinson, M. D., 1873; Washington L. Atlee, M. D., 1874; William Goodell, M. D., 1875; Thomas M. Drysdale, M. D., 1876; Henry H. Smith, M. D., 1877-79; Albert H. Smith, M. D., 1880-81; Horace Y. Evans, M. D., 1882; William M. Welch, M. D., 1883-84; Richard J. Levis, M. D., 1885-86; J. Solis-Cohen, M. D., 1887-88; W. W. Keen, M. D., 1889-90; John B. Roberts, M. D., 1891-92; De Forest Willard, M. D., 1893-94; J. C. Wilson, M. D., 1895-96, and James Tyson, M. D., the present incumbent. The present officers, besides President Tyson, are as follows: Edward Jackson, M. D., first vice-president; S. Solis-Cohen, M. D., second vice-president; Collier L. Bower, M. D., treasurer; John Lindsay, M. D., secretary; Elwood R. Kirby, M. D., assistant secretary; Drs. W. M. Welch (secretary), H. St. Clair Ash, Thomas H. Fenton, F. P. Henry and W. Joseph Hearn, censors; Drs. Henry Beates, Howard F. Hansell, Joseph S. Gibbs, Charles W. Burr and T. Mellor Tyson, directors; and Drs. A. A. Eshner, Thomas G. Ashton and A. O. J. Kelly, committee on publication. The membership of the society now numbers nearly seven hundred, making it by far the largest and most powerful organization in the city.

The American Medical Association is not the only national association that has been organized in Philadelphia. Several others have originated here. The American Surgical Association, founded by Dr. Gross, has already been mentioned. The Association of American Physicians is another, a limited body for "the advancement of scientific and practical medicine," organized largely by those who were not in sympathy with the course taken by the American Medical Association in regard to the Congress of 1887. Its first session was held in 1886, Dr. Francis Delafield of New York and Dr. Wier Mitchell being, respectively, its first and second presidents. It aims to be "an association in which there will be no medical politics and no medical ethics," but one devoted to purely scientific and practical medicine. The Congress of 1876 produced another national society, which was organized in Philadelphia on September 6, of that same year. This was the American Academy of Medicine, the design of which was to draw together those of the profession who were alumni of some classical, scientific or medical institution, and to advocate a higher general education for physicians, preparatory to professional study. Dr. Traill Green was the first president. The present period has been prolific of such movements. Philadelphia has also been the chief headquarters of the State Society, and all movements connected with medical activity in this State, so that the medical history of Pennsylvania must always give its metropolis the very largest predominance.

Societies purely local claim the chief interest, and the present period abounds in these, which are nearly all of a specialist character. There are the Pathological Society, the Obstetrical Society, the Medico-Legal Society, the Neurological Society, the Laryngological Society, the Medical Jurisprudence Society and the Association of Hospital Physicians. Indeed, except the Northern Medical Association, which traces its organization to so ancient a date as December 5, 1846, at the Northern Dispensary, and which has had an influential career in that section of the city, the alumni associations of the colleges, the women's societies, the smaller clubs, quiz associations and the like, whose number is large, are all special societies devoted to some particular branch of research or practice, or to merely social entertainment.

The oldest and largest of them is the Pathological Society, which has exercised more influence on the profession of the city than all the others, either special or general. This society, as has been said elsewhere, is the second of that name, the one founded by Gerhard being the first; the present society being founded by Dr. S. D. Gross at the "Hospital Building, Spruce street, above Eighth," on October 14, 1857, not long after his arrival from the West. It proposed "the cultivation and promotion of the study of Pathology, by the exhibition and description of specimens, drawings and other representations of morbid parts," and was an actively working body, from its very beginning. The first officers chosen were Dr. Gross as president; Drs. La Roche and Stillé as vice-presidents, Dr. Addinell Hewson as treasurer, Dr. Da Costa as secretary, and Dr. T. G. Morton as assistant secretary, and the first specimen was exhibited by Dr. S. Wier Mitchell. The members of the society down to about the opening of the civil war were: Drs. D. Hayes Agnew, C. S. Boker, J. H. Brinton, J. M. Da Costa, J. T. Darby, James Darrach, Emil Fischer, W. S. Forbes, S. D. Gross, S. W. Gross, A. D. Hall, G. C. Harlan, R. P. Harris, Edward Hartshorne, Henry Hartshorne, Addinell Hewson, H. Lenox Hodge, William D. Hoyt, George H. Humphreys, James Hutchinson, John K. Kane, W. V. Keating, W. Keller, René La Roche, James J. Levick, Samuel Lewis, E. Livezey, J. F. Meigs, S. W. Mitchell, Geo. R. Moorehouse,

T. G. Morton, William Moss, J. H. Packard, R. A. F. Penrose, T. B. Reed, Albert H. Smith, Francis G. Smith, Alfred Stillé, Ellwood Wilson and J. J. Woodward, not including corresponding members, of whom there were ten.

Its successive presidents have been: Samuel D. Gross, M. D., LL. D., D. C. L., Oxon., LL. D. Cantab., elected in 1857; René La Roche, M. D., elected in 1858; Alfred Stillé, M. D., elected in 1859, '61 and '62; Edward Hartshorne, M. D., elected in 1860 and '63; J. M. Da Costa, M. D., elected 1864, '65 and '66; John H. Packard, M. D., elected in 1867-8; S. Wier Mitchell, M. D., elected in 1869; John Ashhurst, Jr., M. D., in 1870; James H. Hutchinson, M. D., 1871 and '72; William Pepper, M. D., 1873, for three years; H. Lenox Hodge, M. D., 1876; S. W. Gross, M. D., 1879; James Tyson, M. D., elected in 1882 and '83; E. O. Shakespeare, M. D., elected in 1884; J. C. Wilson, M. D., 1885 and '86; F. P. Henry, M. D., 1887 and '88; Henry V. Formad, M. D., 1889-90; Arthur V. Meigs, M. D., 1891 and '92; J. H. Musser, M. D., 1893.

"On the evening of the 29th of September, 1857," said President Hutchinson, then the oldest elected member, in his annual address in 1873, "twenty-seven gentlemen, all of them, with scarcely a single exception, either at that time distinguished, or having since become so, met at the office of Dr. J. M. Da Costa for the purpose of organizing the Pathological Society. The meeting was called to order by the selection of Professor Samuel D. Gross as chairman and of Dr. Da Costa as secretary. At this meeting little was done beyond appointing one committee to make a draft for a constitution, and another to select a place of meeting. You are probably aware that permission to use one of the lower rooms in the building formerly called the Picture House, and now occupied by the Historical Society of Pennsylvania (j), was granted by the managers of the Pennsylvania Hospital, and that the society continued to meet there for nearly two years, or until March 13, 1867, when, after proper consideration, it was determined that the interests of the society would be advanced by a removal to our present hall. . . . . . Anyone who will take the trouble to read the minutes of the early meetings of the society will find that an enthusiasm for the study of morbid anatomy was at once developed by its establishment, which continued until the outbreak of the late rebellion, when the society, in common with many other scientific bodies, suffered severely. For not only did the army draw off at once many of our most active members, but there was an inability on the part of those who remained to divert their thoughts from the all-absorbing topic of the war. We, therefore, find that the meetings during 1861, 1862, 1863 and 1864 were very poorly attended, and that the specimens exhibited were almost wholly derived from the Pennsylvania Hospital. Indeed, on many occasions, no quorum was obtained, and there can be no doubt that the society would have ceased to exist but for the determination of a very few of the members, to whose exertions, during that very trying period of its history, I believe, we owe, in large measure, the fact that we celebrate to-night its sixteenth anniversary. The interest in pathology, which had slumbered during the war, was again aroused at its close, from which time our minutes afford, in the main, satisfactory evidence of the progress of our society." In 1865 a curator was added to the list of officers, and in 1869, a recorder, and by 1876 there were 162 active members. Various changes and additions have been made, but a general characterization of its work since then has been made by one of its late presidents in his address in 1889. "At one time in the history of this society," said he, "there was a tendency to cultivate the study of histology to the exclusion of everything else. Frequently the only part of a specimen presented here was to be found under the microscope, the tumor of which it was a sample being considered so unimportant in comparison with its minute structure that it was thought unnecessary to exhibit it. It seems to me that there is now a tendency to go to the opposite extreme. For example, at a very recent meeting several specimens of carcinoma were presented, in none of which had there been a microscopical examination. The tendency referred to is not confined to this society, and is doubtless one result of the present intense interest in bacteriology."

The other leading societies are all special, except the Northern

Medical Association. This society is next to the oldest of the medical societies of Philadelphia, the College of Physicians being of greater age. The society was organized in 1846, and has existed from that to the present, notwithstanding the customary ups and downs peculiar to the periods through which it has passed. Since its reorganization in 1884 it has been unusually successful and active; its membership is rapidly increasing, and it soon promises to attain the proud position it held in its youth, as the most prominent of the successful medical societies of Philadelphia.

Its constitution and by-laws were adopted on January 7, 1847. Dr. Wilson Jewell seems to have been one of the most active in the proceedings.

On February 18, 1847, the society elected delegates to the American Medical Association, and this measure was annually repeated until 1874, after which year the American Medical Association refused to receive delegates from any other than regularly organized county societies.

In 1848, delegates were sent to aid in the formation of the State Medical Society. The first annual oration was delivered by Dr. Arnold Naudain, at the hall southeast corner of Seventh and Callowhill streets, January 7, 1848, the members of the College of Physicians and of the Philadelphia Medical Society being invited. The second oration was delivered by Dr. Isaac Remington, January 6, 1849, at the hall northeast corner Eighth and Buttonwood streets.

Until January 27, 1881, when the association moved, with the Northern Dispensary, to 608 Coates street, the meetings had been regularly held at 603 Spring Garden street, the old hall of the dispensary. In 1883, on December 14, the Philadelphia Clinical Society was organized, and the Northern Medical Society became amalgamated with it, but in 1884, on May 29, it was reorganized under its original name, and has continued in a flourishing condition to the present time.

On December 5, 1896, was the commemoration of the semi-centennial of the existence of the society.

The Northern Medical Association was the first to admit women in the days when they were striving for admission to the County Medical Society.

The following is a list of the presidents since 1846: 1846, Arnold Naudain; 1847, Thomas H. Yardley; 1847, Nathan L. Hatfield; 1847 to 1853, Benjamin S. Janney; 1854, Nathan L. Hatfield; 1855, M. B. Smith; 1856, J. F. Lamb; 1857, Nathan L. Hatfield; 1858, Wm. Mayburry; 1859, Levi Curtis; 1860, Jos. R. Bryan; 1861, Lewis P. Gerhard; 1862, Owen Osler; 1863, Alfred M. Slocum; 1864, John Rhein; 1865, Chas. F. Wittig; 1866, J. Henry Smaltz; 1867, Robt. Burns; 1868, E. B. Shapleigh; 1870, Wm. M. Welch; 1871, James Collins; 1872, L. P. Deal; 1873, Nathan L. Hatfield; 1874, E. I. Santee; 1875, J. Solis-Cohen; 1876, Chas. K. Mills; 1877, S. R. Knight; 1878, L. B. Hall; 1879, Edw. R. Stone; 1880, E. E. Montgomery; 1881, James B. Walker; 1882, Henry W. Rihl; 1883, J. T. Eskridge; 1884, Nathan L. Hatfield; 1884, Robert H. Hess; 1885, Philip Leidy; 1886, H. C. Paist; 1887, Silas Updegrove; 1888, Geo. W. Vogler; 1889, Jos. S. Gibb; 1890, James Collins; 1891, Chas. P. Noble; 1892, I. P. Strittmatter; 1893, Daniel Longaker; 1894, Samuel Wolfe; 1895, H. B. Nightingale; 1896, E. B. Gleason; 1897, P. N. K. Schwenk.

The present officers of the Northern Medical Association are as follows: President, Dr. P. N. K. Schwenk; vice-president, Dr. Thomas Schriner; secretary, Dr. John Gordon Ross; treasurer, Dr. John W. Millick; corresponding secretary, Dr. H. Paist; librarian, Dr. Robert Hess; censors, Drs. H. Rihl, David Longaker, Robert Hess, Silas Updegrove, Thomas Shriner.

After the Pathological Society came the Obstetrical Society, which was organized in 1868, with Francis Gurney Smith as president. Its successive executives have been Drs. Robert P. Harris, William Goodell, A. H. Smith, John S. Parry, John H. Packard, L. D. Harlow, E. L. Duer, R. A. Cleemann, B. F. Baer, T. M. Drysdale, Theophilus Parvin, W. H. Parish, W. H. Githens, B. C. Hirst, W. H. Parish and E. E. Montgomery. In 1877 the Medico-Legal Society was organized at Twentieth street and Ridge avenue, for practical protective purposes of a professional and semi-legal character, and has, since the correction of the abuses it attacked, taken on a more purely professional character along medico-legal lines. The Medical Jurisprudence Society, devoted purely to medico-legal science, was organized in 1884 by Dr. Henry Leffmann, Mr. Hampton L. Carson and others, with Dr. S. D. Gross as its first president. In 1879 Drs. S. D. Gross, Agnew, Levis, Hewson, T. G. Morton, W. H. Pancoast, J. H. Brinton, Packard, S. W. Gross and Mears organized the Academy of Surgery, which has had a successful career. In 1880 Dr. J. Solis-Cohen and others organized the Laryngological Society, and Dr. Solis-Cohen was made its first president, and in 1883 Dr. C. K. Mills and others formed the Neurological Society, of which Dr. S. Wier Mitchell was made the first executive. The Association of Hospital Physicians and Surgeons of Philadelphia was formed in 1892 for the purpose of giving professional visitors to the city every facility for attending hospital clinics. The Pediatric Society of the present year is the most recent organization. Besides these special societies there are numerous clubs for social purposes.

While the societies and colleges have a certain similarity in their influence upon the profession, both locally and nationally, the third great branch of medical activity differs widely from both of them. The hospitals and their natural allies, the dispensaries, are more and more becoming the great laboratories of the medical fraternity. From the professional point of view, the hospitals are the foundation of all medical activity, without which there could scarcely exist either colleges or societies. "Where the hospitals are, there the other institutions are also," may be said of any city, and the fact is faithfully illustrated in the progress of medicine in Philadelphia. There can be no doubt that the Pennsylvania Hospital of 1751 was the foundation of this city's great medical career, and that the advance of the present period is due to the large number and capacity of the hospitals. And yet there was a time when this relation was not appreciated by the profession. Fortunately, its importance was recognized by a far-seeing surgeon-physician almost a century and a half ago, and the fact that Philadelphia is a great hospital center is largely due to Dr. Thomas Bond. Hospitals arise from various motives. The compassion of Christian communities for the bodily and spiritual condition of the afflicted is one of their most fruitful sources. It is an interesting fact that the desire to help the mentally diseased was the motive of the earliest efforts in this direction. The Friends made the first attempt at a hospital proper in 1709, though it was not immediately successful, and their lead has been followed since by Episcopalians, Roman Catholics and almost every other religious body of any prominence in the city. These denominational institutions have been governed by benevolent and religious motives; but few of them grant free admission to all applicants. In consequence, each one has its special excellence. Charitable motives prevail in denominational institutions; the desire for public safety, as regards health, controls the hospitals founded by the city, state or nation. In some cases, the medical profession has been given opportunities to make the hospitals contributory to medical advancement, as great laboratories for the education and research of physicians and surgeons. Sometimes interest in special diseases produces a special hospital, like the Wills, the Orthopædic or the Rush. Sometimes residents and citizens of foreign birth are so numerous and so affluent as to be able to provide a hospital for those of their own race. A grand example of this mode of origin is furnished by the German Hospital. The ever-present necessities in connection with child-birth have given rise to hospitals for women and children. Those believing in exclusive systems of medicine have hospitals proportionate to their strength locally. But the hospitals most intimately connected with the medical profession at large, and most influential, are those in which facilities for research or instruction have gained a place in the policy of the management. Such is the case in the oldest hospital—the Pennsylvania, which is the great type of the general hospital. Such is also the case in the great Philadelphia Hospital, connected with the Almshouse, and such, even to a greater degree, is true of those splendid institutions connected with the colleges and specialist schools. The highest type of the latter class is the Polyclinic, which is a great hospital, wholly devoted in its plans and methods to purposes of study and research, under the direction of distinguished specialists. The Pennsylvania Hospital, while resembling them all in policy, shares the advantage of financial aid from the commonwealth. The Pennsylvania, although it, like nearly all the other hospitals, began by private subscription, found it necessary to call upon the Provincial Assembly for aid in the erection of its first building, though this necessity has been resorted to but seldom in later years. As decade followed decade for a full century, it became evident to the more thoughtful observers that general hospital capacity in Philadelphia was not keeping pace with increase of population in any degree comparable with that of European cities. Then the Hospital of the P. E. Church, St. Joseph's and a few other denominational and other hospitals arose. After the close of the war the city increased so rapidly that the need for hospital facilities became still more urgent. In 1872, during the great removal of the University to West Philadelphia, it was decided, through the influence of Dr. William Pepper, to take radical measures, so far as the University Hospital was concerned, and to appeal for state aid. Philadelphia had always received and treated a large proportion of the sick and injured from all parts of the state, and it was rightly argued that the state should bear part of the burden of their support. The fact that the hospital for which state aid was requested was a part of the University was also a strong argument in favor of granting it. The appeal was successful, and the first payment was made late in 1872. Other institutions rightly claimed the same support, and from that date many of them, especially those of the schools, have received it. In fact, it is now the policy of the state to set aside appropriations for this purpose and, in consequence, Philadelphia compares favorably with all other cities in the capacity of her hospitals.

The Pennsylvania Hospital and the Philadelphia Hospital, on account of their age and size, have been the great clinical hospitals, outside of those associated with the colleges. One of the most instructive object lessons in the medical history of Philadelphia is afforded by a visit to the three clinical amphitheaters of the Pennsylvania Hospital, in which students have been taught since the time of Thomas Bond. The first is situated in the rotunda, almost in the cupola of the main building. The second, built in 1869, is a fine circular structure connected with the northern and southern pavilions. The third is contained in the fine Garrett Memorial Building and was formally opened on April 23, 1897. "From the room that preceded the one we inaugurate," said Dr. Da Costa, who has been a worthy successor of all of whom he speaks in his address, "from the old rotunda, from the newer building in which, until now, successive generations of eager students assembled, have gone forth lessons that have stamped themselves into the professional mind. . . . In the rooms that were anterior to this, here stood and taught those who were not unworthy successors to Rush, who, for thirty years, was the most conspicuous medical figure in this hospital, as, indeed, by his learning, captivating eloquence and ardent zeal, he was the most conspicuous figure in the profession in the United States; and to Physick, the dignified surgeon, who, bringing with him into our century the appearance and manner of another time, stood before his class with his hair powdered and clubbed, their idol, as in his cultivated voice he gave admirable illustrations of the conservative surgery of which he was the great exponent. In those rooms taught John K. Mitchell, the versatile and gifted, with the eye of genius foreseeing the part minute organisms play in the production of disease; George B. Wood, as methodical and accurate in his statements at the bedside as everywhere in his respected career; William Pepper, clear in his descriptions and consummate in unraveling obscure processes; William Gerhard, take him for all in all, the greatest observer and clinician America has produced; John F. Meigs, inheriting with his famous medical name, an interest in this hospital from the illustrious and inimitable teacher whom also it was our boast to have had on our list, and showing here the same skill and kindness that made him the most sought after physician in the community. In the old rooms also have been heard the voice of Barton, the pride of his colleagues, whose ability and ingenuity remained a tradition for long years, joined to regret for the early retirement from a profession in which, still young, he attained the first rank; of Norris, the truthful, honest, conscientious gentleman and teacher; of Joseph Pancoast, the brilliant surgical artist, devising processes that seemed to be the result of intuition, and practicing, long before it was taught, a kind of antiseptic surgery, of which he himself did not recognize the importance or wider application; and of Agnew, the most esteemed man of our day in the American profession, cool, skillful, daring, yet of the soundest judgment, and a clear, concise, admirable teacher. Thus from the days, one hundred and thirty years ago, when Bond enthusiastically, with the full approbation of the managers, introduced clinical teaching into the Pennsylvania Hospital, and therefore on this continent—for it was in this hospital that the first bedside instruction in medicine was given—up to our time there has been a succession of men bestowing publicly their best thought and experience without reward, or idea of reward, on those who were to come after them. . . . The traits of the many distinguished teachers that have been connected with the hospital, and the influence of the character of the hospital itself, have made, indeed, a great school of both Practical Medicine and Surgery, developing on rational lines."

Clinical instruction in the Philadelphia Hospital began, so far as is known, with the first obstetrical clinic in the city, as early as 1770. But, for the period extending from that time until 1861, nearly a century, it had to make an almost continuous fight for existence, and its final success was probably most largely due to the efforts of the University medical school. In 1872, Drs. Rush, Kuhn, and Clarkson sought to enlarge its means of clinical instruction, for, says Dr. Agnew, in 1862, "It was then the most extensive hospital on the continent, containing about three hundred and fifty persons, and must unquestionably have contained much disease of an interesting and instructive character." The revolution interrupted the teachings of this hospital, and it was not until 1803 that they were resumed under Drs. James and Church. It was in 1807 that Dr. James secured the green room for the inauguration of clinical lectures outside the wards. Students increased rapidly in the next two or more decades, and many of the ablest men of the profession were among the lecturers. By 1834 Jefferson men were equally active in this direction, and it was about this time (r)

(r) The final removal from the old Almshouse was begun July 7, 1834.

that the removal of the hospital to "Blockley township," across the Schuylkill river, was made. This change made the transfer of students from Ninth and Tenth streets one of the interesting features of their course. "The transportation," says Dr. Agnew, "was no inconsiderable item. Long lines of omnibuses (for there were then no street cars) were stationed about Ninth and Chestnut streets on Saturday mornings, and in a few minutes crowds of students, full of life and excitement, were stowed away—not seated —in glorious, good-natured confusion; and at the usual salutation of the knight with the whip, 'all right,' were whirled away at a spanking speed, some to the South street ferry, to be carried over on a boat which has long been suspected as one of Charon's—and is, so far as the transportation of spirits is concerned, not untruly; others by the Market street bridge. Some of my very pleasant recollections of college life, in 1837, are associated with those weekly trips so admirably calculated to relieve the tedium of town, and regale the lungs with more invigorating air. The lecture room was situated in what is now the lunatic department, and only recently abandoned. It was the most capacious and finely arranged amphitheater in the country, and capable of seating from seven to eight hundred persons. Until 1845, this hospital continued to be the great clinic school of the country, annually opening its exhaustless treasures of disease to crowds of educated, zealous inquirers after medical knowledge." A trivial incident which occurred on June 30, 1845, was the indirect cause of the cessation of clinics at the Philadelphia Hospital for nine years. It is thus described by Agnew in his Medical History of the Philadelphia Almshouse:

"The resident physicians were boarded at the table of the steward where, as I understand, in consequence of the want of due formality and decorum in the destruction of an unfortunate cockroach, which had rashly taken a near cut across the table instead of going around, these gentlemen became indignant, and demanded of the managers to be transferred to the table of the matron. Their refusal to comply with this request determined a unanimous resignation, leaving the hospital unprovided with any medical assistance. The evening of that day Drs. Horner and Clymer attended and prescribed for the sick. Here was a *casus belli*, and the managers promptly passed a resolution of dismissal. . . . . What great results proceed from small and unlikely causes. Who would have ever thought that the official existence of a medical board composed of the ablest men in their various departments on the continent, could have depended on the life of a contemptible cockroach! In this manner the doors of the Philadelphia Hospital, as a school of instruction, were sealed for nine years." These were the days of political management at their worst. In 1854 several attempts were made to revive the clinical teaching, and the efforts of Drs. Henry H. Smith and J. L. Ludlow were finally successful. Early in October a train on what is now the West Chester Railway carried the students to the hospital. In the winter of 1856-57 the clinics were again closed. The students appealed to the managers, and late in 1858 ten lecturers were appointed. The old managers were removed in 1859, and a new medical staff appointed, among whom was Dr. Robert Luckett, who afterward became the chief leader of the exodus of Southern students. In 1860 the wards were thrown open to free clinical instruction, and in 1861 the present lecture room, which, in the words of Agnew, "for elegance and convenience has no superior," was constructed. This was used for thirty-one years, when it was thoroughly remodeled on modern plans. "Nothing remains of the former hall," said the president of the medical board, Dr. Roland G. Curtin, in his opening address, "but the old stone walls, which have been renewed in appearance by the stucco covering. . . . The facilities for clinical instruction in this hospital are excelled by only about four hospitals in the world, and by none on this side of the Atlantic. This hospital embraces what in New York is called Bellevue Hospital or the City Hospital, and Charity Hospital, which is associated with the Almshouse, criminal institutions, and others that are under city control. . . . . I have made a calculation that in thirty-one years fifteen to twenty thousand students have attended clinics in the old clinic room. This teaching has had much to do with making Philadelphia the medical center of the United States. . . . The attendance on the Philadelphia Hospital clinics is from all countries. I have seen on the benches Turks, Roumanians, Africans, Canadians, Bermudans, Brazilians, Chilians and Japanese—male and female— old style, new style and eclectics. Old students are welcome, and are admitted on an equal footing without fee, and receive the best practical instruction we can give. . . . 'Old Blockley' is honored all over the land and in many foreign countries by the teaching that has been given here by such lights as Benjamin Rush, Gerhard, Pennock, Gross (father and son), Pancoast the elder, Ludlow, Agnew and others who have gone to their reward; and among those now living who have long since retired from the staff, by Stillé, Da Costa, Penrose, Pepper, Wood, Tyson, Osler, the younger Pancoast, and many others who might be mentioned if time permitted. They gave their valuable time without pecuniary compensation to the poor of Philadelphia."

Clinical instruction in these two great institutions first began to be supplemented by the schools when Jefferson began her struggle for existence, in 1825. The early clinical facilities of this institution were, however, of a very primitive character, although they were the starting point of the present Jefferson College Hospital. The difficulties the women had to contend with to gain entrance to clinics led to the opening of their hospital during the early years of the war, and the removal of the University early in the seventies occasioned the rise of its great hospital. In April, 1877, the present Jefferson Hospital was formally transferred by the Building Committee to the Trustees of the College. The Medico-Chirurgical and Polyclinic hospitals have risen within the present period. From the foregoing, it is evident that Philadelphia affords unusual facilities for that most important supplement to medical teaching—post-graduate service in a general hospital.

The Pennsylvania Hospital staff has enrolled a most notable list of physicians since its organization in 1751. It embraces the following: Drs. Lloyd Zachary, Thomas Bond, Phineas Bond, William Shippen, John Morgan, Cadwalader Evans, Charles Moore, Adam Kuhn, Thomas Parke, James Hutchinson, William

Shippen, Jr., John Jones, Benjamin Rush, John Foulke, Caspar Wistar, Philip Syng Physick, Benjamin S. Barton, John Redman Coxe, Thomas C. James, John Syng Dorsey, Joseph Hartshorne, Thomas C. James, John C. Otto, Joseph Parrish, Samuel Colhoun, John Moore, Thomas T. Hewson, William Price, John Wilson Moore, Samuel Emlen, John Rhea Barton, John K. Mitchell, Benjamin H. Coates, Thomas Harris, Charles Lukens, Hugh L. Hodge, William Rush, Jacob Randolph, George B. Wood, George W. Norris, Thomas Stewardson, Jr., Charles D. Meigs, Edward Peace, William Pepper, William W. Gerhard, George Fox, Joseph Carson, John Neill, Joseph Pancoast, Francis Gurney Smith, James J. Levick, John F. Meigs, Edward Hartshorne, Addinell Hewson, William Hunt, Thomas G. Morton, J. M. Da Costa, D. Hayes Agnew, James H. Hutchinson, J. Aitkin Meigs, Richard J. Levis, Arthur V. Meigs, Morris Longstreth, John H. Packard, John Ashhurst, Jr., Morris J. Lewis and Richard H. Harte, the present staff being: Drs. J. M. Da Costa, Arthur V. Meigs, Morris J. Lewis, James C. Wilson, Thomas G. Morton, John Ashhurst, Jr., Richard H. Harte, W. Barton Hopkins, and the Pathologist, Henry M. Fisher, for the Pine street main hospital; and Drs. Fisher, Frederick A. Packard, Joseph Leidy, J. Allison Scott, Walter D. Green, Robert G. Le Conte, Joseph M. Spellissy, John H. Gibbon, George C. Harlan, Peter N. K. Schwenk, Alex. W. MacCoy, J. Montgomery Baldy, A. R. Moulton, Henry B. Nunemaker, Eli E. Josselyn, Horace Phillips and Thomas S. K. Morton, for the out-patient department; and seven resident physicians. The staff of the Hospital for the Insane includes Dr. John B. Chapin, four assistant physicians, one resident, and a consulting gynecologist. The present plant of the Pennsylvania Hospital has grown up around the old original structure, which still remains, occupying the square at Eighth and Pine streets. This structure was the east wing, built in 1754; the west wing was added in 1796, and also the central building. In 1841 the Department for the Insane was opened in West Philadelphia, and in 1869 the second clinic hall addition was built. In 1875 the Nurses' Training Department was organized, and eleven years later the Picture House (j) was made their "Home;" in 1892 the present fine structure was erected for their use. The out-patient department grew out of the dispensary service, and in 1892 its present building outside the grounds on Spruce street was secured. The first memorial pavilion was begun in 1892, and the cornerstone laid in 1893. These pavilions are three in number, and with the magnificent clinic hall just completed, and the Nurses' Home, give the Spruce street side five imposing structures, the middle one being connected with the central building. The old Hospital for the Insane is equally well provided with buildings, on its extensive and beautiful grounds in West Philadelphia, which are models for their purpose. This institution must always be associated with the name of Dr. Thomas S. Kirkbride, whose devotion to it, from 1840 to his death in 1883, has caused the institution to be popularly known as "Kirkbride's." He was a native of Bucks County, born in 1809, and was a graduate of the University Medical School in 1832. This institution, under the management of Dr. Kirkbride and his successor, Dr. Chapin, is world renowned for its skillful treatment of the mentally diseased. The crowning addition to the historic old Pine street hospital is the Garrett Memorial Building, in the northeast corner of the grounds, facing Eighth and Spruce streets, and containing the great clinic hall, opened in 1897. Over 26,000 patients are annually treated in the hospital proper, and over 550 in the Department for the Insane.

The other great clinical school, the Philadelphia Hospital, has had a staff of equal eminence. Beginning with Drs. Thomas Bond and Cadwalader Evans, in 1768, at the old Spruce and Tenth street grounds, they are as follows: Drs. Adam Kuhn, Benjamin Rush, Samuel Duffield, Gerardus Clarkson, Thomas Parke, George Glentworth, D. Jackson, James Hutchinson, (z) Wilson, Caspar Wistar, J. R. Rodgers, Michael Leib, John Morris, Samuel P. Griffitts, N. B. Waters, William Shippen, (z) Cumming, (z) Pleasants,

(j) The picture house was built in 1816 for Benjamin West's picture, "Christ Healing the Sick." It was removed in 1892-3. The picture is in the old clinic hall.

(z) The Christian names of Drs. Wilson, Cumming and Pleasants are omitted in the chronological list of the members of the Medical Boards of the Philadelphia Hospital, contained in the reports of that institution.

Samuel Clements, Jr., William Boyce, Samuel Cooper, John Church, Thomas C. James, John Proudfit, Philip S. Physick, Charles Caldwell, Elijah Griffiths, Benjamin S. Barton, Samuel Stewart, John Rush, James Reynolds, Isaac Cathrall, Peter Muller, John S. Dorsey, Nathaniel Chapman, Joseph Parrish, Joseph Klapp, Thomas T. Hewson, Joseph Hartshorne, Samuel Colhoun, W. P. C. Barton, William E. Horner, Samuel Jackson, John K. Mitchell, Richard Harlan, Hugh L. Hodge, S. G. Morton, Jacob Randolph, William W. Gerhard, Joseph Pancoast, William Ashmead, N. Stuardson, Robley Dunglison, Edward Peace, Meridith Clymer, John Rhea Barton, William Gibson, J. V. O. Lawrence, Charles B. Gibson, John Moore, Henry Neill, Nathan Shoemaker, Chas. Lukens, B. Ellis, F. S. Beattie, C. W. Pennock, W. D. Brinklé, R. M. Huston, James McClintock, W. H. Gillingham, J. L. Ludlow, W. F. Mayburry, Chas. P. Tutt, Robert Luckett, J. M. Da Costa, O. A. Judson, George J. Zeigler, Alfred Stillé, J. S. De Benneville, Edward Rhoads, William Pepper, H. C. Wood, James Tyson, J. M. Keating, E. T. Bruen, J. C. Wilson, John Guitéras, Roland G. Curtin, S. J. McFerran, J. T. Eskridge, W. G. McConnell, Jos. F. Neff, John H. Musser, William Osler, F. P. Henry, J. M. Anders, W. E. Hughes, S. Solis-Cohen, Eugene L. Vansant, F. A. Packard, Judson Daland, Samuel Wolfe, Julius Salinger, S. D. Gross, D. Hayes Agnew, R. J. Levis, Edward L. Duer, R. S. Kenderdine, J. W. Lodge, W. H. Pancoast, F. F. Maury, John H. Brinton, Harrison Allen, Samuel W. Gross, N. L. Hatfield, J. William White, William G. Porter, A. A. McDonald, W. S. Janney, George McClellan, A. S. Roberts, W. Joseph Hearn, C. H. Thomas, A. W. Ransley, Lewis W. Steinbach, John B. Deaver, Edward Martin, Orville Horwitz, Ernest Laplace, J. M. Barton, J. Chalmers Da Costa, Alfred C. Wood, R. A. F. Penrose, John Wiltbank, W. B. Stroud, Lewis Harlow, G. J. Ziegler, J. S. Parry, George Pepper, J. V. Ingham, J. R. Burden, Jr., E. E. Montgomery, J. B. Walker, S. S. Stryker, G. W. Linn, M. B. Musser, W. H. Parish, Clara Marshall, E. P. Bernardy, Hannah T. Croasdale, Theophilus Parvin, Donnell Hughes, E. Richardson, B. C. Hirst, E. P. Davis, W. E. Ashton, R. H. Hammill, George I. McKelway, J. W. West, R. C. Norris, J. M. Fisher, W. F. Haehnlen,

Elizabeth L. Peck, Chas. K. Mills, H. C. Wood, Roberts Bartholow, F. X. Dercum, J. H. Lloyd, Wharton Sinkler, C. H. Bradfute, E. O. Shakespeare, G. E. de Schweinitz, Geo. M. Gould, C. A. Oliver, Louis Duhring, H. W. Stelwagon, J. A. Cantrell, C. J. Seltzer, James Tyson, R. M. Bertolet, Jos. Berens, H. F. Formad, W. M. L. Coplin, E. B. Sangree, A. Ghriskey, L. Henley, J. H. Benton, S. W. Butler, D. D. Richardson, A. A. McDonald, Philip Leidy, William H. Wallace, G. M. Wells, Daniel E. Hughes, S. Wier Mitchell, Andrew Nebinger and James Simpson. The present staff embraces the following: Drs. Tyson, White, Mills, Curtin, Hearn, Steinbach, Musser, Stelwagon, Dercum, de Schweinitz, Deaver, Hirst, Henry, Martin, Lloyd, Davis, Sinkler, Anders, W. E. Hughes, S. Solis-Cohen, Vansant, Horwitz, Laplace, Ashton, Cantrell, Cattell, W. B. Jameson, Barton, Seltzer, Geo. M. Marshall, Hamill, McKelway, F. A. Packard, R. C. Norris, J. C. Da Costa, S. Wolfe, J. L. Salinger, Guitéras, A. A. Eshner, Sangree, Oliver H. Toulmin, Haehnlen, A. C. Wood and Elizabeth L. Peck. It is of interest to note that the clinical lecturers immediately before the war were Drs. J. L. Ludlow, Caspar Morris, Joseph Carson, J. B. Biddle, J. Aitkin Meigs, J. M. Da Costa, Henry H. Smith, D. Hayes Agnew, John Neill, R. P. Thomas, W. S. Halsey, R. J. Levis, R. A. F. Penrose, Wilson Jewell and E. McClellan.

This great hospital, always a part of the Almhouse, has grown from the time of its first wards, set apart for the sick, at Spruce and Tenth streets, step by step, until it now occupies the great building forming the northeast side of the vast quadrangle of Almshouse structures at the southwest corner of Thirty-fourth and Pine streets. It is three stories high, with dormer roof, and is 540 feet by 63 feet in dimensions. Aside from the Children's and Insane Departments, there are the Pathological Department, first really organized in 1860, the Neurological in 1877, the Ophthalmological at the same date, the Laryngological in 1890, and the Nurses' School, which now, since 1884, has a fine new building. The annual average of cases within the hospital proper is about 8,000.

The college hospitals—if Jefferson's and the Woman's small early building be excepted—have practically all arisen during the present period. Their staffs are, as a matter of course, composed of members of the corresponding college faculties' staff. In the case of Jefferson, rooms were rented in an adjoining building in 1843 for the use of patients treated in the clinic, and it soon grew to a capacity of about a score of beds, and remained at this stage for about twenty years. Then arose the project of the University Hospital, which, with other circumstances, prompted a similar enterprise by the Alumni Association of Jefferson. In December, 1872, the project was set on foot. Subscriptions were secured and an appropriation of $100,000 was voted by the state on April 9, 1873. Dr. E. B. Gardette was made chairman of a committee to secure the present site near the college. This was completed in March, 1876, and on September 17, 1877, the new structure was formally opened. Since that time it has been a most valuable adjunct to the college. It is not the intention to make any comparison between the college hospitals, nor to enter into the details of their development. It is to be taken for granted that these great undertakings are not only the equals of any similar institutions, but leaders in all the highest developments of modern hospital service. Jefferson now averages about 1,500 cases annually in her hospital, and over 95,000 in the dispensary service. The University Hospital has a similar average in the hospital proper, but not so large a dispensary service. The latter institution was suggested in 1871 by Dr. H. C. Wood, W. F. Norris and William Pepper, on the occasion of the proposed removal of the University from Ninth street and the vicinity of the Pennsylvania Hospital, on which the University depended so largely for clinical material (k). It is true the University, by its removal, became contiguous to the Philadelphia Hospital, but the latter institution, at that time, had not the prestige and excellence of the former, so that the new hospital was intended, in a large measure, to replace the Pennsylvania Hospital, so far as the University School was concerned. Under the chairmanship of the Hon. Morton McMichael, the alumni of the medical school were rallied about the project, and it was proposed to raise $700,000.

(k) The University also had rooms rented for the use of chronic cases previous to this.

Dr. Pepper was made chairman of the commission, and early in 1872 decided to ask for State aid. It was urged that New York, with a million people, had 6,325 free beds in hospitals, but Philadelphia, with nearly three-fourths her population, had only 1,100. Other arguments in favor of the project were urged, and on April 3, 1872, the state granted an appropriation of $100,000, to be paid when $250,000 had been raised, a feat which was accomplished by November following. On May 18 the City Councils voted the University five and one-half acres as a site for the hospital. Other subscriptions and grants from the state were received, and on July 15, 1874, the hospital was opened for patients. Since that date its development has been worthy of its vigorous beginning. The Woman's Hospital began with a house on North College avenue, in 1861, when Dr. Ann Preston saved the college from extinction by her foresight in opening this institution. Over $382,000 has been raised for the hospital and Nurses' School, and the entire service includes about 4,000 cases annually, including the dispensary service. The Alumnæ Hospital of the college is at 1212 South Third street, and was first proposed about 1892, but was not opened until October 31, 1895. It averages over a thousand cases a year, including dispensary service. The Medico-Chirurgical Hospital averages over 1,200 cases annually, with about 40,000 accident and dispensary patients. It began in a small way in 1881-2 with the college at the southeast corner of Broad and Market, opposite the Broad Street Station, and has gradually increased its new plant, both on Cherry and on Eighteenth street, until its development has been such that it takes rank with the other college hospitals. Like the Medico-Chirurgical College, the Polyclinic began, not only with, but as, a hospital in 1882, in its days of small things. In its fine new building it now averages about 800 cases annually, not including a dispensary service of about 77,000 a year. These are all large institutions, with a complex development so extended and ramifying that they are models of the most highly organized hospital management. They may be considered offshoots of the Pennsylvania and Philadelphia hospitals, in that they were prompted by the inadequacy of those institutions. State aid has made them all, in a sense, State institutions also. They all include in their equipment, schools for the training of nurses, and, for the most part, an ambulance service, as well as a multitude of other details too numerous to consider here. They are all general hospitals, with dispensaries, in which the various specialties are fully provided for. Few of the public, and not all of the profession, realize the extent of these institutions and the great part they play in the welfare of the city, because their life is so merged with that of the institution to which they are attached. It will be seen from their dates of organization that this great series of hospitals has arisen practically in the present period, and that, like their two great prototypes, they are the work of the profession.

Other general hospitals arose through the instrumentality of the great religious bodies, which began to realize, even before the civil war, the necessity for larger hospital accommodation than was furnished by the Pennsylvania and Almshouse or Philadelphia hospitals. This work began to be felt about 1850, and the first who attempted to fill it were the Roman Catholics, who founded St. Joseph's in 1849, a hospital which now receives patients averaging over 1,600 annually, not including a dispensary service of over 14,000 cases. It has a large four-story structure, of the conventional hospital type of those days, that is, a central building, with two wings of similar architecture, connected with the main building by structures of almost equal size. It fronts on Girard avenue, between Sixteenth and Seventeenth streets, and is under the care of Sisters of Charity. It had the honor to be one of the first, if not the first, of the hospitals to open its doors to the soldiers during the war, and had its share of them during the whole of that conflict. Its growth has been gradual from the first. Its present staff consists of Drs. Robert B. Cruice, Geo. M. Marshall, A. G. Bournonville, Geo. R. Morehouse, John H. Packard, Henry Morris, M. T. Prendergast, C. K. Mills, S. L. Zeigler, E. E. Montgomery, Jos. Siler, G. G. Davis, H. B. Allyn, John S. Miller, W. H. Baker, G. F. Baker, Jas. McKee, W. Krusen, F. H. Maier, B. K. Chance, C. L. Felt, M. M. Franklin, Henry J. Walcott, H. P. Fisher and A. M. Harrison. St. Joseph's Hospital was followed in

1866 by St. Mary's, at Frankford avenue and Palmer street, near the Delaware. St. Mary's Hospital was established in July, 1866. The hotel at the corner of Frankford road and Palmer street was purchased for the institution at a cost of $30,000; repairs, $15,000. In 1892 a wing was added at a cost of $25,000.

Dr. James Cummiskey was its first medical director; Dr. Andrew Nebinger second; Dr. J. H. Grove third; Dr. W. V. Keating fourth; Dr. P. S. Donnellan fifth, and Dr. J. V. Kelly its present medical director.

It now accommodates over 100 patients. It has done much work for the poor, and has an able staff. It has educated three resident physicians annually since its foundation.

Its chief benefactors were Francis Drexel ($71,000), Mrs. A. Glass, Mr. O'Neill and Leandro de la Cuesta. A bequest of the latter provides an income of over $1,000 annually.

From 1875 to 1877 the following hospitals were founded: St. Christopher's Hospital for Children, at Huntingdon and Lawrence streets, with a capacity of 50; St. Vincent's Home and Maternity, at Seventieth and Woodland avenue, a private institution in West Philadelphia, and St. Agnes' Hospital, containing 213 beds, at Broad and Mifflin streets, organized in 1888. From the above it will be seen that two of the Roman Catholic hospitals are in the northern section of the city, and that their greatest growth has been within the present period.

St. Agnes' Hospital was founded by Dr. Andrew Nebinger, under Rev. Mother Agnes, the Superior of the Order of St. Francis. It was dedicated in May, 1888. Dr. Nebinger was its chief benefactor. Other large benefactors were: Mr. John Carew, Mrs. Catharine Horstman and the Drexel family. It occupies an entire square at Broad and Mifflin streets. St. Agnes contains 213 beds. The *personnel* of the establishment, aside from the medical staff, is composed of 36 sisters, 12 postulants, 4 lay nurses, 4 male "help," and 12 male attendants. According to the last report there were admitted during the year 1,738 patients, and 4,826 cases were treated in the dispensary. According to the original plan, there is one wing yet to be added. The hospital has a training school for nurses, from which eleven were graduated last year. The training school committee consists of Drs. William H. Parish, A. A. Stevens, Edward Martin, B. Franklin Stahl and A. O. J. Kelly. Dr. Michael O'Hara is the present medical director. Former directors were: Drs. A. Nebinger, J. H. Grove and W. V. Keating. The present medical staff is composed of Drs. M. O'Hara, J. P. C. Griffith, A. A. Stevens, B. F. Sthal, A. O. J. Kelly, A. W. Ransley, W. J. Taylor, E. Martin, E. Laplace, W. W. Keen, J. H. Grove, W. H. Parish, John C. Da Costa, M. O'Hara, Jr., J. N. Rhoads, F. M. Perkins, E. G. Rehfuss, C. A. Oliver, L. P. Smock, D. B. Kyle, C. S. Means, F. X. Dercum, G. A. Muehleck, M. V. Ball and R. Wilson, with ten others for dispensary work and four residents. The cost of the hospital is about $40,000 annually. Sister M. Barromeo is sister in charge.

The Hospital of the Protestant Episcopal Church came next after St. Joseph's, and it also, as its name implies, is a church institution, and, therefore, with no other object in view than that of healing the sick and injured and training nurses to care for them. Bishop Potter led in the founding of this hospital. On March 14, 1851, a meeting of clergy and laity was held, at which plans were laid and a committee of eleven appointed to carry them out. Drs. Caspar Morris and William Keith were the physicians on this committee. Soon after the corporators of the institution were presented with the old Leamy mansion, surrounded by six acres of land, and on December 11, 1852, the hospital was opened. It continued to occupy the Leamy mansion for ten years. On May 24, 1860, the cornerstone of the new building, facing Lehigh avenue, on the corner of Front street, was laid. It is now composed of a large central structure, with several wings, or "pavilions," connected with the main building by covered passages. The general plan is said to have been suggested by the Hôpital Lariboisière of Paris. In reality, it was for a long time composed of three great and almost equal structures, which have been added to, as found advisable, from time to time. One of its principal features is a magnificent ward, or rather wing, for incurables, a memorial to the late George L. Harrison, whose family has contributed nearly half a million dollars to its building and maintenance. It was one of the hospitals which cared for soldiers during the war, and was, with the Pennsylvania, St. Joseph's and "Old Blockley," the only general hospital of that time. "It is just a century since the first effort for the establishment of the Pennsylvania Hospital was made," said Bishop Potter, in his appeal in 1851, "and it may be hailed as a not inauspicious omen that, without design, this epoch has given birth to a new attempt. . . . . . In that whole period the charity of Philadelphia for the sick has lain dormant, or been imperfectly applied by isolated and individual effort, with the single exception of the endowment of the Wills Hospital for the Blind and Lame; whilst the increased density of the population, the introduction of steam, the establishment of manufactories and the extension of railroads have added incalculably to the necessity for some provision applicable to all classes of sickness and accident." The earliest medical board recorded in the reports is that of 1854, and includes Drs. Deacon, Hunt, Biddle, Reese, Bernard Henry, A. Hewson, West, Drayton, Wiltbank and Stocker. In 1860, when the new buildings were started, the bishop said: "It is not in our own estimate only that the necessity exists. St. Joseph's has been organized under the patronage of the Church of Rome, within the last few years, while two other institutions, struggling to maintain a feeble existence, the one in the southwest and the other in the northwest portions of the city plot, indicate that others have been equally impressed by this necessity. An effort is now being made to plan on a broader foundation an hospital especially devoted to the treatment of diseases of children." These statements show the position which this hospital was intended to occupy in the northeast quarter of Philadelphia. By the beginning of the present period the medical staff consisted of Drs. Herbert Norris, Wharton Sinkler, H. B. Hare, Frederick P. Henry, John Ashhurst, W. S. Forbes, Samuel Ashhurst and John H. Packard, with eight members of the dispensary staff, four resident physicians, a curator of the museum and a superintendent, Dr. Samuel R. Knight. The expenses at this time averaged $45,000 annually. This was after a quarter century of progress, when the hospital received a thousand patients a year. Now the average yearly expense is considerably above $100,000, and over 2,800 patients are treated annually. This does not include dispensary patients, the number of which is stated at 33,000 per year. The hospital, as looked at from Lehigh avenue, presents an imposing array of five great structures, united on each story by well-lighted and roomy corridors. The staff according to the last report, consists of Drs. D. J. M. Miller, Caspar Morris, D. D. Stewart, Henry M. Fisher, G. G. Davis, Thomas R. Neilson, H. C. Deaver, Richard H. Harte, G. O. Ring, W. T. Van Pelt and J. S. Gibbs, with sixteen on the dispensary staff, eight resident physicians and a pathologist. The superintendent is Dr. Henry Sykes.

About the time of the founding of the two last-named church hospitals, that strong feeling of nationality, so characteristic of their race, had inspired the Germans of Philadelphia to undertake the establishment of a hospital which, while open to all, should be essentially *German* in its management, and in which the German language should be spoken by physicians and nurses. Attempts to carry out this project were made in 1850 and in 1853, but it was not until 1860 that success attended them and a charter was received. The physicians most prominently connected with its founding were Drs. Tiedemann, Keller and Seidensticker. It was on the 20th of May, 1861, that the William Morris homestead, "Pennbrook," at Twentieth and Norris streets, was purchased for the German Hospital, but the Government had need of it for sick and wounded soldiers, and occupied it from the middle of 1862 to the summer of 1866. The board then obtained control of the property and the hospital was inaugurated, with accommodations for about fifty patients. The institution was most successful, and in 1872 measures were taken to secure the present hospital site, occupying the ground bounded by Girard and Corinthian avenues and Poplar and Twenty-second streets. The removal took place on October 23d of that year, when the main building was erected. In 1874 and in 1884, extensive additions were made, and in 1888 the beautiful Mary J. Drexel Home, which combines a Children's Hospital with a Home for the Aged, of German birth or descent, was built on its grounds; while in 1893 another beautiful hospital wing was finished, the entire group making this great hospital one of the finest and, with its picturesque grounds, one of the most attractive in the State. This is the seat of the United States Marine Hospital Service also, in connection with the Delaware bay and river division of the service. The German Hospital now receives more than 2,600 cases annually, not including about 30,000 dispensary patients. No account of the German Hospital can be complete without a reference to its greatest benefactor, Mr. John D. Lankenau. "The removal of the hospital to its present site was made possible largely through his efforts, and the rapid but substantial developments which the hospital underwent at that time, the increased accommodations, the rebuilding and the erection of new buildings on such a magnificent scale, the introduction of the deaconesses and the consequent change in the administration of the affairs of the hospital, are all due to the untiring, indefatigable energy and, to a great extent, to the personal efforts of this great human benefactor."

The present staff of the German Hospital includes Drs. Adam Trau, L. Wolff, J. C. Wilson, John B. Deaver, G. G. Ross, A. D. Whiting, C. S. Turnbull, A. A. Bliss, Fairfax Irwin (1), Carl Frese and five residents. About the same time as the movement for the establishment of the German Hospital an attempt was made to inaugurate a Charity Hospital. Late in 1857 it seems to have made a start with some difficulty, but was not incorporated until May 13, 1861, when it opened its doors in Buttonwood street, just below Broad street. Among physicians most interested in its welfare in the first decade of its existence were Drs. W. H. Pancoast, H. Y. Evans, A. M. Slocum, H. St. Clair Ash, H. Leaman, W. M. Welch, E. I. Santee, L. K. Baldwin, A. H. Fish, N. Hatfield, T. E. Ridgeway and J. M. McGrath. Afterward it was removed to 1802 and 1832 Hamilton street, and in August, 1893, it was again removed to a four-story building at 1831 Vine street, in which are annually treated about 7,000 cases, including dispensary patients. Its present medical staff includes Drs. H. St. Clair Ash, J. H. Lopez, Justus Sinexon, G. E. Stubbs, A. F. Chase, A. B. Hirsh, W. J. Pennock,

(1) Marine hospital service.

Edwin Lippincott, G. A. Sulzer, F. Eft, J. H. Boyd, C. P. Franklin, S. F. Wilson, M. Franklin, J. D. Moore and N. H. Saxman.

The Germantown Hospital dates from September 3, 1863, and was first suggested by Dr. James E. Rhoads. Drs. James Darrach and Owen J. Wister were also among the first to become interested in the project. It began as a dispensary in the Town Hall, and met with such encouraging success that, six years later, a patient of Dr. Wister's, Mrs. P. E. Henry, offered to add a cottage hospital. The offer was accepted, and the dispensary and hospital were installed in their present quarters in 1870. Improvements and additions rapidly followed, and to such an extent that the hospital, which opened with twelve beds, now has an annual average of 560 cases, with a dispensary service of nearly 8,500 cases. Drs. A. F. Müller, R. W. Deaver, C. A. Currie and W. N. Johnson are the hospital staff. The dispensary staff numbers six, and there is one resident physician and four consultants.

Five years after the Germans began their work another group, prompted by that beneficence which is so actively exerted, so far as those of their own race are concerned, founded a hospital, because, as stated in the preamble to its constitution, "it is the duty of Israelites to take care of the suffering and needy ones among them, and as the sick are especially objects of charity and public solicitude, and since there is no institution now in existence within the State of Pennsylvania under the control of the Israelites, wherein they can place their sick, and where these can enjoy during their illness all the benefits and consolations of our religion; we, the subscribers, and our successors, associate ourselves under the following constitution to carry out the benevolent views proposed at a meeting of the District Grand Lodge, No. 3, of the I. O. B'nai' Berith, held at Philadelphia, on the 14th of August, 5624." The incorporation was obtained in 1865, with the privilege of establishing an institution that should be a "hospital and home." The result has been that in the thirty-two years since that date there has grown up a great establishment on the Olney road, near York road, with its fine group of buildings for the hospital proper, the home, the dispensary and other purposes, which, with its extensive grounds in that beautiful suburban region, make it one of the leading hospitals of the city. All patients whosoever, except, of course, cases of contagious disease, are admitted, and the annual average is now nearly 700, with nearly 1,400 dispensary cases. The present medical staff consists of Drs. B. B. Wilson, Thomas G. Morton, L. W. Steinbach, John B. Roberts, W. H. Teller, Adolph Feldstein, Thomas Betts, S. Solis-Cohen, W. A. Cross, F. X. Dercum, Isaac Leopold, E. A. Jarecki, P. A. Trau and two assistant physicians. Like the other leading hospitals, it also has its own training school for nurses, and all the appointments of a first-class institution.

From this extreme northern part of the city we now turn to West Filbert street and Powelton avenue, at Thirty-ninth street, where, about five years after the foundation of the Jewish Hospital, another hospital was instituted under the auspices of a religious denomination. Enclosed by these streets and Saunders avenue were the extensive grounds of an institution of learning, known popularly as the "Old Institute," and owned by the Rev. Dr. E. D. Saunders. Whether or not the great controversy in the Presbyterian Church, which had divided that sect into the "old and new schools," had delayed the erection of a Presbyterian Hospital, it is a fact that the Presbyterian Alliance of Philadelphia determined to found a great charitable institution as a memorial of the reunion of the two bodies. The first General Assembly after the reunion met in Philadelphia in May, 1870, and the resolution of the Presbyterian Alliance of Philadelphia, above referred to, was adopted in September of the same year. The Rev. Dr. Saunders offered his entire college property for the use of the new charity (n). An organiza-

---

(n) The object of the charity intended as a memorial of the reunion of the old and new schools was not specified by the Presbyterian Alliance. The suggestion that it should take the form of a hospital was first made by a well-known physician of Philadelphia, Dr. R. M. Girvin, as appears in the following extract from a letter written by the Rev. Dr. E. D. Saunders to Prof. F. W. Hastings, February 25, 1871: "In all the plans which presented themselves to my mind for the final disposition of this beautiful grove for a charitable institution, there was not the first thought of a hospital. Dr. Girvin, who originated the idea, is a member of the Princeton congregation; you, with whom he had the encouraging consultations before he approached me on the subject, are an elder in the Princeton church; and the one, whose opposition or lack of cordiality even, would have wholly prevented my action, is a member of the Princeton church," etc. Dr. Saunders in this portion of his letter, was endeavoring to show how largely the

tion was effected on April 3, 1871, with Rev. George W. Musgrave as president, and a formal transfer of the property was made at the grounds on July 1st. The "Old Institute" was thus converted into the Presbyterian Hospital, with beds for forty-five patients. Over $350,000 was raised the first year, and in 1875 the first of the numerous new buildings of this great institution was erected. Now it has property worth about $800,000 and an endowment of $1,250,-000.

On the old college grounds are now eight fine structures, all but two of which are known as "wards"—two for men, a surgical and a medical; two for women, likewise; one for children, and one for emergencies and accidents. Besides this plant, the hospital owns a valuable tract of fifty-three acres, near Devon, sixteen miles from Philadelphia, on which are the Richardson and Cathcart homes, the former for convalescents of both sexes, the latter for incurables. Neither of these homes receives free cases. The Presbyterian Hospital handles annually above 1,800 cases, not counting about 2,500 in the out-patient department. Its medical board includes Drs. Oscar H. Allis, H. R. Wharton, William G. Porter, De Forest Willard, D. F. Woods, John H. Musser, R. G. Curtin, S. S. Stryker, Robert M. Girvin, E. L. Duer, George Strawbridge, C. H. Burnett, W. E. Hughes and H. W. Catell, with four others for Devon and seventeen for the dispensary staff. This great institution, as it now exists, is almost entirely a development of the present period.

In 1880, when John B. Stetson, the hatter, began his Union Mission and Hospital in the northeastern part of the city for his employés, the hospital post was a mere dispensary; but, in 1891, when he opened its new building on Fourth street above Columbia avenue, it had become a large institution with twenty members on its medical staff, and Dr. Thomas H. Fenton as medical director.

Its present staff, according to the last report, is as follows: Department of Internal Medicine and Pædiatrics—Physician, John H. Dripps, M. D.; assistant physician, E. G. Hawkes, M. D. Department of Surgery—Consulting surgeon, John H. Packard, M. D.;

---

movement was "Princetonian," and incidentally refers to Dr. Girvin's admirable suggestion.

surgeon, W. H. Noble, M. D. Department for Diseases of Women —Consulting surgeon, Howard A. Kelly, M. D.; surgeon, Chas. P. Noble, M. D. Department for Diseases of the Ear, Nose and Throat —Emeritus surgeon, Carl Seiler, M. D.; consulting surgeon, Harrison Allen, M. D.; surgeon, Chas. B. Warder, M. D.; assistant surgeon, Lewis S. Somers, M. D. Department for Diseases of the Eye —Assistant surgeon, Isaac Leopold, M. D.

It was reserved for a physician, Dr. Scott Stewart, a trustee of St. Paul's Methodist Episcopal Church, to take the initiative in founding the Methodist Episcopal Hospital on South Broad street. He provided the funds for the institution in his will in 1877, about six years after the opening of the Presbyterian Hospital. It is an interesting and somewhat anomalous fact that every member of the staff of this hospital must, in accordance with a provision of Dr. Stewart's will, have received the degree of Bachelor of Arts, as well as that of M. D.

Dr. Stewart's bequest not being operative until his sister's decease, it was not until February 14, 1885, that a charter was secured, and the same month Drs. H. C. Wood, D. M. Barr, J. S. Pearson, C. K. Mills, S. D. Risley, S. Harlow and A. C. Deakyne were elected as an advisory board. Numerous difficulties having been overcome, on July 8, 1887, a lot about 400 by 500 feet, bounded by Broad, Wolfe, Thirteenth and Ritner streets, was purchased. The plan provided that an administration building should front on Broad street, with three large pavilions on each side. So far only one pavilion has been erected, but this fine structure and the large administration building present an excellent idea of the future appearance of the hospital when its plans are completed. Already it compares favorably with any similar institution in Philadelphia. The present medical staff is as follows: Drs. R. C. Norris, T. S. Westcott, G. E. Shoemaker, W. R. Hoch, J. H. Lloyd, W. C. Hollopeter, J. P. C. Griffith, John B. Roberts, H. R. Wharton, R. G. Le Conte, E. W. Holmes, G. E. de Schweinitz, B. A. Randall and S. S. Kneass, with a dispensary staff of eleven. At present the annual average of cases is about 650, with over 3,200 out-patients. The annual expense of the hospital is about $35,000.

The Temple, the great Baptist Church at North Broad and Berks streets, under the guidance of Rev. Russell H. Conwell, followed in 1891, with the next general hospital, located on North Broad and Ontario streets. The Samaritan Hospital, as it is called, is so far small, with only a bed capacity of about 20 or 25, in an old residence building, but it is doing an excellent work, especially in its ambulance and dispensary service, and undoubtedly has an assured future as one of the great denominational hospitals of the city. Dr. E. S. Coburn is physician in charge.

The most recent general hospital is a small, but excellent, one for colored people, at 1512 Lombard street, not far from the Polyclinic, called—in honor of a distinguished member of the African race—the Frederick Douglass Memorial Hospital and Training School (for nurses). It was founded in 1895, and has a medical staff of twenty-three, including some of the best known names in the city. Dr. N. F. Mossell is chief of staff. It originated in a demand for trained colored nurses, and, in consequence, especial attention, unusual in so small an institution, is given to the training of nurses. The hospital was opened in a neat three-story brick building, and its two years' work has proved that it has supplied a long-felt want.

Since none of the general hospitals receive maternity cases, it has naturally resulted that the special hospitals are mostly devoted to obstetrics and the diseases of women and children. In that long period from the founding of the Pennsylvania Hospital to about the year 1850, when the denominational hospitals began, the need of institutions for the care of indigent women during confinement was widely felt, and was first supplied by the Lying-in Charity in 1828, and a little later by the Preston Retreat. The Philadelphia Lying-in Charity was instituted in 1828 by Dr. Joseph Warrington as a society for aiding indigent maternity cases in their own homes, and is the oldest institution of the kind in this country. A more formal organization was made on November 22, 1831, at a meeting attended by Drs. Beattie, Jewell, Spackman, Steward, Ash, Watson and Warrington. Incorporation was secured May 7, 1832, and, on November 12, the first annual meeting, at which forty-two cases were reported, was held. Dr. Dewees was made president and Dr. F. S. Beattie chairman of the medical board, with Dr. Harper Walton as secretary. The city was divided into six districts, with two physicians and three managers to each, the physicians being Drs. Robert Stewart, George Spackman, F. S. Beattie, E. Y. Howell, G. S. Schott, C. B. Matthews, T. F. Ash, H. Walton, J. G. Nancrede, W. Jewell, J. Dunott and J. Green. In 1844 the Nurses' Society united with the Lying-in Charity, and in 1850 a Nurses' Home was secured at the southeast corner of Eighth and Race streets. The first real headquarters of the Lying-in Charity opened July 2 of that year. In a certain sense it was an ally of the Philadelphia dispensary obstetrical service during these early years and endeavored to supply a want not provided for by the other hospitals of that date. In 1860 the managers secured a new home for the Charity at the southeast corner of Eleventh and Cherry streets, where its present beautiful four-story structure stands, as what may be called a highly organized school of obstetrics and gynecology. There have been many eminent physicians connected with this excellent institution, but when, in 1852, Dr. Warrington announced Dr. Ellwood Wilson's appointment as his senior assistant, the Lying-in Charity acquired him to whom the institution owes its most interesting development, and a debt of gratitude for long years of service as its chief. Next to Wilson, Dr. Albert H. Smith, who was elected a member of the staff in 1863, was the most active contributor to the success of the Lying-in Charity. Dr. Oliver Hopkinson, Jr., W. R. Wilson and G. M. Boyd, with four residents and six dispensary physicians, constitute the present staff.

When the Lying-in Charity had been in existence for about seven years, Dr. Jonas Preston made a will, in 1835, in which he said: "It has long been my opinion that there ought to be a Lying-in Hospital in the City of Philadelphia for indigent married women of good character, distinct and unconnected with any other hospital," and gave property for its founding. It has now had a career of over sixty years and has a capacity of fifty beds.

Preston Retreat, as it is called, is located at Twentieth and Hamilton streets. The names of Drs. William Goodell and Joseph

Price will always be associated with the excellent work of this noble charity. Dr. Richard C. Norris is the present physician in charge.

In February, 1873, three of the obstetrical staff and some of the ex-residents of "Blockley" (the Philadelphia Hospital), believing that a special institution should be formed to receive and help a large class of unfortunates who were about to become mothers, opened the Maternity Hospital at 734 South Tenth street, which was incorporated on January 2, following. The first year it received 69 cases, and year by year there was a gradual increase, until 1885, when the number of cases, for the first time, exceeded one hundred. During the year ending September 30, 1896, 161 permits for admission were issued. This institution and the Lying-in Charity are associated with the Midnight Mission, which cares for the mother until childbirth occurs; then, when mother and child are strong enough, they are sent to "The Sheltering Arms," and later the Children's Aid Society, or interested friends, directs them to a home in the country, "or to some other place of security and self-support." Two members of the Board of Governors of the Maternity Hospital deserve special mention on account of their self-sacrificing devotion to its interests. These are Dr. J. W. White, the first president of the board, and Dr. James V. Ingham. The latter has, for many years, been identified with this noble charity, and has probably done more for its welfare than any other individual. The Maternity medical staff includes Drs. W. C. Goodell, L. J. Hammond, L. S. Smith and D. T. Lainé, with Drs. Stillé, Penrose, Mitchell, Starr, Duer, White, Williams and Oliver as consultants.

The northeastern part of the city was once the site of one of the earliest hospitals for diseases peculiar to women and children amongst the poor. This was the Gynecological Hospital, created in July, 1874, and opened at 1624 Poplar street. Its medical board were Drs. J. J. Reese, J. A. McFerran and Theodore H. Seybert. In the same part of the city arose the Gynecean Hospital, incorporated January 10, 1888. This was an outgrowth of the work of the old Philadelphia Dispensary on Fifth street, and has the same aims as the last mentioned hospital.

It was founded by Dr. Joseph Price, opened in 1880, and incorporated January 10, 1888. Its first site was the corner of Twelfth and Cherry streets; later it occupied a house on Cherry street, and, finally, four or five years ago, was removed to 247 North Eighteenth street. While under Dr. Price's management the work of the institution was largely among private patients. Its present staff consists of Drs. C. B. Penrose, J. M. Baldy, J. B. Shober, R. G. Le Conte, L. S. Smith, M. O'Hara, Jr., H. D. Beyea, Norton Downs, W. F. Atlee, J. M. Da Costa and H. C. Bloom.

In 1883 Dr. Howard A. Kelly founded the Kensington Hospital for Women. In 1887 it was incorporated, and after ten years of successful growth averaged over 400 cases annually. It has a new building of forty-five-bed capacity, erected in 1897, at 136 Diamond street. Its medical staff includes Drs. C. P. Noble, surgeon-in-chief, H. A. Kelly, W. H. Parish, John B. Roberts, W. W. Keen, H. A. Wilson, C. B. Penrose, James Tyson, C. K. Mills, R. P. Harris, H. E. Applebach, W. E. Parke, E. H. Byers and several assistant physicians.

WEST PHILADELPHIA HOSPITAL FOR WOMEN.

Origin: This hospital was started because of the realized need of a hospital under the care of women physicians in this section of the city.

Dr. Elizabeth H. Comly-Howell was the one most actively interested in the establishment of the hospital, and it was at her call that the ladies met who formed the Board of Managers.

History: The hospital was opened July 15, 1889, at the northeast corner of Forty-first and Ogden streets. It occupied a private house and accommodated ten patients. The parlor was used as a dispensary. The hospital was incorporated January 18, 1890. For the first few months the hospital was under the care of a physician in charge, but in 1890 two internes were appointed, one to serve in the house and the other to have charge of the out-practice. In April, 1891, 4035 Parrish street was purchased and the hospital moved there, as the original quarters had become very cramped. This change gave eighteen beds. In the spring of 1894, there not being sufficient room for the nurses, 4048 Ogden street was purchased. The second and third stories were used for the nurses, and the first floor as a dispensary. The dispensary now being moved from the main building, a ward was opened on the first floor with a capacity of seven beds. Alterations were made on the second floor, by which were secured a fine operating room, finished in tile; an etherizing room and a surgical ward adjoining. The management was somewhat altered during this year, a trained nurse being appointed as superintendent of the hospital. In 1895 the roof to the main building was raised so as to give the full height of ceiling to the third floor rooms. Additions were made to the back buildings, a new diet kitchen built, and the laboratory and lavatory arrangements improved. Accommodation was made for 28 patients. In 1896 a lot adjoining the hospital was purchased, giving space for a nice garden, from which fresh vegetables are supplied. A house adjoining the dispensary was rented and opened in July as a maternity house, with seven beds. This gave a total bed capacity of thirty-five. In the spring of 1897, 4046 Ogden street, which had been used as a maternity, was purchased.

Training School for Nurses: This was opened July, 1890. The first nurse commencement was held October 25, 1894, at which time four nurses received diplomas. Fourteen nurses have graduated from the school.

Original Medical Staff: Physician in charge, Dr. Elizabeth L. Peck.

Attending Physicians, Drs. Elizabeth H. Comly-Howell, Ida E. Richardson and Elizabeth L. Peck.

Ophthalmologist, Dr. Amy S. Barton.

Pathologist, Dr. Marie K. Formad.

Consulting Physicians, Drs. Anna E. Broomall, Hannah T. Croasdale, Jas. B. Walker, W. W. Keen, John H. Musser, J. B. Roberts.

Clinicians, Drs. Elizabeth H. Comly-Howell, Elizabeth L. Peck, Emily Waterman-Wyeth, A. Helena Goodwin, Anna P. Sharpless.

Present Medical Staff: Attending staff, Drs. Ida E. Richardson, Elizabeth L. Peck, A. Helena Goodwin, Mary W. Griscom.

Assistant Physicians, Drs. Frances Hatchette, Lida M. Stewart, Margaret F. Butler, Anna P. Sharpless.

Laryngologist, Dr. Emma E. Musson.

Ophthalmologist, Dr. Mary Getty.

Pathologist, Dr. J. Dutton Steele.

Consulting Physicians, Drs. Anna E. Broomall, Hannah T. Croasdale, Amy S. Barton, Elizabeth H. Comly-Howell, Jas. B. Walker, Chas. H. Burnett, W. W. Keen, John B. Roberts, Thos. G. Morton, Chas. K. Mills, John H. Musser, Jas. Tyson, William Pepper.

The District Nurse Society, now the Visiting Nurses' Society, was begun March 2, 1886, somewhat after the plan of the similar society in Manchester, England, and has done a good work supplementary to the above lines. It has a central office at 1340 Lombard street and two branches in Huntingdon and Carver streets. The Children's Hospital was opened in November, 1855. It was first begun on Blight street, near Pine, east of Broad street, with Drs. T. Hewson Bache, F. W. Lewis, R. A. F. Penrose, the elder Pepper and J. F. Meigs as its medical staff. In 1865, after two removals, its present building on Twenty-second street, below Walnut, was erected, and was opened in February, 1867. Since its establishment in that situation, its growth and development have been rapid and varied. It now has a capacity of ninety-seven beds, and a country branch for thirty-two patients. The annual average is about 700 cases, with from 5,000 to 7,000 dispensary cases.

Besides the above mentioned institutions there are special hospitals devoted to the treatment of such affections as the following: Diseases of the mind and nervous system, diseases of the eye, hospitals for the treatment of deformities, hospitals for incurables, etc. The oldest of these is the beautiful Friends' Asylum for "those deprived of their reason," in one of the most picturesque situations to be found near Frankford, about ten miles from Philadelphia. In 1813, the year that Dr. Rush died, its founders proposed a hospital where "the insane might see that they were regarded as men and brethren." Its eighty acres of lawns and gardens make a park of rare beauty. To its other buildings has been recently added a new Nurses' Training School—Elmhurst.

In this connection may be mentioned the immense plant of the great State Hospital for the Insane at Norristown, which is only incidentally Philadelphian. Philadelphia, however, furnishes about two-thirds of its 2,000 inmates. The institution was founded eighteen years ago. Its medical staff consists of Drs. D. D. Richardson, A. W. Wilmarth, G. W. McCaffrey, Alice Bennett, S. J. Taber, Mary Willits, Florence H. Watson, William C. Posey, E. M. Corson, Edward Martin, O. Horwitz, E. W. Holmes, Isaac Ott and S. P. Gerhard. Thus, with this state institution, the Pennsylvania Hospital for the Insane, and the Friends' Asylum, Philadelphia has long generously provided for the most unfortunate of her afflicted, although provision for the greater number has been made in the present period. It is doubtful if any other city can show a longer and brighter record in this department of medical and charitable interest.

Just twenty years after the Friends established their Frankford asylum for the mentally afflicted, there was completed, on Race between Eighteenth and Nineteenth streets, a hospital for the indigent blind and lame, under the direction of the Board of City Trusts, to which this duty was entrusted by a bequest of the late James Wills. The Wills Hospital, as it is called, was undertaken on May 24, 1831, when the bequest was received by the Mayor, and the first building was completed in 1833. Extensions have been made from time to time, until the institution now handles over 13,000 cases annually. Indeed, it has grown to be not only a great eye hospital, but a great school of ophthalmology, somewhat as the Lying-in Charity is a school of obstetrics and gynecology. This arises from the fact that, without design, from the first the treatment of eye diseases has been so prominent a feature of the institution as to give the hospital its popular name. Among the surgeons whose long and skillful service has made a world-wide reputation for Wills Hospital, are: Drs. Littell, Hall, Harlan, Keyser, Norris, Goodman, McClure, Strawbridge and T. G. Morton. The first surgeons were Drs. Isaac Parrish, S. Littell, Isaac Hays and George

Fox, and the first physicians, Drs. George Spackman, Fredk. Turnpenny, P. B. Howell and R. Stewart. Its present staff, according to the last report, is composed of Drs. Conrad Berens, Frank Fisher, G. C. Harlan, Eward Jackson, P. D. Keyser (o), W. W. McClure, W. F. Norris, Charles A. Oliver, Samuel D. Risley, William Thomson, ten assistant surgeons and two resident surgeons. Its greatest growth has been during the last twenty-seven years, and its services are entirely gratuitous.

Exactly twenty years after Wills Hospital was completed, "a number of bright, enlightened and progressive physicians and surgeons of Philadelphia," says Dr. Laurence Turnbull, in a recent address, "felt the necessity of organizing in the profession a new mode of classifying and treating diseases, with facility and greater success by means of specialties, after the plan of the Vienna Hospital, each physician selecting the department for which he, either from study, inclination or experience, was best fitted." Drs. O. H. Partridge, Joseph Klapp and others among these physicians, in 1853, proceeded to establish what was then called "The Western Infirmary," their organization being effected in May, 1854. Its first location was over a drug store at the northwest corner of Pine and Seventeenth streets, with two rooms, but the facilities there afforded soon proving inadequate, the infirmary was removed to Lukens place, on Christian street, between Fifteenth and Sixteenth. In 1858 the title was changed to "Western Clinical Infirmary and Hospital for Incurables," and after two other removals on Lombard street, Dr. Laurence Turnbull was chosen manager, and, in 1886, took the lead in securing its present site at the southeast corner of South Broad and Catherine streets, where were soon erected its present fine buildings. The hospital now averages about 300 cases annually, from 1,000 to 2,000 accident cases, and an out-patient service of over 8,000. Its present staff includes: Drs. George McClellan, Edward Martin, C. H. Frazier, Charles Wirgman, A. E. Roussel, G. B. Massey, B. C. Hirst, John B. Shober, W. B. Atkinson, E. P. Davis, Lewis Brinton, J. M. Taylor, F. D. Castle, W. C. Posey, E. L. Vansant, A. W. Watson, H. W. Stelwagon, two residents and

---

(o) Since deceased.

one clinical assistant. Its name has again been changed to "Howard Hospital and Infirmary for Incurables," and, as has been seen, its greatest development has been wholly within the present period.

Fourteen years after Howard Hospital was projected, Drs. T. G. Morton, H. E. Goodman, D. Hayes Agnew, S. D. and S. W. Gross and G. W. Norris, together with others, non-medical men, proposed to found the first regular chartered institution in this country for the relief of deformities, such as distortion of the spine, club-foot, knock-knee, affections of the joints, contraction of tendons and muscles and the like. In October, 1867, the step was decided upon, and in December the Philadelphia Orthopædic Hospital was incorporated on plans similar to those of the great foreign institutions for the treatment of deformities. A building was secured at 15 South Ninth street, then opposite the University. In 1870 there was added the department for nervous diseases, and in February, 1872, a new home at North Seventeenth and Summer streets was secured. It then took its title, "Orthopædic Hospital and Infirmary for Nervous Diseases," and on March 19, 1887, its present fine building was opened. The present medical staff consists of Drs. T. G. Morton, W. W. Keen, G. G. Davis, S. Weir Mitchell, Wharton Sinkler, M. J. Lewis, G. R. Morehouse, R. G. Le Conte, W. J. Taylor, J. M. Spellissy, T. S. K. Morton, J. M. Taylor, G. Hinsdale, J. K. Mitchell, F. X. Dercum, J. H. W. Rhein, G. E. de Schweinitz, B. C. Hirst, C. W. Burr, D. B. Kyle, W. J. Freeman and two residents. The annual average is now nearly 400 cases, with about 3,800 clinical cases. This institution, too, is largely the product of the present period.

In 1872, the same year in which the Orthopædic Hospital moved to Summer street, a number of temperance workers and philanthropists met early in the year to devise some method of helping the inebriate, from the point of view of treating him "both as an invalid and a sinner," without considering him as the subject of hereditary disease. The result was the Franklin Reformatory Home for Inebriates, organized on April 1, 1872. As over eighty per cent of inebriates require medical treatment, it is in a true sense a hospital. Its excellent home is situated at 911-15 Locust street, and its annual average of cases is above 200. The medical staff includes Drs. E. E. Graham, M. H. Williams, W. E. Hughes and W. C. Posey. Five years later, 1877, the Protestant Episcopal City Mission, which had been organized seven years before, opened its department for consumptives. This consists of the House of Mercy for Men, at 411 Spruce street and the Women's Home for Consumptives, at Chestnut Hill, the oldest and largest institution of the kind in the State. Over 2,300 cases have been treated since their organization, and the annual average of cases reaches about 170. During the same year, on May 4, 1877, the Philadelphia Home for Incurables and Cancer House was organized, and now, after twenty years, has an average of about eighty patients. So many applicants were cancer cases that a cancer annex has been established. The home, with its several structures, is located at Forty-eighth and Woodland avenue (Darby road), and its medical staff consists of Drs. C. P. Turner, W. C. Dixon, W. W. Keen, De Forest Willard, E. L. Duer, C. S. Turnbull, C. W. Burr, D. B. Kyle, S. W. Morton, Harry Toulmin and Isaac Leopold. This institution and the Episcopal Homes for Consumptives had been in operation thirteen years when Drs. T. J. Mays, L. F. Flick, Charles W. Dulles and others secured the incorporation of Rush Hospital for Consumption and Allied Diseases on September 15, 1890. It was designed to meet demands that the Episcopalian homes, with all their capacity, could not meet, for, says Judge Ashman, in '94, "in every year more victims succumb to this disease in the City of Philadelphia than have fallen in battles which have become historic." At first it was located at the northeast corner of Pine and Twenty-second streets, but in July, 1895, it secured its present extensive grounds at the northwest corner of Thirty-third and Lancaster avenue, where it undoubtedly has a great future before it, and where it is already doing an excellent work. Its medical staff consists of Drs. Alfred Stillé, R. G. Curtin, Harrison Allen, T. J. Mays, J. P. C. Griffith, S. Solis-Cohen, T. M. Tyson, W. R. Hoch, B. A. Randall, Charles W. Dulles and Joseph McFarland, with two physicians for the out-patient department. When this institution moved to Thirty-third street, in 1895, the colony part of the Pennsylvania Epileptic Hospital and Colony Farm was chartered, and the following year was merged with the St. Clement's Church Hospital, which had been organized in 1886. The hospital is located at Cherry and Claymont streets, and the farm at Oakbourne, in Chester County. These institutions are doing an excellent work. The present medical staff includes: Drs. S. Weir Mitchell, J. M. Da Costa, T. G. Morton, J. W. White, G. E. de Schweinitz, C. H. Burnett, S. W. Morton, H. Shoemaker, G. E. Shoemaker, H. A. Slocum, W. C. Posey, A. A. Bliss, W. G. Spiller and A. F. Witmer.

The City is represented in the Municipal Hospital for Contagious Diseases, mentioned in connection with the boards of health and quarantine service; the State by the Norristown institution, already mentioned, and the Nation by the United States Naval Asylum and Hospital on the old Pemberton estate on the Schuylkill, at Gray's Ferry road and Bainbridge street. This was bought for the Government in 1826 by Dr. Thomas Harris, a Pennsylvanian and a naval surgeon. As an institution which has sheltered many of the defenders of our country it has an historic interest, which, however, is chiefly national. Its hospital department, established in 1868, has a capacity of 100. In addition to these institutions there are private enterprises innumerable in almost every line of medical activity, many of these institutions being of the first order in the excellence of their work. The dispensaries of the city, from the foundation of the old Philadelphia and the Northern dispensaries down to the present, have increased to such an extent that it would be impossible to mention them all in a work of this sort. Indeed, every department of the medical activity of Philadelphia, during the twenty years since the Medical Congress of 1876, has increased at a rate far beyond that of any former period of equal length.

Philadelphia, during the present year, has witnessed two events of national significance, which may fitly close the story of the present period, as well as that of her medical career of nearly two and a half centuries. One of these is the semi-centennial anniversary of the foundation of the American Medical Association in Philadelphia, the fifth meeting of that body held in this city. In his opening address of that event on June 1, 1897, at the Academy of Music, President Senn gave to Philadelphia the following tribute: "It is appropriate," said he, "that you should have selected Philadelphia as the place of meeting at this time. It was here that the organization of our association was completed half a century ago. Philadelphia is near and dear to every American citizen, as it is the birthplace of the greatest and most prosperous of nations in the world. It is here that, on July 4, 1776, the most precious document in the possession of the American people—the Declaration of Independence—was signed, read and approved by the representatives of a people who cared for freedom, liberty and independence. It was here that the sweet music of the liberty bell was first heard, the reverberations of which reached from the Atlantic to the Pacific and from the Great Lakes to the Gulf of Mexico, and which has continued and will continue to echo and reëcho over our vast and free country for all time to come. It is a source of congratulation to every and all honest and progressive practitioners of medicine that that document, which was the means of planting a free government upon the virgin American soil and creating a new nation, was signed and heroically defended by America's greatest physician—Benjamin Rush. The bloody struggle for independence by a united, patriotic people and its great success culminated in the foundation of the great Republic of the United States, which, in time, gave the medical men an opportunity to establish American medicine upon a free American soil. It required a long time after the permanency of our government was assured for our professional ancestors to appreciate this opportunity and to take the necessary steps to secure adequate facilities for our young men to obtain a satisfactory medical education in this country and to create a medical literature of their own. Foreign textbooks were used and European universities continued to be the Mecca for American students who sought a higher medical education. The country was new, its resources limited, its inhabitants represented different customs and nationalities, and the number of qualified practitioners limited. It is, therefore, not surprising that the organization of the profession, the establishment of institutions of learning and the foundation of an American medical literature met with many difficulties, which it required years to correct and remove. Philadelphia has a special charm for every practitioner of medicine who has the interest and welfare of his profession at heart, as it has been, and still remains, the center of medical education and medical literature in this country, besides being the birthplace of the American Medical Association."

Previous to this event a meeting was held at the national capital to celebrate the fame of another Philadelphian, who must always take rank with Benjamin Rush, the physician, namely, Samuel Gross, America's most famous surgeon. For the first time in American history a statue of a member of the medical profession was erected among those of the patriots, statesmen and warriors whom the nation has delighted to honor. The project was carried to completion by the Alumni Association of Jefferson Medical College, of which he was the most distinguished member, and by the American Surgical Association, of which he was the founder. On May 5, 1897, there was unveiled, with ceremonies of a national character, a bronze statue, nine feet high, mounted on a red granite pedestal of a height of eleven feet, and bearing the name "Samuel D. Gross," surrounded by a wreath, underneath which is inscribed: "American physicians have erected this statue to commemorate the great deeds of a man who made such an impression upon American surgery that it has served to dignify American medicine."

Nearly a month later, when President Senn delivered his opening address at the Philadelphia Academy of Music, he made an appeal for the Rush Monument Fund, which has been progressing at a snail's pace since it was proposed in the National Association in 1884, with hope of unveiling a statue to Rush at the Congress of '87. "See to it," said he, "that the capital city will soon be graced by a magnificent statue of the idol of the American profession, the patriot-physician, and one of the greatest benefactors of our country—Benjamin Rush." On Friday, June 4, 1897, a resolution was passed providing for the raising of $100,000 for this purpose by the American Medical Association. So when, in future years, the visitor at Washington beholds the first two statues erected to American physicians, and reads the names—Benjamin

Rush and Samuel D. Gross—he may realize the truth of the words of one of the most famous of Philadelphia's living physicians, the poet-novelist: "In new lands, peopled by the self-selection of the fittest, by those who have the courage of enterprise, and the mental and moral outfit to win for it success, the physician is sure to take and keep the highest place, and to find open to him more easily than to others, wealth, social place and, if he desires it, the higher service of the state. In New England the clergy were for a long time dominant. In New York then, as now, commercial success was the surest road to social position. South of us it was the land-holder who ruled with undisputed sway. But in this city—I may say in this state—from the first settlement until to-day, the physician has held an almost unquestioned and somewhat curious pre-eminence." But if that visitor were to come hither and become familiar not only with the city's medical past, but with the spirit and achievements of the present, he would realize that it is fitly expressed in other words from the same pen:

> "A grander morning floods our skies
> With higher aims, and larger light;
> Give welcome to the century new,
> And to the past a glad good-night."

CHAPTER VI.

MEDICAL AND SURGICAL APPLIANCES.

The earliest invention by a Philadelphian, of which we have been able to find any record, was the Bond splint, invented by Thomas Bond (1712-1784), for the treatment of fractures of the lower end of the radius, and still much used for that purpose. He also invented an œsophageal forceps for the extraction of foreign bodies from the œsophagus.

Benjamin Rush (1745-1813), in his book on the "Diseases of the Mind," describes his famous "tranquillity chair," and a less known apparatus which he termed a "gyrator." Dr. T. G. Morton, in the "History of the Pennsylvania Hospital," gives an account of these two appliances, accompanied by an illustration of the "tranquillizer." The latter "was supposed to control the impetus of the blood toward the brain, and by lessening muscular action, or reducing motor activity, to reduce the force and frequency of the pulse." The "gyrator," on the other hand, was designed for use in "torpid madness." The head was placed at the greatest distance from the center of motion, and, on revolving the "gyrator," the blood, by the centrifugal action, was caused to go to the head and accelerate the action of the heart from seventy to one hundred and twenty beats in a minute.

Philip Syng Physick (1768-1837, "the Father of American Surgery," invented many surgical instruments and appliances. In the performance of his first lithotomy he divided the internal pudic artery, occasioning very alarming hemorrhage, which he had much difficulty in checking. He found that he was unable to ligate the artery with the ordinary means, without enclosing in the ligature a quantity of surrounding tissue. To overcome this difficulty, under similar circumstances, he invented his forceps and needle, which were subsequently used in the ligation of other vessels, as well as the internal pudic. In 1795, he invented an instrument for the performance of internal urethrotomy, consisting of a lancet, concealed in a canula. The canula was to be pushed down to the stricture, and then the lancet was to be thrust forward so as to effect its division. After this a catheter or bougie was to be inserted to keep the opening patulous.

In 1796, he invented his "bougie-pointed catheter" under the following circumstances: A case of retention of urine was brought to the Pennsylvania Hospital. Dr. Physick found he was unable to introduce a catheter, and that the introduction of a bougie was not followed by any flow of urine. He then fastened the point of a bougie upon the extremity of an elastic catheter, and this contrivance he succeeded in introducing into the bladder, with immediate relief to his patient.

In the Medical Repository, 1804, Vol. I, p. 127, there is a very interesting account of the performance of his celebrated seton operation for ununited fracture. The operation was performed on December 18, 1802, at the Pennsylvania Hospital. The patient was a sailor, 28 years old, who had sustained a fracture of the humerus, twenty months previous to the operation. Dr. Physick says that he had himself been a witness to the unsatisfactory results of the ordinary method of treatment of these cases, which consisted in sawing off the fractured extremities of the bone, thus reducing the part to the condition of a recent compound fracture, and that he had consequently determined to treat this case by an entirely different plan. He passed a silk seton between the ends of the bone and left it there, with a view, he says, "of exciting inflammation and suppuration until granulations should arise on the ends of the bone, which uniting, and afterward ossifying, would form the bony union that was wanting." On the 4th of May, 1802, the seton was removed, and on the 28th of May the patient was discharged from the hospital, "able to move his arm in all directions as well as he could before the accident."

In Randolph's memoir of Physick, he tells how, in 1830, he was attending a man in a remitting fever. He says: "A few days after my first visit, in riding past his door in company with Dr. Physick, feeling very uneasy about the condition of my patient, I requested the doctor to step into the house and see him with me and give me the benefit of his advice." Dr. Physick complied with his request, and recognized in the patient the man upon whom he had first passed a seton for ununited fracture of the humerus, twenty-eight years previously. The man died, and Randolph secured his humerus, which showed, at the place of fracture, the bone perfectly consolidated by a mass of callus, in the center of which there was a hole, showing the place through which the seton had passed.

In the Philadelphia Medical Museum, 1805, Vol. I, p. 307, Bishop, the instrument-maker, describes a modification of the ordinary curved bistoury, which Dr. Physick had devised for use in the operation for fistula in ano. Dr. Physick had the instrument made with a silver guard to prevent the edge from cutting any part of the sinus during its introduction into it. This guard was detachable, after it had been introduced, by a very simple mechanism, consisting of a button, which was pressed forward. It thus combined the advantages possessed by both the sharp and the blunt pointed bistoury.

In the Philadelphia Medical Museum, 1805, Vol. I, p. 186, Bishop describes Dr. Physick's improved lithotomy gorget. It was made so that the beak and the blade were separable from one another. This permitted a fine edge to be given to that part of the blade which was contiguous to the beak, the object being to facilitate division of the prostatic gland and neck of the bladder. In January, 1809, Physick first performed his operation for the cure of artificial anus, which consisted in getting rid of the septum by placing a ligature around it for seven days, and then establishing communication between the two portions of the bowel by an incision with a curved bistoury.

In the Eclectic Repertory, 1816, Vol. VI, p. 389, there is a letter from Dr. Physick, in which he speaks of the delay in the healing of wounds because of the ligatures in use. He says: "Several years ago, recollecting how completely leather straps, spread with adhesive plaster and applied over wounds, for the purpose of keeping their sides in contact, were dissolved by the fluids discharged from the wound, it occurred to me that ligatures might be made of leather, or of some other animal substance, with which the sides of a blood-vessel could be compressed for a sufficient time to prevent hemorrhage, and that such ligatures would be dissolved after a few days and would be evacuated with the discharge from the cavity of the wound." He requested Dr. Dorsey to try such a ligature on a horse, and the result justified his anticipations. The letter goes on to say that, acting on Dr. Physick's suggestion, Dr. Hartshorne had used ligatures made of parchment on some of the arteries, after an amputation of the thigh, and they were found dissolved at the first dressing. Dr. Dorsey, with Dr. Physick's assistance, used French kid ligatures with success in several cases. He experimented with different substances to ascertain which would withstand the solvent power of pus for the longest time, by applying the material over the surfaces of ulcers. Buckskin and kid dissolved first, then the parchment, lastly the catgut. Fearing that the leather might dissolve too soon in tying large vessels, he intended to request Dr. Dorsey to use leather, impregnated with the varnish used in making elastic catheters. In his letter he makes the suggestion that perhaps tendon would be found more durable than any of the materials above mentioned.

In the American Journal of the Medical Sciences, 1828, Vol. I, p. 262, Physick describes his tonsillotome. This instrument he first had made with a view of amputating the uvula in a particular case, but its success for that purpose led him to apply the same principles to the construction of an instrument for the removal of the tonsils. He acknowledges that the primal idea of his instrument was derived from Bell's instrument for the amputation of the uvula. Physick's instrument was composed of a straight, flat piece of steel, with an oval opening in its distal extremity, which was designed to receive the tonsil. To the plate, there was attached a knife, fitted in lateral grooves, which could be pushed forward after the tonsil had been fitted into the opening in the plate, and would then amputate the projecting part. Physick also used an original form of toothed forceps to draw the tonsil from its bed. Randolph attributes to Physick the improvement in the treatment of coxalgia, by a curved splint, combined with absolute rest.

Dr. Physick has often had ascribed to him the credit of being the first to suggest washing out the stomach in cases where poisons had been swallowed. In the Eclectic Repertory for October, 1812, he published an account of this method, as he had employed it in the treatment of two children suffering from laudanum poisoning, and he there stated that it was original with him, but in a subsequent communication to the same journal he acknowledged that the invention of this method of treatment belonged to Dr. Alexander Munro, Jr., of Edinburgh, who published an account of it in his inaugural thesis in 1797. Doctor Physick states that he was ignorant of Dr. Munro's priority of invention until he, since his first communication to the Eclectic Repertory, had received a copy of Munro's Anatomy, in which it was mentioned. Physick was, however, the first to actually put this treatment in practice.

Physick modified Desault's apparatus for the treatment of fracture of the femur by carrying the outer splint all the way up to the axilla, thus securing counter-extension more in the line of the body, and preventing lateral inclination of the pelvis.

Dr. James Hutchinson (1752-1793) modified Physick's modification of Desault's apparatus still further by attaching a block to the splint, which enabled extension to be kept up, and by securing the splints with tapes, enabled the part to be seen without the labor necessary in the removal of the eighteen-tailed bandage, which had formerly been used to retain the splints in position.

Dr. Joseph Hartshorne (1779-1850) invented an apparatus for the treatment of fractured patella, consisting of a tin splint, with straps and buckles to go above and below the fragments, and secure them in apposition.

He also devised a method for the treatment of fractures of the femur, in which counter-extension is made against the perineum at the upper end of the inside splint, and extension is made by a movable footboard, worked with a screw. By this arrangement the outer splint could be detached from the inner one without disturbing the extending or the counter-extending force.

Dr. Joseph Parrish (1779-1840) invented an aneurismal needle, consisting of a handle and stem, and a number of needles of different curves, each having an eye near the extremity, and which could be secured or detached from the stem of the instrument.

In 1800, he first conceived the idea of treating epididymitis by firm pressure, evenly applied. He accomplished this by means of a narrow roller.

John Syng Dorsey (1783-1818) was the inventor of a splint for the treatment of fractured patella. It was made of wood, and extended from the tuberosity of the ischium to the heel. Attached to it were strips of muslin to go above and below the fragments, which could be brought together by tying the strips.

William Gibson (1788-1868) was the first to introduce the use of the inclined plane for the purpose of making counter-extension in the treatment of fractures of the femur. He modified Hagedorn's apparatus for the treatment of this condition, extending the two splints on the outside of the thighs up to the axillæ.

He invented the Gibson head bandage for the treatment of fractures of the jaw.

Charles Delucena Meigs (1792-1869) invented a much-used form of ring pessary.

John Rhea Barton (1796-1871) originated the bran dressing for fractures of the lower extremity. It was applied by placing a mackintosh over the bottom and sides of an ordinary fracture box. In the bottom of the box a layer of bran was spread, on which the limb was placed after the reduction of the fracture. The remaining space in the box was then filled in with more bran.

He was the first to attempt to connect the fragments in a case of fractured patella, by silver wire. The patient, however, did not survive long after the operation. He invented the bandage for the head which bears his name; likewise the Barton handkerchief bandage for making extension in fracture of the lower limb.

William E. Horner (1793-1853) invented an instrument which he termed an awl, for passing ligatures around deep-seated vessels. He modified Desault's apparatus for fractured femur, by substituting padded splints for the plain splints with junk bags, and by attaching the counter-extending band to the upper end of both splints.

Hugh Lenox Hodge (1796-1873) also used a modification of Desault's apparatus for the treatment of fractures of the femur, which consisted in doing away with a counter-extending band altogether, and using instead a long outside splint, with an iron hook, extending over the top of the patient's head, at its upper extremity. He placed adhesive strips across the patient's chest and then connected them with the hook by a longitudinal strip, thus making counter-extension.

He invented a lever pessary, also an obstetric forceps.

S. D. Gross (1805-1884) was the inventor of many ingenious devices. Probably the most important of them was his horseshoe tourniquet, by which pressure could be exerted over directly opposite points on a limb. In the treatment of fracture of the femur he used a long fracture box, with a fenestrated footpiece, and with two crutches, one for the perineum and one for the axilla, attached to its two outer sides.

For the treatment of fractures at the condyles of the humerus he devised a tin case, extending from the axilla to the metacarpophalangeal articulations. He also originated a tin splint for use in fractures of the tibia. A very useful invention of his was a foreign body extractor, for use in the ear and nose. Dr. Gross designed an apparatus for the transfusion of blood, which is very largely used. He was also the inventor of a bullet probe, a blood catheter, tracheal forceps, an artery forceps, urethrotome and a fenestrated forceps, for use in the operation for artificial anus.

Dr. Joseph Pancoast (1805-1882) was the first to use pins subcutaneously to unite the fragments in ununited fracture. His apparatus for the treatment of coxalgia was simple in design and of great service.

Dr. George Fox (1806-1882) was the inventor of the apparatus for the treatment of fractured clavicle which goes by his name. It consisted of a wedge-shaped pad, to fill in the axilla, with tapes attached to each angle; a ring made of muslin stuffed with hair, to encircle the arm at the shoulder, and a broad sling. The ring was slipped over the arm of the sound side, and the pad placed in the axilla of the injured side, and maintained in position by tying the tapes to the ring. The arm was then placed in the sling, the wrist suspended to the ring by the front tapes, and the elbow carried upward and backward and secured to the ring by the tapes attached to the upper and lower parts of the posterior portion of the sling.

Dr. Henry Horner Smith (1815-1890) invented an apparatus for the treatment of ununited fractures of the lower extremity, by means of which the ends of the bone at the point of fracture were kept in a position which caused them to rub against one another, whilst the bone was kept in correct position.

Dr. D. Hayes Agnew (1818-1892) devised a well-known splint for fractured patella. It was made of board, about thirty inches long, somewhat convex on its upper surface, in its long axis. On each side, a short distance above and below the middle, there were placed wooden pegs. Overlapping adhesive strips were placed above and below the injured bone and attached to the screws. When the latter were rotated they tightened the strips and brought the fragments together. Agnew's apparatus for the immobilization of the hip-joint, while permitting locomotion, has been much used. He devised anterior and internal angular splints for the treatment of fractures of the humerus. He also invented a retractor for holding aside the peritoneum during operations on the iliac arteries; a mackerel-billed forceps for dividing the pedicle of a uterine polyp; a flexible spiral wire probe; a blood catheter; a urethral dilator, with three blades, for use in the female urethra; a toothed artery forceps; an intercostal artery compressor, and the special instruments required for use in his operation for the radical cure of hernia.

Dr. John Neill (1819-1880) invented an apparatus for the treatment of factures of the leg, consisting of a long fracture box, in which the leg was placed, and extension and counter-extension applied by adhesive strips attached to the upper and lower portions of the leg, and connected to corresponding parts of the box. He also modified Desault's splint for fracture of the femur, by attaching a double cord to the extending and counter-extending bands, and bringing the ends over the upper and lower extremities of the outside splint, so that extension and counter-extension could be made simultaneously by twisting the rope.

Dr James J. Levick (1824-1893) originated the treatment of sunstroke by rubbing the patient with ice.

Dr. Richard J. Levis (1827-1890) invented a wire loop for the withdrawal of the lens in cataract operations; a notched director for the division of the constricting band of a hernia; a phimosis forceps, and an apparatus for the treatment of fractured patella, which consisted in a splint to go behind the knee, a band to cross the limb above the upper fragment, and a strap passing down from this band to a stirrup, which was placed under the foot. He also modified Malgaigne's hooks by dividing them into two halves, longitudinally, and then introducing the hooks some distance apart. He likewise invented an apparatus for producing extension in fracture of the femur; a metallic splint for fractures of the lower end of the radius, and a tractor for the reduction of dislocations of the digits. The latter consisted of a piece of wood, about eight inches long and somewhat wider than the fingers or thumb. A row of perforations ran down on each side of the piece of wood. The dislocated member is laid on the wood, tapes are passed over it and through the perforations, and wound tight to the tailpiece of the board, and the instrument, when thus adjusted, is capable of exerting powerful traction if pulled.

Dr. Addinell Hewson (1828-1889) was the inventor of a torsion forceps, which consisted of two sets of blades, one set broad and flat for seizing and drawing out the artery, the other much smaller, duckbill-shaped, or curved at the point, and designed for dividing the coats of the vessel. The torsion was applied by rotating the forceps on its axis. He also originated the method of treating wounds with earth, and invented a fracture bed.

Of other Philadelphia surgeons who have invented instruments we may mention: Dr. Isaac Hays, who invented a cataract knife; Dr. S. W. Gross, who invented a coiled silver prostatic catheter, an urethral dilator and an urethrotome; Dr. John Ashhurst, Jr., who invented a bracketed wire splint for use after excision of the knee, and Dr. T. G. Morton, who, in 1866, designed a hospital ward dressing carriage, which received a certificate of award from the U. S. Centennial Commission in 1876. He is also the originator of a method of bringing together the fragments of a fractured patella, with a drill, which is passed through the fragments and then close apposition is maintained by a nut which is run down one end of the drill.

Dr. John H. Packard first called attention to the value of the stage of primary etherization in the performance of minor operations. He also devised a bracketed splint for use in compound fractures of the femur. Dr. Oscar H. Allis invented the ether inhaler which goes by his name; also a bistoury for division of the constricting band of a hernia. Dr. John B. Roberts is the originator of the treatment of fractures of the nasal bones by means of pins. Dr. W. B. Hopkins has introduced a modification of Charrière's artery compressor, by increasing the number of points by which the pressure is exerted; also a very useful gouge forceps, for use in trephining, and a vertebrated saw for the removal of plaster bandages.

Among the surgical appliances invented by Philadelphians should also be named Bonwill's surgical engine, especially of service in dentistry, but also capable of application in many surgical operations. Kolbe and Osborne's orthopedic appliances are of national fame. Gemrig and the firm of Lentz and Sons have added many valuable instruments to the surgeon's armamentarium.

CHAPTER VII.

THE PUBLIC MEDICAL LIBRARIES OF PHILADELPHIA.

The appreciation of the value of a public medical library by the profession itself is measured by the character and scope of the works contained in it, and by its accessibility to readers and inquirers after information. So it happens in Philadelphia that, although there are three medical libraries which deserve consideration as available for professional use and consultation, only one is generally referred to when mention is made of public libraries— the Library of the College of Physicians of Philadelphia; those of the Pennsylvania Hospital and of the Philadelphia Hospital being more restricted in their use, and less accessible, on account of the more private character of the hospital regulations as to hours and the provisions by which they are governed.

The Library of the Pennsylvania Hospital antedates the other two, having had its origin in the colonial period of American history, while that of the College of Physicians was first spoken of as a possible creation nearly twelve years after the Declaration of Independence, and that of the Philadelphia Hospital seventeen years later. As a matter of historical record, therefore, it becomes our duty, in chronicling the rise and progress of public medical libraries in Philadelphia, to give precedence of mention to the one which was established at the earliest date, even though it has not risen to the first rank in prominence, either for purposes of consultation or in practical usefulness to the medical profession of this city and vicinity.

It has frequently been a matter of discussion and consideration among the thinking members of the profession in Philadelphia whether it would be possible, at any time, to consolidate the two libraries, inasmuch as their catalogues, when compared a few years since by a careful observer, exhibited a remarkable absence of duplication of titles of books; but no such action has ever been attempted, even if ever seriously contemplated.

In addition to the medical libraries already mentioned, there is a by no means insignificant collection of medical works of great value scattered through the shelves of the great general libraries of Philadelphia, as the Philadelphia Library and the Mercantile Library. The former, in its main building and in its Loganian branch, contains several thousand volumes of valuable old medical works of the sixteenth, seventeenth and eighteenth centuries. It is greatly to be regretted that such gems as some of these undoubtedly must be, or, at any rate, such works of intrinsic value as many of them are, should be buried, or at least hidden, almost beyond the contemplation, if not the search, of the medical reader. Several of the medical societies of Philadelphia have accumulated a number of books, periodicals and pamphlets for reference and the use of their members, but none of them have as yet risen to the dignity and importance of distinct medical libraries, deserving detailed description in an account of the public medical libraries of Philadelphia.

I.—The Medical Library of the Pennsylvania Hospital.

The foundation of this library was laid in the year 1762, fourteen years before the signing of the Declaration of Independence, and eleven years after that of the hospital itself, in the presentation by Dr. John Fothergill of a work on "Materia Medica," by William Lewis, F. R. S., through Mr. William Logan, a manager of the institution, while on a visit to Europe. It was expressly stated that this volume was presented "for the benefit of the young students in physic who may attend under the direction of the physicians." The same donor shortly afterward gave to the hospital a variety of models, anatomical and other pictures, etc., valued at about $350, which were placed at Professor Shippen's service in his course on Anatomy.

Soon after this, that is, in 1763, pecuniary considerations, looking toward the establishment and maintenance of a library, were entertained and adopted. At that time there were no resident physicians, so-called, their duties being performed by apprentices, and these, in consideration of their services to the hospital, were exempted from paying the fee required of all medical students attending there, by resolution then adopted by the managers. This fee was six pistoles, a sum fixed and suggested by the attending physicians of the hospital, and by them recommended to be used for defraying the expenses of a future medical library, instead of being given to the physicians and surgeons of the hospital, as was then the custom in Great Britain.

Inaugurated in this way, by unselfish relinquishment of fees to which these physicians were fairly entitled, according to the usages of those times, the library soon began to grow, receiving gifts of books from friends at home and abroad; among the noteworthy ones from the latter source being two large volumes on Materia Medica, forwarded by Benjamin Franklin in October, 1770. The only other works added in any quantity to the library prior to the Revolution are entered upon the hospital's books as received at the end of 1774, from England, as "a trunk of books," which, it is presumed, were presented to the library as the results of a direct appeal to friends in England, on behalf of the young medical students attending lectures in Philadelphia from "the neighboring provinces," to whom such works were not otherwise accessible.

Then came the momentous struggle of the Revolution, during which both hospital and library had a hard battle for existence, in the depreciation of the currency and in the turmoil and military occupation and movements of those agitating times. For fourteen years the books added to the library did not average one a year, and only one pamphlet was received in all those years. To show how great was the depression of the currency at that time, one volume, purchased in 1780, which, in ordinary times, would have cost one pound fifteen shillings in gold, was purchased for one hundred and thirty-five pounds five shillings, which was equivalent to the same amount.

The first systematic catalogue of the library was prepared under the supervision of several prominent medical men, and issued in 1790, and contained the titles of 528 works. The apothecary of the hospital was the librarian at this time, acting under rules adopted in the latter part of 1789. Another catalogue was prepared and issued in 1795. In the meantime books had been purchased for the library in Great Britain, and a number of others had been received from friends in that part of the world as donations, notably from Dr. J. C. Lettsom. Strict rules as to loaning books, and in regard to the return of missing volumes, were adopted at this time, with something more direct than a hint that the apprentices or residents were responsible for the loss of a number of books missing from the library, for which they were called upon to pay before relinquishing their services at the hospital.

In the year 1800 the library, having grown beyond the capacity of a few bookcases, was removed to a room of its own, on the first floor, which it occupied for forty-seven years, when the large new room, specially arranged for it, on the second floor, was opened as its future home, which, for half a century, the library has occupied.

A donation of 142 volumes, from Sarah Zane, in the first year of this century, is interesting, as probably exhibiting the style, or rather the dimensions, of books at earlier periods, if we may accept these as indicative of the characteristic literature of two or three centuries previous, when quartos and folios largely predominated, as they did in this collection.

The transference of the care of the library, in succession, from one apprentice to another—for the apprentices were for a series of years the acting librarians—was quite a formal affair. The apprentices, on assuming these duties, were obliged to give a receipt for all the books in the library, to note the names of all the missing volumes, which were charged to the previous occupant of the position, and the library itself was even closed, and the books, when not returned, were advertised in the newspapers of the day, and lists sent around to all the medical men of the city, in the hope of securing the stray volumes. Such were the rather primitive methods of those days; but Philadelphia was then compact and not widespread, and its corps of physicians could readily be counted on one's fingers and could be easily reached by appeal or direct application. As many as fifty volumes were at one time found to be missing from the shelves, when the incoming apprentice-librarian and the two managers, who superintended the transfer, met to make the formal arrangements for the care of the library. The duties of the apprentices—especially the outgoing librarian—did not, therefore, rest upon a bed of roses, and a sense of future responsibility must have been ever present in the minds of the continuous line of apprentices who successively assumed the duties of book-custodians, while others were acting as unauthorized book-*keepers*. But, perhaps, the acting librarian had some solace from the fact that other labors were simultaneously imposed upon him, for even while having the books under his watchful care he was expected to bleed, cup and leech, when it was necessary to employ such treatment, to dress wounds and assist in the treatment of fractures.

The minutes of the hospital give interesting particulars of the inner life of these hard-worked and thoroughly-occupied young gentlemen of those days, the medical representatives of the apprenticeship system, then, and for many years afterwards, in vogue. Although not strictly relative to the subject in hand—the library proper—it may not be considered inappropriate at this point to state the terms under which these apprentices—the acting-librarians—were admitted to the privileges and the labors of the hospital. The minutes state that each apprentice was to bring with him a single feather bed, which he was to leave in the house; he was to serve five years; give ample security to pay at the rate of one hundred pounds per annum for every day that he was absent from his duties without leave from the managers; he was to fill up his time in study; to look for no indulgence by leave to attend parties of pleasure or places of amusement, nor to be abroad in the evening, nor to receive visits at home. The managers allowed him to attend two courses of medical lectures, selected by themselves, and it was made his duty to return home to the hospital as soon as each lecture was over. Those who were able to follow faithfully this severe course of discipline to the end, doubtless realized at its conclusion some personal gratification in the review of the benefits that had accrued to them, but there must have been a marked degree of personal satisfaction when the long-looked-for day of liberty and emancipation at last arrived.

With the exception of the printing of the first part of a new catalogue of the library, in 1806, by Zaccheus Collins, Richard Wistar, Dr. Thomas Parke, and, particularly, Dr. Joseph Hartshorne, then an apprentice in the hospital (the second part being prepared twelve years later), there was but little increase of the library until 1816, when nearly three thousand dollars were expended in the purchase of books on Natural History and Botany, that had formed part of the library of the late Dr. Benjamin Smith Barton, and nearly two thousand dollars were spent in the importation of books from Europe.

The library was now developing into numerical and scientific importance, and the medical profession of the growing city was also assuming larger proportions, and probably becoming more appreciative of its value as a means of reference. Drs. James and Hewson were requested, in 1822, by the managers of the hospital, to act in conjunction with a "committee to have charge of the library"—the first ever appointed—in looking after its interests. In March, 1824, Mr. William G. Malin was appointed clerk of the hospital and librarian, remaining as such for sixteen years, when he became steward. In 1829 he prepared a new catalogue, showing a total of 5,828 volumes in the library; a supplement to which was issued in 1836. A "Sketch of the History of the Medical Library," by the librarian, was published with the catalogue in 1829. Other items of interest, during the next few years, were the sale of certain works on Comparative Anatomy and Natural History to the South Sea Surveying and Exploring Expedition sent out by the Government in 1837—volumes that could be readily imported from Europe by the library; and, in 1841, a slight depletion in the removal of works treating of the Mind and Mental Diseases, and others, of a general literary character, to the new Hospital for the Insane in West Philadelphia, a branch of the Pennsylvania Hospital.

The library had become crowded by the year 1847, and encroached on the apothecary shop and hall, so that it became necessary to construct a new library-room on the second floor of the hospital, and here it has ever since remained, the ward for females being removed and the room altered, to be devoted to this object.

Five years later, that is, in 1852, Mr. George Ord of Philadelphia presented more than a hundred volumes of great interest to medical and scientific men. In 1855 Dr. Emil Fischer prepared a new catalogue of 750 pages, which received a supplement twelve years later, at the hands of August F. Müller, then librarian.

A charge of three dollars a year for the use of the library was made in 1867, by resolution of the managers, and of twenty-five dollars for the life-use of the same and for attendance on the medical and surgical practice of the house.

The interesting and valuable work, "The History of the Pennsylvania Hospital, 1751-1895," prepared by Drs. Thomas G. Morton and Frank Woodbury, states that the additions to the library of the hospital to 1893 bring up the aggregate number of volumes to 14,892.

At this present date (October, 1897) the hospital library contains 405 folios, 1,874 quartos, 11,206 octavos and 1,481 duodecimos, a total of 14,966 volumes; but such a classification is rather fanciful in these later days, when many of the duodecimo volumes are with difficulty distinguished from small octavos. There has not been any regularly appointed librarian in recent years, the clerk performing that duty.

II.—The Library of the College of Physicians of Philadelphia.

When the College of Physicians was founded, thirteen years before the expiration of the eighteenth century, there was no mention on the minutes of the prospective library, which in after years was to be, perhaps, its chief adornment. In the spring of the following year, by-laws were proposed, a section of which contained, as a heading, the word "Library," without any additional words to give it vitality. The library was not then even in an embryonic state; it was only a possibility of the future, for which the worthy founders of the college thought it scarcely necessary, in its total absence, to make provision.

About half the medical profession in Philadelphia were founders or fellows in the first year of the existence of the college; but then the whole number of medical men in the city at that time was scarcely more than fifty. The best portions of Philadelphia at that period of its history, as to respectability of the population and desirability of residence, were those situated low down, in the vicinity of the Delaware River. Fifth street seemed to be almost the western limit, for only one of the fellows lived beyond it, and almost all the others were residents of Water, Front and Second streets. The early fellows and founders were apparently the cream of the profession, being the leading teachers and practitioners of the city, a number of whom were already distinguished, and their names have been handed down to us for preservation of their enduring reputation. The University of Pennsylvania was then in Fourth street, below Arch, and here the College of Physicians held its meetings and laid the foundation, in 1788, for its future library.

In June, 1788, and at almost every meeting thereafter, to the end of 1789, the library occupied the attention of the fellows of the college, and particularly of a committee of three, appointed to report upon its organization and formation. These were Drs. John Jones, Samuel Powel Griffitts and Caspar Wistar. After the usual appeal for donations of books, which seems an essential feature of all such enterprises, the corner-stone of the library, if we may so call it, was laid, by the presentation of a few medical books by Dr. John Morgan, early in 1789, before the college had had time to procure a bookcase for their reception. It was not until 1792 that the care and custodianship of a distinct officer seemed to be required, when Dr. Nicholas H. Waters voluntarily assumed the position of librarian.

In 1789 it was determined that the papers read before the college should be collected, as soon as possible, in a Volume of Transactions, which, however, did not make its appearance until 1793; but, in the meantime, the college had made itself, its objects and its literary needs known to the profession in all parts of the country, in a letter addressed "to the most respectable medical characters in the United States"—but to only one hundred of these —but with the good result, after the issue of the Transactions, of bringing the college into literary affiliation with all similar works and with medical journals, although these, all told, at that time were not numerically strong. At a meeting in the summer of 1789 the college appointed a committee—Drs. Jones, Parke and Wistar—to make out a list of books to be purchased in Europe; but more than a year elapsed before they were received from Amsterdam, voyages in those days being long and transportation tardy. Upon the death of Dr. John Morgan, in 1790, about a dozen folio and quarto volumes—the works of Hippocrates, Galen, Morgagni and Harvey—came into the possession of the library. The single case, which contained the whole library of the college, became, at the end of the year 1791, too small to accommodate any other than the bound volumes, and the unbound ones had not even found room anywhere in the college, being kept at the home of the secretary.

In January, 1793, the library was removed to the room of the American Philosophical Society, but the fellows were allowed to take out books only once a month, at the regular meeting, and were rigidly fined if delinquent in their return. Dr. Michael Leib was elected librarian in 1792-93, but it is not stated how long he served in that capacity. From this time on to the close of the century, the library, although frequently mentioned in the minutes, did not make much progress numerically, nor did it receive many donations from the private collections of local medical men, or additions by importation from abroad. The funds of the college were limited, and the professional zeal of the fellows was absorbed in active labors in behalf of the sufferers from the yellow fever epidemic of 1793. The interest in the library soon revived, however, and before the occurrence of the next epidemic of the same disease—that of 1797—and its successor of 1799, new books had been received from Amsterdam; the Medical Society of London had forwarded its Transactions, and a number of European Latin and French medical journals had been subscribed for. The three yellow fever epidemics gave the college an opportunity to collect and publish the experiences of its fellows and of the profession at large, bearing particularly on the nature and origin of the disease.

The library, at the beginning of the nineteenth century, found itself feeble, tardy in increase, with only occasional donations, and annual appropriations of sixty pounds from the college that were sometimes merely nominal, not being paid out of the treasury, as ordered. It was, indeed, another illustration of a good resolution that was not carried out. The only memorable donation was that of Dr. William Currie, in 1800, of twenty volumes, ten of which were Adrianus Spigelius "De Humano Corpore." The bookcase, although apparently crowded with books, contained also a few pathological specimens; the minutes show that one of the meetings of the college was made sensational by the effort to trace the purloiner from it of the heart of an extra-uterine fœtus.

Dr. John Coakley Lettsom, founder of the Medical Society of London, and one of the originators of the Royal Jennerian Society, and the first one to forward vaccine lymph to this country, an associate fellow of the college, in 1803 forwarded from England, for the library, a few valuable books.

From 1805 to 1815, during part of which period the war of 1812 was uppermost in the minds of all Americans, both college and library languished, and there was little in the work or progress of either to excite admiration or enthusiasm. Few new fellows were added to the list, although the initiation fee, formerly fixed at $26.67, to help along the library, was now placed at $15. After 1815—for five years—both college and library showed a greater degree of vitality, although donations and purchases were still infrequent, only one donation, that of a Spanish work on Tifus Icterodes, by Moreno, being received during that period, and the chief purchase being of ten volumes of the Edinburgh Journal for six pounds five shillings. The imperfection of the previous catalogue of the library was so fully recognized that a new one, prepared by Drs. Parke and J. W. Moore, was issued early in 1819.

The college always met "at early candlelight," but a number of years elapsed before anything important was entered on its minutes relative to the progress of the library. It is presumable that funds were not available for its further increment or that times were not so prosperous as to warrant private or personal expenditure in this direction. To us of the present day it would seem an impossibility that more than thirty years could have gone by without any material growth of the library, and that at the end of that period—that is, in January, 1835—the first regularly appointed committee on the library—Drs. J. W. Moore, William S. Coxe and Simon A. Wickes—reported that "it is in a bad condition and going to decay." In June of this same year this committee presented to the college the first annual report of their well-directed labors, which gave the fellows an accurate idea of the character and number of the volumes in the library, showing that the books were chiefly ancient and inconveniently placed for reference, and that for a whole year not a single volume had been called for. The college could hardly boast of the possession of a library; it was merely a foundation on which to build in the future, for the college was now within two years of its semi-centennial, and all told there were but 31 folio volumes, 67 quartos and 193 octavos, making a total of 291.

In 1836 the Kappa Lambda Association of the United States, which had published twelve volumes of the "North American Medical and Surgical Journal," was dissolved, and all its private papers, proceedings, etc., were deposited in the library of the college. The annual reports showed for a number of successive years a continuous unanimity of expression of the fact that a single volume and a few pamphlets had been added to the library during the year, and that but little reference had been made to it by readers or inquirers. It is difficult to realize in these modern days of enlightment and research that the library could have been so woefully neglected, but this was probably due to the fact that the books comprising it were not of such recent publication as to provoke inquiry or that the exchange system was then imperfect and other medical journals not regularly received.

In October, 1840, an effort was made to interest the college, the Philadelphia Medical Society and the Philadelphia Medical College in a proposed "Medical Hall Association of Philadelphia," in which a library—the library—was to be placed, and books donated or deposited by medical contributors to add numerical strength and

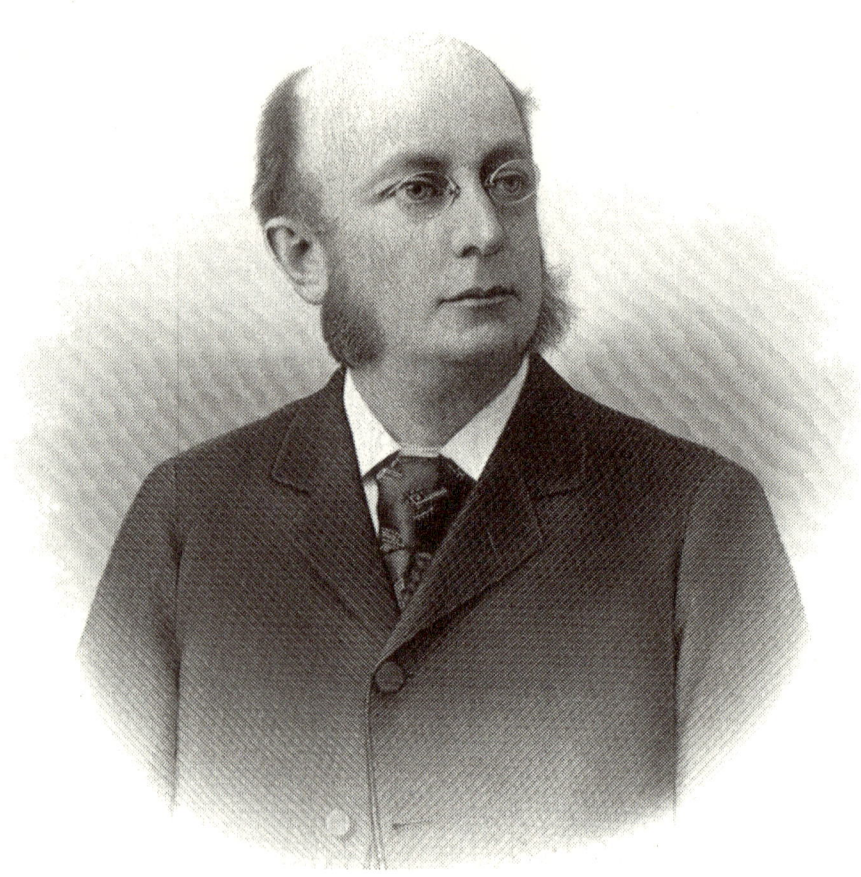

Goodspeed Bros. Publishers, Chicago.

J. C. Wilson

public importance to it. Of the three institutions named, the college alone survives. The expense of the undertaking was of itself sufficient to throw a damper upon the fruition of the project, and the plan was soon abandoned.

In 1844 Dr. John C. Otto, being about to leave Philadelphia, sold his valuable library to the college for two hundred dollars, but there seems to have been no room for the books at the college, as they were deposited in a room over Dr. Hodge's office at Ninth and Walnut streets. In June of this year the library committee presented to the college some important suggestions as to the election of a librarian, the arrangement of hours for access to the library, and its future development, cataloguing, etc.; and yet one hour, twice a month, one of these two hours being that of the monthly meeting of the college, was considered ample for the literary needs of the fellows; but then the same report stated that the library was "useless for want of care and arrangement, and its benefits entirely lost to its members," and the bookcase containing it stood on the first landing of the staircase.

An important step was taken in 1845, when the college library, now numbering nearly 600 volumes, was removed to the Mercantile Library building; a new catalogue was finished in January, 1846, and several hundred volumes were deposited by the Philadelphia Medical Society, when it suspended its existence in 1846, which were finally donated to the college in 1850, but under stipulations as to their use by members of the society, who were not fellows of the college, that were not acceptable to the latter. The strange upshot of this affair was the return of the books to the Philadelphia Medical Society, and their sale by the latter for about four hundred and fifty dollars, which amount was handed over to the College of Physicians, and invested by the college for the purchase of new books; and this culmination of the original transfer of the books took place nearly a quarter of a century after their first deposit in the library.

An effort was made in 1847 and 1848 to make the library more accessible, by giving every fellow a key to the room but not to the bookcases, except when the college was in session; but, as this semi-liberality did not go far enough, keys to the cases were left in the table-drawer. The medical journals were within reach, however, and the fellows took them home so often to read, and forgot to return them, that a new order of things, after a while, became necessary, although how long this defective system referred to had existed is not stated on the minutes

New interest in the library was stirred up in 1852, so that a large collection of odd journals and pamphlets were gathered from shelves on which they had been collecting dust for several years. The bookcases began to feel the weight of these accessions, and the future care of the library soon passed into responsible hands, after the alteration of the by-laws in 1854, by the annual election of a librarian; so that the secretary of the college, who had been temporarily acting as such, and the committee on the library, must have been greatly relieved.

In 1854 the library was removed, and the college changed its meeting-place to the Spruce street house, a portion of the Pennsylvania Hospital in which Benjamin West's great picture, "Christ Healing the Sick," had its abiding place. This would have been an appropriate time, if such a plan was ever feasible or desirable, for this library and that of the Pennsylvania Hospital, when they were in such near proximity and propinquity, to be carefully compared, catalogued and consolidated; but the college library could not, under such conditions, be left permanently on the hospital grounds, to be tied down by strict hospital regulations as to its use for purposes of consultation.

Interest was rapidly centering in the library; Dr. T. Hewson Bache was elected librarian in January, 1855, under the new by-laws; hundreds of medical journals were contributed to complete defective sets, and more than a hundred volumes of these were bound and placed on the shelves, while donations of books came in, in large numbers, from the fellows, notably Dr. Alfred Stillé, Dr. Samuel Lewis, who afterward became one of the library's greatest benefactors, and Dr. Moreton Stillé, personally, and a few months later from his estate. The library now contained about 1,700 volumes, a total which was soon increased, as by report made in January, 1857, to 2,155 volumes. In the fall of 1857 Dr. Thomas F. Betton of Philadelphia gave his own library and that of his father, Dr. Samuel B. Betton, to the college, comprising a large number of valuable and curious works. This was the first large addition which the library had ever received by donation. The Betton library amounted to 1,265 volumes.

A change in the location of the college, by its proposed removal to Thirteenth and Locust streets, was agreed upon on May 1, 1859. At the same time a communication was received from the widow of Professor Thomas D. Mütter of Jefferson Medical College, then recently deceased, offering to deposit his library with the college, to remain as a permanent gift, in connection with his pathological museum, when a permanent building for its reception should be constructed by the college. Dr. Henry Bond, during this year, also left as a legacy a number of valuable works for the library; so that when the annual summary was made, it was found that the library contained nearly 4,000 volumes. Early in the next year Drs. T. H. Bache (librarian), Ruschenberger, West, Lewis, R. P. Thomas and W. F. Atlee were appointed a committee to prepare a new catalogue, but, by some mysterious fatality, their labor of many months was brought to naught by the loss or destruction of the completed manuscript in some way that could never be explained.

In 1862 twenty-three fellows of the college subscribed for the purchase of 192 volumes of *"Theses"* submitted to the Faculty of Medicine of Paris for twenty-five years previous to and including 1846. In the latter part of 1863, by the death of Dr. Isaac Remington, the library became the possessor of 195 volumes, in addition to numerous pamphlets and journals. Dr. Walter F. Atlee succeeded Dr. Bache in 1863 as librarian, the latter having entered the military service of the War of the Rebellion. The library was soon after removed to its new quarters at Thirteenth and Locust streets, which it occupies at present. It then numbered about 4,500 volumes. The librarians successively elected were: Drs. C. S. Baker in 1864, J. H. Slack in 1865, Robert Bridges in 1868, and Frank Woodbury in 1881, on the resignation of the latter.

The Lewis Library, as it has since been called, was founded in 1864 and 1865 by the addition of about 2,500 volumes to the general library, the gift of Dr. Samuel Lewis of Philadelphia. This valuable collection greatly enriched the college library, and the additions since made to it by the generous donor have given it still greater importance, and it remains as an enduring monument to his memory.

In 1866 another donation of great literary value was made to the college by Mr. George Ord of Philadelphia, comprising a collection of voyages and travels, non-medical dictionaries, classical writings, etc., appraised in value at $4,000, for which, however, the college had to pay $350 for collateral and other taxes.

By April, 1866, the total number of volumes in the library was 12,448, and so important for reference had it become that, at the suggestion of Dr. G. B. Wood, president, who offered also to make a personal gift of five hundred dollars to meet the additional expense, the duties of the librarian were increased, and the library was to be open daily from 11 to 3 o'clock. Dr. Bridges was elected librarian and a new catalogue put into an active state of preparation. In February, 1870, an important Russian work on Lithotomy, containing plates, 23x30 inches, was presented to the library by Bujalsky, a Russian surgeon.

Dr. Francis West, in 1869, left, by will, several hundred volumes to the college library, and Dr. Charles D. Meigs, in like manner, gave it, early in 1870, ninety-two volumes on Midwifery. The college, in 1871, determined to keep the library open in the evening, but the attendance was so slight that it did not seem a justifiable procedure to continue doing so.

Serial literature has been one of the important features of this library, and private subscriptions, as far back as the year 1870, took organized shape for the regular purchase of medical journals, in the establishment of a fund, voluntarily contributed by a number of the fellows, constituting themselves "The Journal Association of the College of Physicians." Up to the present time their continued efforts, supplemented by donations of periodicals and transactions from fellows, medical editors and others, have been very serviceable to the library in this direction.

In 1871 the college determined to purchase the pamphlets and MSS. formerly belonging to Dr. Charles Caldwell of Lexington, Kentucky. In 1872 the accumulated interest of the fund given by the Philadelphia Medical Society was paid over to the library committee for the purchase of books. In 1874 a fixed annual appropriation was determined upon for the use of the library, and Dr. Thomas Stewardson acted as librarian during the summer vacation. In 1876 a committee of the County Medical Society was appointed to confer with the college on the practicability of extending the privileges of the library to its members; but the college considered that under existing regulations ample facilities were already afforded members and the medical profession for using it, when properly introduced. In November, 1877, the college was authorized, on the death of Dr. Joseph Carson, to select from his library whatever books they needed.

In May, 1879, the hall committee was authorized to make important changes in the library, by the addition of an intermediate fire-proof floor, and in June of the same year the library committee was authorized to dispose of portions of the Ord Library, which interfered with the growth and extension of the general library. In the summer of this year Dr. S. Hazlehurst acted temporarily as librarian.

The choice of books in the library of Dr. George B. Wood, deceased, was given to the college by will, and a number of valuable books were added to the library from this source.

In November, 1880, Dr. S. Weir Mitchell gave one thousand dollars to the library fund, for the establishment of a competent journal fund, or for other disposition of that sum if the college preferred. The "Weir Mitchell Library Fund of the College of Physicians of Philadelphia" was thus created. In January, 1881, the library committee was authorized to employ annually a male or female assistant to the librarian to prepare and continue the card catalogue and to assist the librarian. Miss Emily Thomas was appointed, early in 1881, to prepare and continue the card catalogue. The librarian was also allowed an assistant to perform the more mechanical duties. The Ordinances of the College were amended in April, 1881, so as to define more clearly the duties of the librarian. In June of the same year the library committee was authorized to present to the library of the Medical Department of the University of Pennsylvania, duplicates in its possession of the books of the late Dr. G. B. Wood. Thanks were extended to Dr. M. F. Wickersham for the donation of rare and valuable medical books. In January, 1882, the library committee was authorized to sell the whole of the Ord Library, and five hundred and fifty dollars were realized from this procedure. At the same meeting a large number of works belonging to Dr. William Furness Jenks were presented by his widow, in pursuance of his expressed wish, and he was enrolled on the list of benefactors of the library. In March, 1882, Dr. S. Weir Mitchell forwarded another check for one thousand dollars for purposes already stated—the increase of the number of journals, or for any other use to which it might be preferably employed. In June of this year the college accepted the deposit of the library of the late Dr. H. Lenox Hodge.

Dr. Woodbury resigned the position of librarian in September, 1882, and Mr. Charles Perry Fisher, who had been his assistant, and who was recommended by him as his successor, was appointed acting librarian in October of the same year. The Ordinances and By-laws were amended in November of the same year, prescribing the duties of the honorary librarian and the assistant librarian, and of the library committee. Dr. James H. Hutchinson was elected honorary librarian, a position which he held until his death in December, 1889. Rules were adopted for the government of the library, which was, for a while, kept open in the evening. Mr. Fisher was nominated by the library committee in February, 1881, and at once assumed the duties of librarian, which he has exercised with zeal and fidelity up to the present time.

In April, 1883, another effort was made to throw the library open to the whole profession, but the council reported adversely as to its feasibility. In September of that year, thanks were tendered Earl Kimberly, in appreciation of his courteous gift of an almost complete set of Hygienic Reports of India. In June, 1884, the college accepted the special deposit of the Samuel D. Gross library, by the Philadelphia Academy of Surgery, which was received in October of the same year, under a mutual agreement as to its use and the expense of its maintenance. A permanent deposit of it was made in April, 1885, and the proposition was accepted that in the event of the dissolution of the Academy, this library should become the absolute property of the college. In November of this year Dr. Alfred Stillé presented 695 volumes to the library. A motion was adopted at the same meeting looking to the union of the library of the college with that of the Pennsylvania Hospital, but at a subsequent meeting was reconsidered and indefinitely postponed. Dr. I. Minis Hays made a donation of 901 volumes to the library; and in November of this year, in accordance with the wishes of his father, lately deceased, presented an excellent portrait of Professor William Potts Dewees. At this meeting Dr. S. Weir Mitchell presented a very valuable collection of works on Hysteria and other nervous diseases; and Dr. Samuel Lewis four beautiful examples of Incunabula and an editio princeps of Asellius of 1627; also a quarto illustrated volume of distinguished professors of the University of Edinburgh.

In January, 1886, Dr. J. M. Da Costa presented 100 volumes of valuable medical works, and Mr. (now Dr.) George I. McKelway 166 volumes. In June of this year the widow of Dr. J. F. Weightman presented 512 volumes to the library, chiefly on ophthalmological subjects. The library of the Obstetrical Society was accepted as a permanent deposit. In December of this year Dr. S. Weir Mitchell presented to the library a high case clock.

At the January, 1887, meeting a marble bust of Dr. Joseph Pancoast was presented by Dr. W. H. Pancoast; and one of the late Dr. Joseph Parrish by Dr. Joseph Parrish. Mr. Richard Wood presented, for his mother, a portrait of the late Dr. George B. Wood. It was ordered that a thousand dollars, presented by Mr. William Weightman, be invested for the purchase of books on Ophthalmic Surgery, to be added to the collection given by the widow of his son, Dr. J. F. Weightman. In February of this year Dr. Hunter McGuire presented an original letter from Dr. Benjamin Rush, in regard to the disease from which George Washington's mother suffered; this was ordered to be framed. In May, Mrs. Mifflin Wistar presented fourteen volumes of MSS. notes, by Dr. Caspar Wistar, of the lectures of Drs. Gregory, Monro, Black and Hunter. In November the library of the late Dr. N. Archer Randolph, 466 volumes and 144 pamphlets, was presented, and Dr. Samuel Lewis gave a complete copy in Latin of Blegny's Zodiacus Medico-Gallicus, 1680-1686, the first medical journal ever published.

In February, 1888, Dr. S. Weir Mitchell announced the purchase and presentation to the library by him of a valuable collection of letters, autographs and official documents accumulated by the late Dr. W. Kent Gilbert of this city. These were afterward collected into four large folio volumes, in which they were skillfully mounted. The college has also in its possession a large bound volume of manuscript archives (1787 to 1847) of priceless value to it, as associated with important events in its history. In May, 1888, it was stated that the Lewis Library now contained over 10,000 volumes. In October of this year Dr Samuel Lewis presented a valuable collection of pamphlets, principally from the collection of Sir Richard Owen.

In June, 1889, the Philadelphia Academy of Surgery was granted permission to deposit in the Samuel D. Gross Library the books of the late Dr. Samuel W. Gross, on the same conditions which governed the original deposit. In January, 1890, Dr. J. M. Da Costa presented 413 rare volumes, purchased by him from the sale of the Hewson Library. In March, 1890, subscriptions were invited from the fellows for the purchase of the new "Dictionnaire Encyclopédique des Sciences Médicales," which was to be published in a hundred volumes. Dr. Frederick P. Henry was at this meeting elected honorary librarian, to succeed the late Dr. Hutchinson. Dr. Henry has occupied this position, by successive election, up to the present time. At the December meeting of the College the death of Dr. Samuel Lewis was announced, and tributes paid to him as a great benefactor of the library. The library at this meeting received a gift of five thousand dollars from the widow of Dr. Lewis Rodman, to found a "Lewis Rodman Library Fund," the income of which was to be expended in the purchase of books.

In March, 1891, Mr. Samuel Clarkson, a descendant of Dr. Gerardus Clarkson, presented ten thousand dollars for the library, to be invested as the beginning of a library endowment fund. At the February, 1892, meeting it was reported that the southeastern room downstairs had been arranged as a stack-room for books.

In March, 1893, Dr. William Osler presented, on behalf of Dr. Awdry of Berkeley, England, a locket containing a lock of hair of Dr. Jenner, who had been, ninety-one years before, refused by the college an election as associate fellow. In May, 1893, through the liberality of Dr. S. Weir Mitchell, some interesting Incunabula were presented to the library. These books, printed prior to the year 1500, are forty-two in number, and include Abana, Petrus de, 1490; Albertus Magnus, 1473-1499; Argelata, P. de, 1499; Arnoldus de Villa Nova, 1475-1497; Averrhoes, 1498; Avicenna, 1486; Celsus, 1481-1497; Cermisonius, 1480-1491; Crescentius, 1486; Corbejensis, Ægidius, 1494; Gazius, Antonius, 1491; Glanvil or Glanvilla, 1483-1485; Grunpeck de Burckhausen, 1496; Heinricus de Saxonia, 1489; Joannes Canonicus, 1481; Kamintus, 1498; Ketam or Ketham, Joannes, 1498; Leonicenus Nicolaus, 1498; Magninus Mediolanensis 1482; Montegnana Bartholomeus, 1487-1497; Moses Maimonides, 1489; Publicius, J., 1490; Regimen Sanitatis Salernitanum, 1484-1491-1499; Rhazes, 1497; Savonarola, M., 1496; Valastus de Tarenta (circa 1470). This work of the latter, "De Epidemia et Peste," Argentorati, M. Flach, is believed to be the first medical work ever printed. The collection of curious old works also includes three excellently preserved volumes of manuscripts of the thirteenth and fourteenth centuries.

In November, 1893, Dr. Alfred Stillé presented about 500 volumes. In March, 1894, the widow of Dr. D. Hayes Agnew presented to the college the souvenir of gold and brilliants presented him in 1888 by his medical friends on the occasion of the fiftieth anniversary of his entrance into the profession. In May, 1894, a gift of five thousand dollars was announced from Mr. Clement A. Griscom, to establish a "John D. Griscom Book Fund," in memory of his father, a fellow of the college, who died in 1890. In June Dr. R. P. Harris gave 228 volumes.

In June, 1895, another effort was made to have the library

open in the evenings, but this was not carried into effect, past experiences not being favorable to such action. In November, 1895, Dr. S. Weir Mitchell presented, on behalf of the president (Dr. Da Costa), himself and a friend of the college, the original diploma in medicine given by the University of Edinburgh to Dr. John Morgan. In January, 1896, Mr. H. Lenox Hodge presented the library of his father, Dr. H. Lenox Hodge, a deceased fellow, which had been in its keeping since his death. In February, 1896, Dr. J. M. Da Costa presented 114 volumes to the library.

At the April, 1896, meeting, on motion of Dr. F. P. Henry, honorary librarian, a committee (fourteen in number) was appointed to obtain subscriptions from the general public toward a fund for the endowment of the library, but, on his motion, the committee was discharged in January, 1897, as it had failed to make any progress. In May, 1896, the estate of Dr. Lewis D. Harlow deposited with the library papers, etc., relating to the Pennsylvania Medical College and Philadelphia College of Medicine, of which he had been the official custodian. In February, 1897, the estate of Dr. William H. Pancoast, a recently deceased fellow, presented 335 volumes to the library. In April, 1897, a committee was appointed to prepare a memorial to Congress, protesting against the removal from the free list, in the pending tariff bill, of books and philosophical apparatus imported for the use of incorporated scientific bodies.

In October, 1897, Dr. Richard J. Dunglison presented a folio volume containing a large number of diplomas, certificates, etc., of his father, the late Dr. Robley Dunglison, a fellow of the college, collected during half a century, and rich in valuable autographs of distinguished men.

At the present time the library of the college has current numbers of more than six hundred journals on its racks, some of them obtained by subscription by the college, but the greater part by special funds, as that of the Journal Association, and by donations, exchange and the gift of publishers and editors. There are about two hundred donors on the list of contributors of works to the library, in small or large amounts, so that it is now impossible, without invidious distinction, to make a comprehensive list of its greatest benefactors.

The walls and niches of the various rooms constituting the library of the college—six in number—are decorated with oil paintings and numerous framed photographs, engravings and mementos, some of'them curious as well as interesting, of the early and late fellows of the college, and of distinguished members of the profession at home and abroad. There are marble busts of Drs. Samuel D. Gross, Samuel George Morton, N. Chapman, Joseph Pancoast and Joseph Parrish; a bronze bust of Henry J. Bigelow, and plaster busts of Stromeyer, Benjamin Rush and John C. Warren; and oil paintings of Hippocrates, William Harvey, Abraham Chovet, Philip Syng Physick, Benjamin Rush, John Morgan, John Redman, William P. Dewees, William Shippen, Cuvier, Alex. Von Humboldt, Oliver Wendell Holmes, Caspar Wistar, Benjamin Duffield, Thomas Parke, John Foulke, Henry Neill, Thomas C. James, John Hutchinson, Thomas Cadwalader, Gay-Lussac, John A. Monges, George B. Wood, Joseph Hartshorne, Charles Caldwell, W. W. Gerhard, J. Rhea Barton, Robert Hare, Lewis Rodman, Samuel Jackson, Washington L. Atlee, Thomas Cooper, Samuel Lewis, William Hunt, Alfred Stillé, S. Weir Mitchell, Jacob M. Da Costa, James H. Hutchinson, W. S. W. Ruschenberger, D. Hayes Agnew, Joseph Leidy and N. A. Randolph.

A count of the books in the College Library, made in October, 1897, shows that there are 54,097 volumes on the shelves, exclusive of duplicates, in addition to 28,750 unbound pamphlets and 4,903 unbound reports and transactions. As exhibiting the steady growth of the library, it may be stated that since January, 1892, 14,764 volumes have been added to it, and this additional number, in only five years, is greater than the total of the library in 1870, which was then, after eighty years of its existence, only 14,102; and is nearly as great as the total of the Pennsylvania Hospital Library at the present time, that being 14,966 volumes.

Mr. Henry M. Smaltz, in October, 1897, presented to the library 285 volumes of medical books, which are included in the above summary.

III.—The Medical Library of the Philadelphia Hospital.

So far as is known the only published account of this library, up to the present time, is that included in a lecture by the late Dr. D. Hayes Agnew, delivered about thirty-five years ago. The subject of a library was first agitated in 1805, and a room devoted to it in 1808, when the first expenditure was made in its behalf. At first the senior student was the librarian; afterward the apothecary assumed the duties. Money received from house pupils was devoted to the library, and the sum of thirty dollars was charged as a life privilege for the use of the library. In 1818 a catalogue was prepared, showing that there were 1,022 volumes in the library. In 1827, 120 foreign theses were presented by Dr. William E. Horner. Another catalogue was prepared by Dr. E. F. Rivinus, one of the resident physicians. Many valuable ancient works were included in it. Additions were made to the library for a number of years by the proceeds of the sales of clinical tickets, until the whole collection amounted to about 3,000 volumes; but Dr. Agnew's historical sketch did not give a very favorable prospect of its future, inasmuch as the library "has been plundered, by the vandalism to which it has been exposed, of much valuable matter." Drs. C. Pendleton Tutt and J. L. Ludlow, successively, acted as librarian for a series of years, but even at that time the giving out of volumes was placed in the hands of a trustworthy resident pauper.

The librarian of the hospital, since the death of Dr. Ludlow, has been the chief resident physician. Dr. D. E. Hughes, the present efficient occupant of that position, assumed control of the library in the year 1890, and found the books in a bad condition and very imperfectly shelved and catalogued. Since then the library has been moved into a larger room, the books mended, properly classified and shelved and catalogued by title and author. Dr. Hughes reports that the rare works mentioned in the early descriptions of the library are mostly missing, although there are many old and valuable works still on the shelves. The present number of books is 4,612; new ones are constantly being added, and the library is well up to date. In fact, it is a first-class working library for hospital uses.

CHAPTER VIII.

MEDICAL JURISPRUDENCE IN PHILADELPHIA.

The history of Medical Jurisprudence in any city or locality should include some account of the most important teachers and writers on the subject, a description of the methods of instruction pursued in the medical and legal institutions in the community, a history of the societies or other organizations interested in the dissemination of medico-legal knowledge, and some account of celebrated or important cases. These subjects can, however, be considered here only briefly and imperfectly. As Philadelphia was the first medical center in this country, the teaching of medical jurisprudence in America probably began in this city. The earliest knowledge of such instruction in the history of Philadelphia relates to Benjamin Rush.

Dr. Rush was connected with the University of Pennsylvania and the Philadelphia College of Medicine, its predecessor, from 1769 until his death in 1813, during which time he occupied the positions of professor of Chemistry, professor of the Theory and Practice of Medicine, professor of the Institutes and Practice of Medicine and Clinical Practice, and of professor of the Practice of Physic. In his volume of Sixteen Introductory Lectures to Courses of Lectures upon the Institute and Practice of Medicine, etc., published by Bradford & Inskeep of Philadelphia, in 1811, Rush devotes his sixteenth lecture to the study of Medical Jurisprudence. This lecture was delivered in 1810 at the University of Pennsylvania, and in it Dr. Rush dwelt on the subject of Medical Jurisprudence. After enumerating the subjects of Medical Jurisprudence in general, he selects for particular discussion those states of the mind which should incapacitate a man to dispose of his property, or to bear witness in a court of justice; and those which should exempt him from punishment for the commission of what are called crimes by the laws of our country.

Brief reference to the main points of this lecture may not prove uninteresting. He attributes intellectual derangement to three causes: To acute inflammation of the brain, called phrenitis or phrensy; to chronic inflammation of the brain, called mania or madness; and to delirium, which is a symptom only of general disease of the blood-vessels, or of some part of the body connected by sympathy with the brain. His conclusions are that in no stage of phrensy is a person in a condition to dispose of property or contract legal guilt of any kind; that in madness, when it is general, or in its intervals, when these occur after weekly, or even monthly, paroxysms of madness, the person is not in a condition to dispose of property or contract legal guilt; and the same is true where persons depart in their feelings, conversation and conduct in a great degree from their former habits."

Dr. Charles Caldwell delivered a course of lectures on Medical Jurisprudence in the University of Pennsylvania from 1812 to 1813.

In 1819, Dr. Thomas Cooper, who had previously been a judge of the courts of Pennsylvania, and was then professor of Chemistry and Mineralogy in the University of Pennsylvania, reprinted in the "Tracts on Medical Jurisprudence," with notes and additions, the English works of Farr, Dease, Male and Haslem. Ten years later Dr. J. Bell published at Philadelphia an introductory address upon the same subject, and also issued a syllabus of a course of lectures on Medical Jurisprudence in the Philadelphia Medical Institute.

The first American edition of a well-known work on Medical Jurisprudence, by Michael Ryan, was edited with notes and additions by Robert Eglesfeld Griffith, M. D., and published by Carey & Lea of Philadelphia, in 1832. Two chapters of this book were entirely written by Dr. Griffith, who was at that time lecturer on Materia Medica and Medical Jurisprudence in the Philadelphia School of Medicine. He was a well-known writer and teacher, having at one time been a professor in the Philadelphia School of Pharmacy and editor of the American Journal of Pharmacy, at that time known as the Journal of the Philadelphia College of Pharmacy. He was also a professor in the University of Maryland and lecturer in the University of Virginia, and later returned to Philadelphia. At the time of his death in 1850 he was one of the vice-presidents of the Philadelphia Academy of Natural Sciences.

Isaac Ray, M. D., LL. D., author of the great work on the "Medical Jurisprudence of Insanity," was a resident of Philadelphia from 1867 until his death on March 31, 1881. He was an influential and active member of the College of Physicians of Philadelphia and of the Social Science Association, and was one of the guardians of the poor of the city of Philadelphia. While holding this position he gave special attention to the insane department of the Philadelphia Hospital. As lecturer on Insanity in the Jefferson Medical College of Philadelphia he gave the first instruction on insanity given in the Philadelphia medical schools after the time of Rush. His treatise on the Medical Jurisprudence of Insanity has never been rivaled nor approached in this country, and has scarcely been surpassed in any other. In his "Contributions to Mental Pathology," published in 1873, are articles on many medico-legal cases, including the celebrated Hinchman case, several will cases, and an article on medical experts. During the time of his residence in Philadelphia Dr. Ray appeared in numerous important cases in which the question of insanity was at issue.

For many years Dr. John James Reese was one of the foremost medical jurists and toxicologists of Philadelphia. He was born June 16, 1818, and died September 4, 1892. He was educated both in the collegiate and medical departments of the University of Pennsylvania. He was one of the founders and the third president of the Medical Jurisprudence Society of Philadelphia; he was an honorary member of the New York Medico-Legal Society, and was a member of a number of medical societies and associations, local, state and national. He was the author of a text-book of medical jurisprudence and toxicology, which has reached a fourth edition and is used as a text-book in several of the Philadelphia medical colleges. He edited the seventh and eighth editions of Taylor's Manual of Medical Jurisprudence, and was also the author of a manual of toxicology and of numerous monographs and contributions on subjects pertaining to forensic medicine and toxicology, among these being one on "Live Birth in Its Medico-Legal Relations." He also wrote an elaborate review of the trial of Mrs. Elizabeth G. Wharton. This case, one of the *causas celebres* of this country, was tried at Baltimore, and in it were engaged a number of distinguished American experts from Philadelphia and elsewhere. He was professor of Medical Jurisprudence, including Toxicology, in the Auxiliary Department of Medicine of the University of Pennsylvania from 1865 until October, 1891.

The Auxiliary Department of Medicine of the University of Pennsylvania was endowed by Dr. George B. Wood in 1865. The intention of its founder was to supplement by it the regular course of medical instruction by lectures on branches of science, which he deemed necessary to the thorough education of the physician. The branches included in the curriculum of this course were zoölogy and comparative anatomy, botany, hygiene, medical jurisprudence and mineralogy and geology. The course was intended to be free to students and graduates of the Medical Department of the University of Pennsylvania, other students being required to pay a fee of $5 and a special tuition fee for each course or all the courses. The faculty of this department was organized December 16, 1865, and the first course of lectures was delivered in the spring of 1866. For many years the lectures of the course were delivered during the spring months, after the close of the regular medical session, in March or April. As the different departments in the University developed, some of the courses of instruction were transferred to different departments. The courses on Hygiene and Medical Jurisprudence were given in the medical hall or in the laboratory of hygiene.

Professor Reese delivered a systematic course on Medical Jurisprudence, including toxicology, in connection with this department, up to 1891. The terms of the endowment of the department called for a course on Medical Jurisprudence, but this was made by the faculty and by Dr. Reese to include toxicology, and his usual course of instruction included two lectures per week on General Medical Jurisprudence and one on Toxicology. These lectures of Dr. Reese were popular with the students, and were generally well attended.

Dr. Charles K. Mills was appointed May 2, 1892, by the trustees of the University of Pennsylvania, professor of Mental Diseases and of Medical Jurisprudence, with the understanding that he was to fill the chair of Medical Jurisprudence in the Auxiliary Department of Medicine, attendance upon the lectures of this course to students desiring a certificate or diploma being compulsory. The lectures on Medical Jurisprudence, like those on Mental Diseases, were also to be open as a voluntary elective to students of the third and fourth years of the regular medical department. Since 1893-94 they have been regularly rostered as a part of the fourth-year course. In 1896, the course was made a minor elective for graduation and the degree in medicine for students of the fourth year. The lectures delivered by Dr. Mills are on Medical Jurisprudence alone. Instruction in Toxicology is given by the professor of Chemistry in the Medical Department. Since 1894 Dr. Mills has made part of his course clinical, giving the instruction at the Philadelphia Hospital, the material being drawn from the large number of patients under his care in the nervous wards and Insane Department. In these lectures he has been able to illustrate practical points in forensic medicine regarding such subjects as aphasia, epilepsy, hysteria, hypnotism, traumatisms, feigned and factitious diseases, alcoholism, idiocy and imbecility, and insanity in all its phases. Although the lectures on Medical Jurisprudence in the fourth year are elective, they are well attended. Certificates of attendance and proficiency in Medical Jurisprudence are given to the graduates of the Medical Department who have attended a full course of instruction in the Auxiliary Medical Department and have passed satisfactory examinations.

Dr. Henry C. Chapman began to teach the subject of Medical Jurisprudence systematically in the Jefferson Medical College in the winter of 1891, making it a part of the regular winter course, and examining on the same, having previously lectured on the subject during the spring for a number of years. The common course extends over about two months, including two lectures a week, excluding toxicology, which has been taught for at least twenty-five years by the professor of Chemistry in the Jefferson College. Dr. Chapman is professor of Institutes of Medicine, which includes Physiology and Medical Jurisprudence, and Dr. Holland is the professor of Toxicology. Dr. Chapman has published a manual of Medical Jurisprudence and Toxicology, the first edition of which was issued in 1893, and the second edition, containing a brief bibliography, in 1896.

Dr. J. J. Reese was appointed lecturer on Medical Jurisprudence in the Woman's Medical College of Pennsylvania, and continued, until 1892, to deliver a number of lectures on the subject every spring. In 1893, Dr. Charles K. Mills was appointed lecturer on Medical Jurisprudence, to succeed Dr. Reese, and since that time has given a course of lectures on the subject late in the winter or early in the spring. The course includes ten lectures, and is attended by students of the third and fourth years. As it is attended by students of both these years, it is made progressive during the two years, the subject lectured upon one year not being lectured upon the next. The entire course of two years, therefore, covers twenty lectures. Toxicology is not included in the instruction, which is given by the professor of Chemistry.

Upon the organization of the faculty of the Medico-Chirurgical College, a chair of Medical Jurisprudence was embraced in the curriculum, and Abraham S. Gerhard, A. M., M. D., was elected professor of Medical Jurisprudence and of Clinical Medicine. After the death of Professor Gerhard, Spencer Morris, Ph. D., M. D., was elected adjunct professor of Medical Jurisprudence. He delivers twenty-eight lectures during a session. The trustees of this college regard this branch of the curriculum of such importance to its alumni that if the candidate for graduation fails in his final examination to obtain a mark of less than seventy, he is refused the degree of Doctor of Medicine. The successful candidate is given a certificate stating that he has passed the required examination.

The standard English Manual of Medical Jurisprudence, by Alfred Swayne Taylor, has passed through a number of American editions, which have been edited by Philadelphia physicians and issued from Philadelphia publishing houses. An early edition, issued by Lea and Blanchard, in 1845, was edited by Robert Eglesfeld Griffith, M. D., who had also been the American editor of Ryan's Medical Jurisprudence. The third, fourth and fifth American editions of this work were edited by Edward Hartshorne, M. D., the last of these appearing in 1861. The sixth American edition of this work, with notes and references to American decisions, was edited by Clement B. Penrose, Esq., of the Philadelphia bar. The seventh and eighth American editions, issued in 1873 and 1880, were edited by Professor John J. Reese, M. D. Reference has already been made to the original contributions of Professor Reese to the subject of Medical Jurisprudence.

"A Monograph on Mental Unsoundness," by Francis Wharton, LL. D., was published in 1885 by Kay & Bro. of Philadelphia. In the same year, "A Treatise on Medical Jurisprudence," by Francis Wharton, LL. D., and Moreton Stillé, M. D., a volume of 815 pages, was issued by the same publishers. Other editions of this work were copyrighted in 1860 and 1872. The medical portion of this treatise was revised, with numerous additions, by Alfred Stillé, M. D., in 1860. The first volume of the third edition was published in 1872, and the second volume, edited by Samuel Ashhurst, M. D., of Philadelphia, Robert Amory, M. D., of Brookline, Massachusetts, and Wharton Sinkler, M. D., of Philadelphia, appeared in 1873. In 1882 a fourth edition of this standard work was issued, the first volume having for its subtitle, "A Treatise on Mental Unsoundness, by Francis Wharton," while the second volume was edited by Robert Amory, M. D., and Edward S. Wood, M. D.

Moreton Stillé, M. D., was a member of a distinguished family, one of his brothers, Charles J. Stillé, LL. D., having been professor of History, and provost of the University of Pennsylvania, and another, Alfred Stillé, M. D., LL. D., having been for many years professor of the Theory and Practice of Medicine in the Medical Department of the University. The share assigned to Dr. Moreton Stillé in Wharton and Stillé's Medical Jurisprudence "consisted in the articles on the 'Fœtus and New-born Child,' on 'Sexual Relations,' on 'Identity,' and on the 'Causes of Death.' Referring to the manner in which this portion of the work was executed, one of his biographers, Dr. Hollingsworth (a), says: 'The unanimous sentiment of the profession, so far at least as it has been expressed in the numerous reviews that have been written upon it, is that it is a most valuable addition to our medical literature. It certainly occupies a position in advance of all previous works upon the same subject, for much of its information, owing to its being gathered from sources almost entirely unexplored before, is positively novel. Almost every page in it testifies, by its numerous references, to the extended research of the writer in these exotic regions.' "

Dr. J. O. Ordronaux was the author of a treatise, entitled The Jurisprudence of Medicine, which was published in Philadelphia in 1869.

Hamilton's System of Legal Medicine, published in 1894, R. C. McMurtrie, Esq., of the Philadelphia bar, has in the first volume a paper on "The Obligation of the Insured and the Insurer," while Volume II contains a paper on "Aphasia and Other Affections of Speech," by Charles K. Mills, A. M., M. D.

In addition to the editing by Philadelphians of the manuals of Ryan and of Taylor, and the publishing of the works of Wharton, Stillé, Reese and Chapman, many valuable medico-legal papers have been written by Honorable William N. Ashman, John A. Clark, Esq.; Hampton L. Carson, Esq.; Thomas W. Barlow, Esq.; Paschal H. Coggins, Esq.; T. G. Wormley, M. D.; H. C. Wood, M. D.; John Marshal, M. D.; Francis X. Dercum, M. D.; Henry Leffmann, M. D.; James Hendrie Lloyd, M. D.; John B. Chapin, M. D.; W. Duffield Robinson, M. D.; M. V. Ball, M. D., and E. N. Brush, M. D.

An organization known as the Medico-Legal Society of Philadelphia has been in existence since 1871. It was organized in a hall at Ridge avenue and Master street, August 25, 1877, under the name of the Northwestern Medical Association. The name was changed to the Philadelphia Medico-Legal Society, January 2, 1880. It was chartered March 12, 1883, as the Medico-Legal Society

---

(a) Biography of Eminent American Physicians and Surgeons, edited by R. French Stone, M. D., Indianapolis, 1894.

of Philadelphia. Its objects are to disseminate such medico-legal knowledge as will be useful to the membership and will prove beneficial to the community at large; and to effect a close adherence to the code of ethics of the American Medical Association.

The following is a list of its presidents: 1883, C. R. Prall, M. D.; 1884, T. S. Butcher, M. D.; 1885 and 1886, Franklin B. Harzel, M. D.; 1887, William C. Hollopeter, M. D.; 1888 and 1889, Joseph D. Schoales, M. D.; 1890, William F. Waugh, M. D.; 1891, Joseph Martin, M. D.; 1892, Wilson Buckby, M. D.; 1893, William A. Chandler, M. D.; 1894, A. Rusling Rainear, M. D.; 1895, Wm. H. Gominger, M. D.; 1896, A. B. Hirsh, M. D.; and 1897, Wm. H. Ziegler, M. D.

The society meets on the fourth Tuesdays of January, April, July and October, and since its organization a number of papers have been read on medico-legal subjects, as well as others relating to general medicine.

Another society for the dissemination of medico-legal knowledge and the discussion of medico-legal topics, "The Medical Jurisprudence Society of Philadelphia," was organized in 1883 and incorporated in 1888. Much valuable work was done by it during several years, although the meetings were discontinued in 1891. The society was one of the first to agitate for a law establishing a State Board of Medical Examiners. Among the papers read during the active life of the society were the following: "Trial by Jury," by Henry Hazelhurst, Esq.; "The Case of Joseph Taylor," by C. K. Mills, M. D.; "The Trial of Charles Baines for Murder," by H. C. Wood, M. D.; "The Medico-Legal Relations of Idiocy," by Hon. Wm. N. Ashman; "Visiting the Forum of the Whipping Post: Is the Cat-o'-Nine Tails a Success?" by G. M. Bradfield, M. D.; and T. H. Andrews, M. D.; "Live Birth in Its Medico-Legal Relations," by J. J. Reese, M. D.; "Will Contests," by W. E. Rex, Esq.; "Food Laws," by Henry Leffmann, M. D.; "Microscopical Examination of Blood," by Henry F. Formad; "The Trial of Lunatics," by W. W. Carr, Esq.; and "The Insanity of Oscar Hugo Webber," by James Hendrie Lloyd, M. D. The late distinguished Dr. Samuel D. Gross was the first president. The following note regarding the first meeting occurs in his autobiography: "I attended this evening the first regular meeting of the Philadelphia Medical Jurisprudence Society, of which I was elected the first president. A better title would have been the Medico-Legal Society, but that name was already in the possession of another organization, although one for a different object. The new society promises well, as it embraces in its list of membership a number of distinguished physicians and lawyers, stimulated by a desire to work. Dr. John J. Reese, professor of Medical Jurisprudence in the University of Pennsylvania, delivered an excellent and exhaustive address on the testimony of experts, in which he exposed the partisan character of such witnesses, the inadequacy of their testimony, and the positive injury which they often do to the cause of justice. He recommended the adoption of the Prussian system, which consists in the appointment by the government of thoroughly educated men, who sit on the bench with the judges and assist them in trying the case by giving a proper direction to the testimony of the witnesses. In 1868, in an address which I delivered before the Medical Association, as its president, I recommended a similar plan, without any knowledge that it was in force in Germany." The following is a list of the presidents of the society: 1884, Samuel D. Gross, M. D.; 1885, George W. Biddle, Esq.; 1886, John J. Reese, M. D.; 1887, Hon. Wm. N. Ashman; 1888, Chas. K. Mills, M. D.; 1889, John A. Clark, Esq., and Dr. James Hendrie Lloyd, most of the presidents having also first served as vice-presidents. The treasurers were Hampton L. Carson, Esq., and Paschal H. Coggins, Esq. Dr. Henry Leffmann was the first secretary and was succeeded by Dr. Francis X. Dercum. The recorder of the society was Dr. G. Milton Bradfield. One of the most interesting meetings of the society was a joint meeting with the Philadelphia Neurological Society, January 24, 1887. This meeting was presided over by S. Weir Mitchell, M. D., LL. D., and the subject of discussion was "Medico-Legal Questions Concerning Insanity."

A name widely known both in this country and abroad is that of Professor Theodore G. Wormley, M. D., Ph. D., LL. D., one of the most distinguished medical chemists and toxicologists of his day. Upon the resignation of Prof. R. E. Rogers, in 1877, he was elected to fill the chair of Chemistry in the Medical Department of the University of Pennsylvania, which he occupied until his death in 1897. His book upon "Micro-Chemistry of Poisons, Including Their Pathological, Physiological and Legal Relations: Adapted to the Use of the Medical Jurist, Physician and General Chemist, New York, 1867," is a standard work. "Medical Chemistry and Toxicology," was the title of an address delivered before the International Medical Congress, held in Philadelphia in 1876, to which Congress he was a delegate. Professor Wormley was an expert in many important cases involving chemical or toxicological questions. As a witness he was careful, lucid and positive, and great weight was always given to his testimony.

Another Philadelphian eminent for his work in toxicology is Dr. Henry Leffmann, A. M., M. D., Ph. D. Dr. Leffmann was lecturer on Toxicology at the Jefferson Medical College from 1875 to 1883, chemist to the coroner of Philadelphia from 1885 to 1897, and he has also been chemist to the Dairy and Food Commission of Pennsylvania since 1893. He has been port physician of Philadelphia twice, namely, from 1884 to 1887 and from 1891 to 1892. He is the editor of the fourth edition of Reese's text book on Medical Jurisprudence and Toxicology, and has taken part in many well-known medico-legal cases in Philadelphia as an expert for the commonwealth of Pennsylvania. Among these are the Philadelphia case of Alfred Gerson, twice convicted and finally executed for the murder of his wife and mother-in-law; the case of Mrs. Whiteling, convicted and executed for the murder of her children, and the case of H. H. Mudget, alias H. H. Holmes, convicted and executed for the murder of B. F. Pietzel. Dr. Leffmann is Professor of Chemistry and Toxicology in the Woman's Medical College of Pennsylvania.

H. C. Wood, M. D., LL. D., the distinguished medical writer and teacher, has figured in many important medico-legal cases in Philadelphia and elsewhere, usually in cases of a toxicological or neurological character, as the Joseph Taylor case, the Meyer poisoning case in New York, the Johnston case, tried at New Bloomfield, Pennsylvania, and a large number of will contests and questions involving the questions of injuries inflicted upon the nervous system.

Among the medical men of Philadelphia who have most frequently appeared in the courts in recent years are: D. Hayes Agnew, M. D.; William H. Pancoast, M. D.; John Ashhurst, Jr., M. D.; W. W. Keen, M. D.; J. William White, M. D.; Henry R. Wharton, M. D.; Thomas G. Morton, M. D.; Thomas S. K. Morton, M. D.; W. Joseph Hearn, M. D.; W. W. Naylor, M. D.; F. X. Dercum, M. D.; Wharton Sinkler, M. D.; James Hendrie Lloyd, M. D.; C. W. Burr, M. D.; John J. Mitchell, M. D., and J. Chalmers Da Costa, M. D.

The author of this paper has been engaged as a medical witness or in an advisory capacity during the last fifteen years in a large number of cases, cases involving chiefly the questions of insanity, imbecility, mental incompetency and injuries or diseases of the nervous system. Among the most important of these were the William Meredith case, the Ruddach will case, the Wistar will case, the Weaver case, the Joseph Taylor case, the Oscar Hugo Webber case, the Bartley Peak case, the Johnston case and the Elwood Rowan case.

CHAPTER IX.

MEDICAL LITERATURE OF PHILADELPHIA.

There are various methods that might be adopted by the writer upon the medical literature of any town or country. In the first place, he might catalogue chronologically everything that has been published, leaving to the reader to separate the wheat from the chaff. This would be equivalent to grouping in one of the cases of the library of the College of Physicians all the cards on which are catalogued the works of Philadelphians, the books being arranged upon the shelves in a corresponding manner: i. e., with sole reference to their place and date of publication. One need not be a librarian in order to perceive the futility of such a plan. Another method would consist in the enumeration of the works of those who are generally acknowledged to have been the leaders of their day, and many of whom, I venture to say, would have been glad, at the close of their careers, to suppress some of their earlier publications. Those who are at all familiar with the contributions to literature which have emanated from Philadelphia will at once perceive that this method would also partake too largely of the nature of a catalogue. There remains the method which we shall adopt, namely, that of indicating the landmarks in the field of medical literature. The value of the work of a medical writer is not dependent upon its quantity, a single article or a few remarks in the course of a discussion being sometimes more precious than an octavo volume. The aim of the writer of this chapter will, therefore, be to indicate and review those contributions to literature which have been described as landmarks, but which might more appropriately be styled the stepping stones by which we have risen to the "higher things" of the present day.

The oldest Philadelphia medical treatise extant is by Dr.

Thomas Cadwalader, and is entitled An Essay on the West India Dry-Gripes; With the Method of Preventing and Curing that Cruel Distemper. To which is added, An Extraordinary Case in Physick.

Philadelphia: Printed and sold by B. Franklin. M.DCC.XLV.

This book is one of the numerous literary treasures collected by the late Dr. Samuel Lewis, and the copy in the Lewis Library is rendered peculiarly valuable, from the collector's standpoint, by the fact that it is the only one containing the two prefaces, one of which was suppressed. These prefaces were both written at Trenton, New Jersey, on the same day, March 25, 1745, and there is no apparent reason for the suppression of either, still less for the publication of both.

At the present day, the book is only of value to the bibliophile and the antiquarian. From a scientific standpoint, it is, as a matter of course, open to a species of criticism which is always unfair: namely, that of a more enlightened age than that in which the author wrote.

The term Dry-Gripes was undoubtedly applied in the West Indies to cases of lead colic, which were unusually prevalent in that region on account of the practice of distilling rum in leaden stills. Cadwalader, however, does not seem to have regarded his cases as due to lead poisoning, for he says: "I have seen in England two instances of the Success attending the Method here laid down for the Dry-Gripes in the Cholica Pictonum, arising from the Fumes of White Lead; which gives me Reason to hope that by a further Trial of it in Europe, it would be found as beneficial in the latter Distemper as in the former." At the same time, he does not fail to note the occasional occurrence of paralysis, for he remarks: "We frequently observe Persons in the Dry-Gripes to lose the use of their Limbs (the Ancles and Wrists becoming weak and the Balls of their Thumbs sinking)."

It seems highly probable that Cadwalader was describing cases of lead colic without recognizing their true nature. In this connection, it is worthy of remark that he gives the preference to subacid liquors for persons of "weak, relaxed nerves:" such as

Rhenish wine, "Madeira Wine in which Rattlesnakes are infused, sour and weak Punch made with old Spirit," etc.

Fancy a Cadwalader putting rattlesnakes in his Madeira! It is to be hoped that it was of an inferior vintage, and that the good doctor was like the *bon-vivant* of whom Weir Mitchell relates, in his "Madeira Party," that, when dying, he "declined to have his wine whey made out of a famous old Madeira, saying that it was a waste of a good thing on a palate which was past knowing sherry from port."

The "Extraordinary Case in Physick," published in connection with the Treatise on the Dry-Gripes, is a remarkable example of mollities ossium in a woman aged forty, who had previously suffered from diabetes and "intermitting fever." The case derives additional interest from the fact that its study was completed by a careful autopsy performed by Dr. Cadwalader on April 12, 1742.

Between the publication of Cadwalader's treatise and the writings of Rush there is little for the chronicler to record, but that little is not without interest. Dr. Thomas Bond contributed two short papers to the Medical Observations and Inquiries, of which the first is "An account of a worm bred in the liver, communicated in a letter to Dr. John Clephane." The second is also in the form of a letter to Dr. Fothergill, in which the writer reports success from the use of the bark in scrofulous cases, as previously recommended by Fothergill. The account of the worm is too vague to enable one to hazard an opinion as to its nature. It was discharged from the bowel in two fragments, of which the first was the "forepart of an annular worm nine inches long, and an inch in diameter; and in six hours more, the tail and other parts of the body, amounting in the whole to 20 inches in length," were voided. "It was of a red color and filled with blood, after the manner of a leech." That the worm had occupied the liver was inferred from the appearance of that organ post-mortem, as well as from the symptoms observed during the life of the patient. The parasite was sent to Dr. William Hunter, in whose collection Dr. Morgan saw it many years later. The most interesting of Bond's writings is his "Introductory Lecture to a Course of Clinical Observations in the Pennsylvania Hospital, delivered there the third of December, 1766." This lecture is preserved among the archives of the Pennsylvania Hospital and is an eloquent plea in favor of the inestimable advantages of clinical instruction.

In the first volume of the Medical Observations and Inquiries is "A Relation of a Cure Performed by Electricity, from Dr. Cadwalader Evans, Student in Physic at Philadelphia. Communicated Oct. 21, 1754." This case deserves particular mention, not only because it was, probably, the first in which electricity was employed in the treatment of hysteria, but also because the electrician was Dr. Benjamin Franklin. The patient was a woman about 24 years of ago, who had suffered from convulsions for ten years. Finding, she says, that "death was more desirable than life, on the terms I enjoyed it," I "went to Philadelphia, the beginning of Sept., 1752, and applied to B. Franklin." ...... "I received four shocks morning and evening; they were what they call 200 strokes of the wheel, which fills an eight-gallon bottle and indeed they were very severe. On receiving the first shock, I felt the fit very severe, but the second effectually carried it off, and thus it was every time I went through the operation; yet the symptoms gradually decreased, till at length they entirely left me. I staid in town but two weeks, and, when I went home, B. Franklin was so good as to supply me with a globe and bottle, to electrify myself every day for three months." ...... "I now enjoy such a state of health as I would have given all the world for, this time two years, if it had been in my power, and I have great reason to hope it will continue."

There are no comments from B. Franklin, but it is scarcely to be supposed that even he could have been at that time aware that suggestion is far more potent in its action upon the nervous system than electricity in any form.

If Dr. John Redman had left no literary remains except his graduating thesis—De Abortu—it would have amply sufficed to stamp him as a scholar. Of this thesis, the library of the College of Physicians possesses a beautiful copy, which was printed at Leyden and dedicated to William Allen, John Kearsley, whom he styles his Mæcenas ("Mæcenati suo in perpetuum colendo"), Thomas Bourne and Joseph Redman, his brother. It is prefaced by the sentence from Boerhaave: Nulla est quæ pulchriora laborum præmia cultoribus persolvit quam medica sapientia.

At the stated meeting of the College of Physicians on September 7, 1793, Dr. Redman read an account of the yellow fever epidemic which prevailed in Philadelphia in the autumn of 1762. This paper remained in manuscript until 1865, when it was printed by order of the college. It is certainly rare for a posthumous honor of this kind to be conferred upon a medical writer. At the present day, it is a commonly accepted fact that the popularity of a book expires with its author. The chief remaining contribution of Redman to literature is a Defense of Inoculation, which seems to have decided in the affirmative a controversy that had been waged concerning the benefits of that practice.

The inaugural theses of Shippen, Morgan, Kuhn and Rush are, from an historical standpoint, among the choicest works in the library of the College of Physicians, but, in addition, they possess a value which is more or less intrinsic. They were all published at Edinburgh, and, as a matter of course, are in Latin. Their dates and titles are as follows:

Thesis of Dr. William Shippen, Jr., De Placentæ cum utero nexu. Edinburgi: apud Balfour, Hamilton et Neill, 1761.

Thesis of Dr. John Morgan, De Puopoiesi sive Tentamen Medicum inaugurale de Puris Confectione. Edinburgi: cum Typis Academicis, 1763.

Thesis of Dr. Adam Kuhn, De Lavatione Frigida. Edinburgi: apud Balfour, Auld et Smellie, 1767.

Thesis of Dr. Benjamin Rush, De Coctione ciborum in ventriculo. Edinburgi: Balfour, Auld et Smellie, 1768.

Of the above, the thesis of Morgan is by far the most interesting, for it maintains a theory concerning the formation of pus which was corroborated more than a century later by the researches of Cohnheim. This is manifest from the following extract: "Hoc mea speciale habet, pus nempe neque in sanguine neque extra vasi generari, sed in ipsis vasis inflammatis; et vasorum mutationes ab inflammatione inductas, esse causas efficientes quae virtute quadam secretoria, pus e sanguine eliciunt."

Concerning this question, the late Dr. George W. Norris, in his classical work on the Early History of Medicine in Philadelphia, remarks:

"That he was the first to announce this doctrine there can be no doubt. The claim to it has been usually awarded to John Hunter; but Mr. Curry, a teacher of Anatomy of Guy's Hospital, in 1817, after most careful investigation, has adjudged it to Dr. Morgan, who, he says, 'discussed the question in his Inaugural Discourse with great ingenuity, and I can find no proof that Hunter taught, or even adopted, such an opinion until a considerably later period' (London Med. and Phys. Journ., Vol. XXXVIII, 1817). The various views which have prevailed on the origin and formation of pus since that period, form a curious study, and now, after more than a century, Cohnheim (Virchow's Archiv., Vol. XXXVIII) has demonstrated that the white corpuscles do actually escape from the intact vessels, and contribute, to a considerable extent, to the formation of pus."

The most interesting of Morgan's writings, from a medical standpoint, is his account "of a living snake in a horse's eye, and of other unusual productions of animals. By John Morgan, M. D., F. R. S., London, Professor of the Theory and Practice of Physic, Philadelphia" (a).

Dr. Morgan, in this paper, gives an accurate description of a living filaria in the eye of a horse that was on exhibition on Arch street, between Sixth and Seventh streets. He refuses to discuss the question of the path by which the animal gained access to the eye, but refers to several other cases of animal parasites, and mentions having had more than one case of guinea worm (filaria Medinensis) under his care at the Pennsylvania Hospital. He also refers to the worm "bred in the liver of Mrs. Holt in this city about thirty years ago" (b), and mentions having seen it in the anatomical cabinet of Dr. William Hunter ten years previously.

(a) Trans. Am. Philos. Soc., Vol. II, p. 383.
(b) Case of Dr. Cadwalader Evans, above referred to.

In 1878 Dr. Charles S. Turnbull exhibited before the Philadelphia County Medical Society a horse in whose eye a filaria, several inches long, could be plainly seen (c), and stated that this case made the third observed in this country, the first having been reported to the American Philosophical Society, September 26, 1783, by Judge Francis Hopkinson. This is an error. Under the title of "An account of a worm in a horse's eye," Hopkinson describes the same case that was studied by Morgan. Hopkinson's paper apparently antedates that of Morgan, for it appears on p. 183 of the second volume of the Transactions, while Morgan's paper is on p. 383. On closer inspection, however, it appears that Morgan's paper was read on June 5, 1782, and Hopkinson's on September 26, 1783.

There are several other papers by Morgan in the second volume of the Philosophical Transactions, of which the most important is on the "Art of Making Anatomical Preparations by Corrosion." In this method of preparing anatomical specimens he was an adept. He acquired his knowledge of the process from the Hunters, who, in their turn, had been instructed in it by a Dr. Nicholls. Morgan claims the credit of having introduced this method into France, and, doubtless, with justice, for M. Sue, in his Anthropomotie, acknowledges having acquired it from him (d).

This chapter, as announced at its beginning, is not intended as a catalogue of literary productions, but no notice of Morgan's work could be regarded as complete without at least a reference to his "Discourse upon the Institution of Medical Schools in America," and his celebrated "Vindication of His Public Character in the Station of Director-General of the Military Hospitals." The latter is sufficiently discussed in another part of this work, and besides its interest is more of an historical and polemical than of a medical character. The discourse, however, is, to use the words of Norris, a "remarkable production, and should be republished and circulated as an act of justice to his memory. Although the science has advanced immeasurably since that day, his enlarged views of what

---

(c) Medical and Surgical Reporter, Oct. 26, 1878.
(d) Mons. Morgan, Docteur en Médicine de la faculté d'Edimbourg en a donné une description exacte à l'Académie Royale de Chirurgie et c'est de lui que je tiens l'art de préparer ces parties."

is required of a medical practitioner by preliminary education, his high-toned sentiments regarding its practice, honors and emoluments, his recommendations of clinical teaching and hospital instruction, his recital of the years of labor spent by him in preparation for its active duties, in addition to its historical value, all make this now very rare tract worthy of such attention."

Thus we conclude our notice of the works of the most interesting character in the history of Philadelphia medicine. Exception may be taken to this statement concerning Morgan, for, as a matter of course, the impression derived from the study of a character depends, to a large extent, upon the tastes and general mental constitution of the student. We venture, however, to assert unqualifiedly that Benjamin Rush, whose writings we are now about to notice, is the most remarkable character, not only in the annals of Philadelphia medical history, but in those of the entire continent. Such is the testimony of all who have studied the works of this great man, and this notwithstanding the fact that they rise from their perusal bewildered as to his statements concerning the etiology of disease, skeptical as to the diagnosis of his cases, and positively aghast at his therapeutics!

The question whether pleasure and profit may be derived from a study of Rush's writings is one that should be answered emphatically in the affirmative. For beauty and clearness of style, vigorous expression and copious and apt illustration, they are undoubtedly unsurpassed. In addition, they contain numerous references to distinguished men of his time, which will always be read with interest. For these reasons they deserve to be ranked as classics. On the other hand, since they were written before the days of Louis, Laennec, Bright and Gerhard, the reader who consults them with a view of obtaining information concerning the pathology, diagnosis and treatment of disease, must of necessity be disappointed. With reference to the latter, the thought constantly arises that many of his "cures" must have been imaginary, in that his treatment was based upon a mistaken diagnosis. How else can we explain the recovery of the "Methodist minister" in the "inflammatory" stage of consumption, whom he bled fifteen times in the course of six weeks, removing, at each bleeding, not less than eight ounces; or that of the other "citizen of Philadelphia," supposed to be suffering from the same disease, whom he bled eight times in two weeks, and "with the happiest effects?" On this account also it is permissible to question his statement (in his Essay on Old Age) that "Dr. Franklin had two successive vomicas in his lungs before he was 40 years old," and even that Rush himself, between his eighteenth and forty-third years, had "occasionally been afflicted with many of the symptoms" of pulmonary phthisis.

Dr. Rush's principal contributions to literature were the following:

1. Medical Inquiries and Observations, published between 1789 and 1804. In 1805 a second edition in four volumes was printed, and in 1809, a third. The fifth edition ("four volumes in two") was printed in 1818.

2. A volume of Essays, Literary, Moral and Philosophical. They were originally published in various periodicals and were collected in one volume in 1798.

3. Medical Inquiries and Observations on Diseases of the Mind, one volume, 1812.

In addition he published six introductory lectures, "Sermons to Young Men on Temperance and Health," two Essays Against Negro Slavery, and numerous articles in medical journals and in the newspapers, the latter mostly on literary and political subjects, and annotated the works of Sydenham, Pringle, Cleghorn and Hillary.

Scarcely one of the numerous papers contained in the Medical Inquiries and Observations can be read without practical advantage to the physician of the present day, while such essays as the "Natural History of Medicine Among the Indians" and the "Account of the Influence of the Military and Political Events of the American Revolution Upon the Human Body," will always be ranked among the most important of medical classics. In the "Inquiry Into the Relation of Tastes and Aliments to Each Other," there are statements concerning diet which the experience of recent years has confirmed, and suggestions which yet remain to be tested.

Probably the best temperance lecture ever written (the best because both forcible and temperate) is to be found in the "Inquiry Into the Effects of Ardent Spirits," although it is open to question whether Rush's interpretation of the Legend of Prometheus, which is contained in it, is correct. "The Fable of Prometheus," he says, "on whose liver a vulture was said to be preying constantly, as a punishment for his stealing fire from heaven, was intended to illustrate the painful effects of ardent spirits upon that organ of the body."

From an historical point of view the most valuable chapters in the Inquiries and Observations are those on the yellow fever as it appeared in Philadelphia, either in epidemic or sporadic form, from 1793 to 1805 inclusive, and of them all, the most intensely interesting and most pathetic is that in which the writer depicts his state of body and mind during the prevalence of the fever. In making this record he wrote as a philosopher recording his sensations, both mental and physical, but at the same time, and unconsciously, he has told a tale of heroic self-sacrifice that is perhaps unparalleled in medical annals. His daily walks at this time were in the valley of the shadow of death, and his nights were such as to make him long for the morning with its inevitable horrors. There is nothing in the English language more touching than his account of the death of his sister. Surely no one could read it aloud without a voice broken with emotion and eyes suffused with tears. "On the first day of October, at two o'clock in the afternoon, my sister died. I got into my carriage within an hour after she expired and spent the afternoon in visiting patients. According as a sense of duty, or as grief, has predominated in my mind, I have approved and disapproved of this act ever since. She had borne a share in my labors. She had been my nurse in sickness and my casuist in my choice of duties. My whole heart reposed itself in her friendship. Upon being invited to a friend's house in the country, when the disease made its appearance in the city, she declined accepting the invitation, and gave as a reason for so doing that I might possibly require her services in case of my taking the disease, and that, if she were sure of dying, she would remain with me, provided that, by her death, she could save my life."

This passage alone, and there are others like it in his writings, is sufficient to prove that Rush was one of those rare natures in which the finest sensibility is combined with indomitable courage.

From a practical standpoint the most remarkable of Rush's writings is his Defense of Blood-letting, in which he sets forth, as he understood them, the indications for and against bleeding. The student rises from the perusal of this chapter with the half-formed conviction that Rush regarded the blood, as he undoubtedly did the bile, as an excrementitious fluid. It is all very well for Rush and his indiscriminating admirers to say that he did not bleed a patient because of the name of the disease or as a matter of course, but the fact remains that he bled him, and, as a rule, copiously. He refers with approval to the fact that "Dr. Physick drew ninety ounces by weight from Dr. Dewees, in a sudden attack of the apoplectic state of fever, at one bleeding, and thereby restored him so speedily to health that he was able to attend to his business in three days afterwards." Truly a most desirable result, especially for the pregnant women who doubtless imagined, as do their descendants of to-day, that their delivery could not be accomplished in the absence of their favorite accoucheur. The question, however, which arises in the minds of those who wish to profit by Rush's teaching is, what does he mean by such terms as the "apoplectic state of fever?" It is impossible to say, and the fact is that our methods of diagnosis and our entire nosology are so radically different from those of Rush's day that we can learn little or nothing from his statements concerning the indications for blood-letting. For the same reasons we have no just balance in which to weigh his claims of its efficacy, and, therefore, we avoid a discussion which must necessarily be futile. It is in the Defense of Blood-letting that is to be found that remarkable passage, where Rush expresses a hope which, in the light of later events, might almost be called a premonition, of the discovery of anæsthetic drugs: "I have expressed a hope in another place that a medicine would be discovered that should suspend sensibility altogether, and leave irritability or the powers of motion unimpaired, and thereby destroy labour pains altogether."

The work on the Diseases of the Mind appeared in 1812, one

year before the death of the author. It went through five editions, and was for many years the only systematic American treatise upon the subject. Of this work the distinguished English alienist, Dr. Hack Tuke, says that if Rush had written nothing else, it "would have given him an enduring name in the republic of letters." No discriminating reader can peruse the works of Rush without being charmed with his style, the beauty of which is as difficult to define as that of the symphony of a master musician. However hard to define, there is no question as to its source. It is the product of a mind trained in the classics, versed in the literature, and especially the poetry, of the English language, and endowed by nature with an unusual degree of taste, sensibility and imagination.

Contemporary with Rush, there were numerous other writers upon yellow fever, which was naturally, at that time, the most absorbing topic of medical discourse. The most prominent of these lesser lights was William Currie, who was born in 1754. There are conflicting accounts of the latter years of his life. According to Norris, in 1818, he "sank into a state of fatuity and so continued till his death in 1829." On the other hand, Ruschenberger states that Currie "addressed a bright communication, December 6, 1820, to the joint committee of the City Councils on the yellow fever of that year. He became hopelessly childish later, and so continued till his death in 1828." Another error in connection with the history of Currie has been detected, and, so far as possible, rectified by the writer. In the Index Catalogue of the Surgeon-General's office, a thesis, "De Phthisi Pulmonali. Edinburgi: Balfour, Auld et Smellie, 1770," heads the list of Currie's works. It appeared evident that this must be a mistake, since the said thesis was published when its reputed author was but sixteen years old. Besides, it is doubtful whether Currie ever received a degree from any school, and Ruschenberger calls attention to the fact that, in none of his numerous works, did he ever affix the letters M. D. to his name. To settle the question, inquiry was made at the Surgeon-General's office, with the following result:

"Dear Sir:—Replying to your communication of 7th inst., I beg to return thanks for calling attention to an error in the Index Catalogue, under the name of William Currie. You are correct in your supposition that the author of the thesis, De Phthisi Pulmonali, Edin., 1770, was other than Dr. William Currie of Philadelphia, and the error has been noted for correction. This library contains nothing further of the writings of William Currie, who wrote the thesis, nor have we been able to find any note of him except that given in the Edinburgh list of graduates, 1705 to 1845.

"Very truly yours,

"J. C. MERRILL,

"Major and Surgeon U. S. A., Librarian S. G. O."

Currie's principal works are the following:

1. An historical account of the climates and diseases of the United States of America, and of the remedies and methods of treatment which have been found most useful and efficacious, particularly in those diseases which depend upon climate and situation. Printed by T. Dobson, at the Stone House, No. 41 South Second street, 1792.

2. A Treatise on the Synochus Icteroides or Yellow Fever, as it lately apeared in the City of Philadelphia, etc., 1794.

3. Observations on the Causes and Cure of Remitting or Bilious Fevers . . . . and an appendix exhibiting facts and reflections relative to the Synochus Icteroides or Yellow Fever, 1798.

(This appendix may be consulted with great advantage by those interested in the history of the various epidemics of yellow fever in Philadelphia.)

4. View of the diseases most prevalent in the United States of America at different seasons of the year. With an account of the most improved method of treating them; 1811.

In one of his publications, "An Impartial Review," etc., 1794, Currie attacked Rush's doctrine of the autochthonous origin of yellow fever. He argued forcibly in favor of its importation, but, unfortunately for his fame, he became, at a later period, convinced that it might originate in this country. Rush maintained that yellow fever had its origin in decaying vegetable matter, and believed the disease to be non-contagious, while Currie, at one time, held that its sole source was from abroad and was from first to last a "contagionist."

One of the most prolific and also one of the ablest of the medical authors of this country was Dr. Charles Caldwell, who began his literary career while a student at the University of Pennsylvania, by the translation from the Latin of Blumenbach's Elements of Physiology (1795), and terminated it by the completion of his Autobiography a short time before his death in 1853. A list of Caldwell's writings occupies more than seven pages of his Autobiography. It includes biographical memoirs, reviews, orations, criticisms, translations, articles on natural history, phrenology and numerous other subjects. It has been estimated that these various publications would amount to not less than ten octavo volumes of one thousand pages each. Caldwell was a born controversionalist, constantly attacking the doctrines of others or defending his own, and hence the influence of his writings, as he himself acknowledges, was of necessity "limited and evanescent" (e). Of them all, with the possible exception of his Life of General Greene, the only one still read is his Autobiography, and this is far too little known. It is certainly one of the most interesting books in medical literature, containing, as it does, a minute history of a physician who, from his earliest career, was in intimate relation with some of the most distinguished men of his time. It is more correct to say of Caldwell that he enjoyed the hostility of his acquaintances than that he enjoyed their friendship, for his natural element seems to have been hot water. One cannot agree with Yandell in the statements that Caldwell's Autobiography has added nothing to his fame and that he was "everywhere unjust to the memory of his contemporaries." There can be no doubt whatever that it will be read with increasing interest as time goes on, while the interest of his other writings and that of the works of his contemporaries will progressively diminish.

Caldwell was a pioneer in many directions. He was the first to urge through the press the introduction of the Schuylkill water into the city; the first to deliver clinical lectures at the Philadelphia Almshouse; and the first to advocate the use of the trephine in cases

(e) Autobiography, p. 239.

of mania. The latter suggestion, however, was based upon the fallacious teachings of phrenology. The character of Caldwell is well epitomized by the late D. Hayes Agnew in his history of the Philadelphia Almshouse. He was, says Agnew, "a man unquestionably of remarkable intellectual force, combined, however, with such incongruous elements of character as were calculated to defeat the best appointed plans of ambition."

The character and abilities of the early teachers in the Medical Department of the University of Pennsylvania are not mere traditions based upon the hero worship of credulous pupils, but facts that may be proved by reference to the books, and especially the text-books, which, amid their manifold labors, they found the time to write.

In 1811 Prof. Caspar Wistar published his "System of Anatomy for the Use of Students." In 1825 the third edition of this work was published, with notes and additions by William Edmonds Horner, at that time adjunct professor of Anatomy in the University of Pennsylvania. It was, subsequently, "entirely remodeled and illustrated by more than two hundred engravings" by Joseph Pancoast, and reached a ninth edition. In its various forms it maintained its place as a text-book for more than thirty years.

That Wistar was not a mere compiler, but a close observer as well, is proved by the fact that he was the "first writer on Anatomy to describe accurately the extremities of the ethmoid bone, which, previously, had been supposed to belong to the sphenoid, and hence they have ever since been known as the 'pyramids of Wistar.'"

Another successful text-book of the same period is the Elements of Surgery, by the brilliant John Syng Dorsey, which first appeared in 1813 and passed through four editions, two of which were posthumous. It was at one time used as a text-book in the University of Edinburgh. Dorsey also deserves mention on account of his ingenious inaugural essay on the lithontriptic virtues of the gastric liquor. In it he gives an account of his treatment of a case of stone in the bladder by the intra-vesical injection of the "gastric liquor of the hog," and arrives at the conclusion that "in cases of stone of recent date the gastric liquor would, probably, in the course of a few weeks, so far diminish its size as to enable the patient to discharge it through the urethra."

A more voluminous writer than either of the two last mentioned was John Redman Coxe, whose first work, entitled Practical Observations on Vaccination, or Inoculation for the Cow-Pock, published in 1802, when he was but twenty-nine years of age, is sufficient to make his fame enduring. Dr. Coxe is said to have been the first to be successfully vaccinated in Philadelphia, the virus having been sent to him, through Mr. John Vaughan, by Thomas Jefferson. He vaccinated his son, Edward Jenner Coxe, when he was twenty-three days old, and such was his faith in the protective powers of vaccination that he shortly afterward allowed a patient "on the eighth day of an ample eruption of smallpox" to hold the child in his arms for a quarter of an hour. The immunity from the disease was thus proved to be complete.

Dr. Coxe published the "American Dispensatory . . . . comprehending the improvements in Dr. Duncan's second edition of the Edinburgh New Dispensatory" in 1806. It reached a ninth edition in 1831. In 1808 appeared the "Philadelphia Medical Dictionary, containing a concise explanation of all the terms used in Medicine, Surgery, Pharmacy, Botany, Natural History, Chemistry and Materia Medica." A second edition of the Dictionary was issued in 1817. A comparison of Coxe's slender dictionary with the bulky volumes of the same character that have lately appeared, makes it evident, either that his claim to have included all the terms employed in the medical sciences, is erroneous or that these terms have multiplied at a remarkable rate. Dr. Coxe's erudition is perhaps best displayed in his "Inquiry Into the Claims of Dr. William Harvey to the Discovery of the Circulation of the Blood," etc. (1834). In this elaborate treatise he discusses, in a learned manner, a question which has always interested the minds of medical scholars, and especially those of Philadelphia. The writings of William Forbes, J. M. Da Costa, and Henry Chapman, upon the same subject are doubtless familiar to the present generation.

In 1835, Dr. Coxe issued "An Appeal to the Public and Especially to the Medical Public from the Proceedings of the Trustees of the University of Pennsylvania, vacating the chair of Materia Medica and Pharmacy." This pamphlet is, as a matter of course, entirely controversial, and is largely composed of correspondence between the parties at issue.

Dr. John C. Otto is an example of the fact mentioned at the beginning of this chapter, viz., that the value of the work of a medical writer does not depend upon its quantity. To paraphrase a sentence of Horace, Otto was undoubtedly *parcus literarum cultor et infrequens*. Nevertheless, he has immortalized himself by a short article entitled "An Account of an Hemorrhagic Disposition Existing in Certain Families," which appeared in the Medical Repository, Vol. VI, No. 1, 1803. In this brief paper, Otto points out the chief characteristics of Hæmophilia, and especially its hereditary transmission through the females of a family to their male descendants; and recommends the sulphate of soda "in ordinary purging dose, administered two or three days in succession." This, he says, generally stops the hemorrhages. In 1805, Otto published another paper on the same subject in Coxe's Medical Museum, "detailing the history of four fatal cases of hereditary hemorrhage occurring in the family of Benjamin Binny, of Maryland." These papers, says Dr. Isaac Parrish in his memoir of Otto, "were, so far as I am informed, the first which had appeared upon the subject of this singular idiosyncrasy, and gave rise to others from different writers by which many curious facts were developed." In his admirable article on Hæmophilia in Ziemssen's Encyclopædia, Vol., XVII, Immermann says that no general interest was excited on this subject until after a series of cases had been reported in American journals. "The first of these American articles appeared in the Medical Repository of New York and contained an account by Otto of a widespread bleeder family in which the disease could be traced back for nearly a hundred years."

But for this pioneer article, Dr. Otto would only be remembered as the successor of Rush at the Pennsylvania Hospital, to which he gave his services as attending physician for twenty-two years.

Dr. Philip Syng Physick certainly did not acquire his title of Father of American Surgery by the quantity of his writings, for, as stated by Horner, thirty or forty pages of printed type would probably contain them all; nor by their quality, for he left nothing worthy of note in this chapter. His title, which no one disputes, was the legitimate result of his preëminent surgical knowledge and skill, and his impressive teachings in the chair of Surgery of the University of Pennsylvania, which he was the first to occupy.

The works of Dr. William Potts Dewees have been among the most successful that have ever been published in Philadelphia. This was undoubtedly due to their intrinsic merit, for it was not until he was well advanced in years that Dewees was in a position to *impose*, had he so wished, his books upon the medical students of his day. On November 15, 1825, he was elected adjunct to the chair of Obstetrics, at that time occupied by Dr. Thomas C. James, whose failing health rendered such assistance necessary. Dr. Dewees was then fifty-seven years of age. He delivered but one course of lectures (1834-35), but broke down in an attempt to deliver the next and resigned his chair on the 10th of November, 1835.

Writing in 1842, the late Prof. Hugh L. Hodge speaks of the "intrinsic value" of Dewees' System of Midwifery, which, says he, "with all its deficiencies, probably constitutes now, at the expiration of twenty years from its original publication, the best practical book in our profession." The tenth edition of the system was published in 1843.

Dewees' Treatise on the Diseases of Females also went through ten editions and, according to Hodge, was, in its day, "the book for reference in all questions of practice on the important, delicate and difficult subjects which it embraces." It was first issued in 1826, one year after the publication of his Treatise on the Physical and Medical Education of Children. In 1830 he published a work on the Practice of Medicine, which, although it reached a second edition, does not deserve to rank with the works previously mentioned. Dr. Dewees was not a precocious writer. He was well advanced in life before he ventured to offer the results of his large and varied experience as guides to his fellow practitioners, and this is doubtless the chief reason why his works retained their authority for so long a period.

The fame of Nathaniel Chapman is far less due to his writings than to his impressive personality, his ability as a teacher and his genial wit, which combined to make him one of the most remarkable men in the medical history of America. It is perhaps unnecessary to add that he was a gentleman in every sense of the word, a man of honor, to whom the arts of the trickster were utterly alien.

Chapman's most important work is his Elements of Therapeutics and Materia Medica, of which the first edition, issued in 1817, was dedicated to John Syng Dorsey, his successor in the chair of Materia Medica. The subsequent editions were dedicated to the medical students of the University of Pennsylvania. The first edition of this work was essentially composed of Chapman's lectures, as they were delivered to his classes at the University. The later editions were enlarged in accordance with the natural growth of the subject. The work went through five editions and was very popular. L. P. Yandell, in his admirable address on medical literature (f), says that he "remembers well the feeling of relief, not to say delight, with which he turned to them from the dry treatises on Materia Medica and the drier dispensatories which they came to supplant." Chapman's other most important works were "Lectures on the More Important Diseases of the Thoracic and Abdominal viscera," 383 pp., 8vo, 1844; "Lectures on the More Important Eruptive Fevers, Hemorrhages and Dropsies, and on the Gout and Rheumatism," 448 pp., 8vo, 1844; and a "Compendium of Lectures on the Theory and Practice of Medicine."

The interest excited by Chapman's teaching is best manifested at the present day by the elaborate notes of his lectures, which were taken by brilliant students, some of whom subsequently attained the highest honors of their profession. Among such students, were George B. Wood, John K. Mitchell, and John Neill, whose notebooks are preserved in the library of the College of Physicians. Mitchell's notes are models of thoroughness and neatness, but are unfortunately incomplete, although from no fault of his own. He prepared an index and abstract in which the cause of this incompleteness is pithily explained. Its title is the following: "Index to, and

---

(f) Transactions, Internat. Med. Cong., 1876.

Abstract of, My Notes on the Lectures of Professor N. Chapman, year 1816-17, in seven volumes—lost by being loaned."

Samuel Jackson, like Nathaniel Chapman, is chiefly remembered as a great teacher at the University of Pennsylvania, with which he was connected for thirty-six years. His contributions to medical literature are mostly to be found in the medical journals of Philadelphia, and especially in the American Journal of the Medical Sciences. His most valuable papers, from a practical standpoint, are those on yellow fever, and on cholera; the former being contained in the first and second volumes of the Philadelphia Journal of the Medical and Physical Sciences, and the latter in the February and May numbers of the American Journal of the Medical Sciences for 1833. In 1832 he published the Principles of Medicine founded on the Structure and Functions of the Animal Organism. Concerning this work Carson says: "The work of Dr. Jackson performed its mission; it was an elementary book of general scope, and when scores of laborious and systematic compilers had spread their productions broadcast and the student was no longer at a loss for condensed sources of knowledge, the necessity of revising and continuing it no longer existed. From the advance of science, to have revised the work would have been to rewrite it, and he permitted it to be superseded." Dr. Jackson's last paper on a "Rare Disease of the Joints" was published in the American Journal of the Medical Sciences, July, 1870, when the writer was 83 years of age.

The next to follow Dewees as a writer on Obstetrics and Diseases of Women was Charles D. Meigs (1792-1869). It is only with reference to time, however, that Meigs can be said to follow anyone; for, as regards versatility of genius, scope of learning and ability in teaching, he is second to none. Meigs' principal works are the following: The Philadelphia Practice of Midwifery, 1838, 370 pp., 8vo; second edition, 1842, 408 pp., 8vo. Woman, Her Diseases and Remedies, 1847, 670 pp., 8vo. This was written in the form of letters to medical students and is justly regarded as "one of the most original medical works of this country." It passed through four editions. Obstetrics, the Science and the Art, 1849. This, which is a continuation of the Philadelphia Practice of Midwifery, passed through five editions. In 1850 he published a work of 211 pages on Certain Diseases of Children, and in 1854, a Treatise on Acute and Chronic Diseases of the Neck of the Uterus. In 1854, he issued a work on Childbed Fevers, which, like the Treatise on Woman, Her Diseases and Remedies, was written in the form of letters to his class.

Franklin Bache (1792-1864), the great-grandson of Benjamin Franklin, will be remembered on account of his work on the U. S. Pharmacopœia and the U. S. Dispensatory long after the fact that he was Professor of Chemistry in the Jefferson Medical College has been forgotten. In association with George B. Wood, he took an active part in the decennial revisions of the Pharmacopœia from 1830 to 1860 inclusive. The undying gratitude of the profession is due to these distinguished men for this philanthropic labor, for they "neither expected nor received any other recompense than the consciousness of duty performed and public benefit conferred" (g).

Dr. Bache's contribution to the Dispensatory amounted to about one-third of the volume, and was concerned chiefly with the "mineral substances and those resulting from purely chemical processes." This was a lucrative as well as an honorable employment, for, up to the time of his decease, he "had received the proceeds accruing to him from the sale of 79,000 copies."

The contributions to medical literature of Dr. William E. Horner (1793-1853), the successor of Physick in the chair of Anatomy at the University of Pennsylvania, although not numerous, were important. According to the list collected by his son-in-law, the late Prof. Henry H. Smith, they numbered twenty-nine, and appeared, for the most part, in the American Journal of the Medical Sciences. He is best remembered as the discoverer of the tensor tarsi muscle, which has been called in his honor, the musculus Hornerii, although his investigations of the intestinal lesions of cholera are, to the practitioner, of much greater importance. The methods which he employed in these researches were both novel and ingenious. "He first made a minute injection of the mucous membrane and then examined it under water with large magnifying

---

(g) Biog. memoir of Dr. Franklin Bache, by George B. Wood, M. D.

lenses; and afterward on the object-glass of the microscope." By means of this technique he was enabled to demonstrate for the first time that "entire desquamation of the epithelium of the small intestines is a cardinal and especial anatomical lesion in cholera."

Although perhaps somewhat irrelevant, the writer cannot refrain from the statement that the life of Horner affords a remarkable example of the pursuit of knowledge under difficulties. He was of frail physique and, in addition, the extracts from his journal published by Samuel Jackson, show him to have been a man who, while outwardly serene, was, throughout his life, oppressed by the profoundest melancholy. His indomitable will enabled him to achieve a brilliant triumph over obstacles which most men would have found insuperable.

It is a singular fact that there is scarcely a biographical record of Dr. René La Roche (1795-1872), who was one of the most scholarly writers of this city, and a member of numerous learned societies, both at home and abroad. According to Ruschenberger, a memoir of Dr. La Roche was written by Dr. Joseph G. Nancrede, but this is a mistake, for Nancrede died in 1856 and La Roche in 1872. The memoir written by Nancrede, which is to be found in Simpson's Lives of Eminent Philadelphians, was of La Roche's father. The only memoir of this distinguished author that I have been able to find is contained in Vol. XXIV of the Transactions of the American Medical Association, of which it occupies but one page. His work on yellow fever (1855) is, however, a colossal monument to his memory. It has been aptly characterized as a "vast storehouse of observation and research," and is certainly one of the most elaborate monographs in the English language. His work on "Pneumonia; Its Supposed Connection, Pathological and Etiological, with Autumnal Fevers" (1854), is also a "monograph of enduring interest."

Joseph G. Nancrede (1793-1856) deserves mention as the reporter of the first case of Cæsarean section in Philadelphia (American Journal of the Medical Sciences, Vol. 16, 1835). The patient was operated on by Prof. William Gibson, and both mother and child were saved. The latter, as I am informed by Dr. Robert P. Harris, is still living, at the age of sixty-two.

The reputation of Dr. Isaac Hays (1796-1879) as a journalist was so great as to obscure his achievements in other fields, although the latter alone would have sufficed to make him famous. Although he was a worker and an organizer rather than a writer, his contributions to the literature of his specialty (ophthalmology) are worthy of the highest praise. He is said by Alfred Stillé to have recorded the first case of astigmatism published in America, and he was "also the first, it is believed, to observe color blindness as a pathological condition." He edited Lawrence on Diseases of the Eye, Arnott's Elements of Physics, and, in association with Dr. R. E. Griffith, translated the Chronic Phlegmasiæ of Broussais, and the Principles of Physiological Medicine of the same author. His editorial connection with various medical journals will be alluded to under the head of the Medical Journals of Philadelphia.

Dr. Hugh L. Hodge (1796-1873), although the third incumbent of the chair of Obstetrics at the University of Pennsylvania, was, in reality, the first authoritative teacher of midwifery in that institution. James did little to advance the art he taught, and Dewees, as has already been stated, was stricken with apoplexy at the end of his first course of lectures. A better example of the irony of fate than that afforded by the life of Dewees can scarely be found in medical annals. Hodge was elected to succeed him in 1835, and it is no disparagement of his more brilliant competitor, Charles D. Meigs, to say that he justified the choice of the trustees. The aggressive genius of Meigs, his fiery, poetic temperament and his untiring energy were the very qualities most essential to a teacher in a school which, on account of its comparative youth, was obliged to assert itself, and they doubtless contributed largely to the well-earned fame of the Jefferson Medical College. On the other hand, the conservative nature of Hodge, his equable disposition and, using the word in no invidious sense, his self-sufficiency, were more in accord with the traditions of the older institution.

Hodge's *magnum opus* was the Principles and Practice of Obstetrics, with 159 lithographic figures from original photographs and with numerous wood cuts. Of this superb work, there are two editions in the library of the College of Physicians, the first of which was published in 1864, not in 1863, as stated by Goodell in his biographical memoir of Dr. Hodge. The second edition appeared in 1866. On account of his imperfect vision (Goodell actually speaks of him as a "blind man") Dr. Hodge labored under great difficulties in the preparation of this work, which, from title page to colophon, was written under his dictation. To the student of medical history, the most interesting portion of Hodge's Obstetrics is its preface, which contains an admirable account of the rise and progress of obstetric teaching in Philadelphia. The chief remaining works of Dr. Hodge are Diseases Peculiar to Women, 1860; a paper on Fœticide, which had a large circulation; and papers on "Synclitism" and the Mechanism of Labor. His studies in these fields will always be of value to the obstetrician, while his strenuous advocacy of the non-contagiousness of puerperal fever can no longer be productive of harm. George McClellan (1796-1847), the founder of Jefferson College, is better remembered by his deeds than his writings. His principal literary work was a text-book on the Principles and Practice of Surgery, a posthumous work edited by his son, John H. B. McClellan, and published in 1848. The book was in press at the time of McClellan's death, and, as stated by Darrach, his biographer: "The first printed sheet was placed before him during his brief illness, but he was already too much exhausted to notice its contents." Jacob Randolph (1796-1848), almost exactly contemporaneous with McClellan, resembled the latter in the brilliancy of his surgical work and the scantiness of his contributions to medical literature. The frequency of this combination is such as to suggest the thought that great manual dexterity and literary talent are, at least to a certain exent, mutually exclusive. Randolph's publications may be found in the North American Medical and Surgical Journal, the American Journal of the Medical Sciences, and the Medical Examiner, and the most important among them are reports of cases in which the operation of lithotripsy was performed. He was the first to introduce this operation into Philadelphia, and, in fact, to him belongs the chief credit of introducing it into this country. Before the time of Randolph there were but two recorded cases of lithotripsy in the United States. His dexterity in the performance of this delicate operation excited the admiration of the most competent critics, among them George W. Norris, who says that, in his opinion, it was unsurpassed "even by the eminent discoverer of the method himself."

There are names in our annals which inevitably suggest the trite but ever appropriate figure of the beacon light, warning from the shoals of error and pointing "every wandering bark" to the haven of truth. One of the most brilliant among them is John Kearsley Mitchell (1796-1858), whose lectures on the Cryptogamous Origin of Malarious and Epidemic Fevers are to be ranked among the most remarkable contributions to medical literature. As Hirsch remarks, he was undoubtedly "the first to approach in a scientific spirit the nature of infective disease, and particularly in malarial fever." It is true that he was mistaken in regarding the cause of malarial fevers as vegetable rather than animal, and, therefore, his merit, in this connection, must rest upon the recognition of an *organic* cause of the diseases in question. This doctrine he supported by an immense number of facts and analogies, and inculcated with remarkable clearness and eloquence. One rises from the perusal of these lectures, not only delighted with the beauties of Mitchell's style and deeply impressed with the force of his reasoning, but also with a feeling of respect for those medical students of the class of 1846-47, who were his attentive hearers and at whose urgent request the lectures were published. Although the terms "toxine" and "antitoxine" were unknown in Mitchell's day, he was none the less acquainted with the fundamental facts of which they are the symbols. This is manifest from the following: "But when," he says, "organic substances find their way into the tide of blood, and that, too, with vital energies capable of reacting on the elements of the sanguine current, it requires but little acquaintance with physiological and pathological phenomena to induce us to dread the most fearful results."

His statement of the cause of immunity from second attacks of certain infectious diseases comprises, in a few well-chosen words, the antitoxine theory of to-day. "Their germs," he says, "having once reacted in the body, leave behind a poison, or at last an impediment, by which their future reaction is there prevented."

J. K. Mitchell's principal writings were published in 1859 in a single volume, under the editorship of his son, Dr. S. Weir Mitchell. The title of this work is "Five Essays," the subjects of which are: (1) The Cryptogamous Origin of Malarious and Epidemic Fevers; (2) An Essay Upon Animal Magnetism, or Vital Induction; (3) On the Penetrativeness of Fluids; (4) On the Penetrativeness of Gases; (5) On a New Practice in Acute and Chronic Rheumatism. From a medical standpoint, the last of these essays is quite as important and interesting as the first, to which allusion has already been made. It was first published in "Hays' Journal" in 1831, and anticipates by half a century Charcot's observations on spinal arthropathies. Dr. Mitchell was led to regard some disorder of the spinal cord as the origin of rheumatism, by observing pain and swelling of the joints in two cases of spinal disease; the first being a case of Pott's disease, the second a case of curvature of the cervical vertebræ. In both these cases the arthritis was promptly cured by leeches applied to the spine. Dr. Mitchell then treated a number of cases of acute articular rheumatism by means of wet cups to the spine and with most satisfactory results. He gives a table of thirty-two cases treated in this manner, twenty-two of which were cured within eight days. The theory of Mitchell that the cause of rheumatism is to be found in some central nervous disorder has been lately adopted in somewhat modified form by Professor Latham, of England, who announced his adherence to it in the Croonian lectures delivered before the Royal College of Physicians in 1886. At present, the weight of opinion is in favor of the parasitic or infectious theory of rheumatism, but in the absence of direct demonstration of the supposed infectious agent, there is, at least, quite as much to be said in favor of the neuropathic theory, as first advanced by J. K. Mitchell. Mitchell was not only a scientific physician, but a poet. He published a number of lyrics which have been described by a competent critic as "melodious, delicate and graceful," and two poems of greater length and more sustained effort "which show a lively fancy and much ready command and choice of language." Reference to these compositions is here made in order to show the absurdity of the vulgar opinion that nothing "practical" can emanate from the brain of a poet, for if ever there was a "practical" man it was J. K. Mitchell.

John Bell (1796-1872) wrote (1) A Treatise on Baths and Mineral Waters, in two parts, of which Part I contained a "full account of the hygienic and curative powers of cold, tepid, warm, hot and vapor baths, and of sea bathing." Part II: "A history of the chemical composition and medicinal properties of the chief mineral springs of the United States and of Europe." 532 pp., 8vo.

2. A Practical Dictionary of Materia Medica, 479 pp., 8vo.
3. Regimen and Longevity, 42 pp., 8vo.
4. Dietetical and Medical Hydrology, 658 pp., 8vo.

In association with Dr. D. F. Condie he wrote a Report of the College of Physicians to the Board of Health, which contained "all the material facts in the history of epidemic cholera . . . and a full account of the causes, post-mortem appearances and treatment of the disease," 1832. Dr. Bell also edited Stokes' Lectures on the Theory and Practice of Physic, Andrew Combe's Treatise on the Physiological and Moral Management of Children, and several other works.

David Francis Condie (1796-1875) was the author of one of the earliest and most successful works on the Diseases of Children. This "practical treatise" was published in 1844 and reached a sixth edition in 1868. It was superseded by the well-known work by Meigs and Pepper on the same subject. In addition Condie published several addresses and a biographical notice of Henry Bond, M. D., and edited Watson's Lectures on the Practice of Physic, Churchill on the Diseases of Women, Carpenter on the Use and Abuse of Alcoholic Liquors, and Barlow's Manual of the Practice of Medicine.

George B. Wood (1797-1879) is chiefly remembered as the author of a text-book on the Practice of Medicine, which, for many years, was *facile princeps* among works on this subject. It is a monument of erudition and a model of literary style. "It became a favorite text-book for students, not only in this country, but also in Great Britain. The time-honored University of Edinburgh was one of several foreign medical schools in which it was officially approved and adopted. It passed, during its author's life, through six editions." The first edition of this great work was published in 1847, three years before Wood was transferred from the chair of Materia Medica and Therapeutics to that of the Theory and Practice of Medicine, the latter having been vacated by Nathaniel Chapman. In attempting to estimate the difficulties encountered by Wood in the composition of this colossal work, it must be remembered that, in his day, there was neither Index Catalogue nor Index Medicus, and that, even as late as 1885, the library of the College of Physicians contained only 1,700 volumes. An author such as Wood was obliged to found a library, which was naturally selected with the greatest care, and it is partly through the gradual absorption of such precious hoards that the collection of the College of Physicians has attained its present size and value. Wood's work on the Pharmacopœia and the Dispensatory, in association with Dr. Bache, has been already mentioned. Of the latter, 120,000 copies were sold during Dr. Wood's life. In addition to these *magna opera*, he published two volumes of Memoirs, Lectures and Addresses, several of which are upon historical subjects. It is probably remembered by few that Dr. Wood was also a poet, or, rather, a versifier, for, according to Henry Hartshorne, his principal metrical work, entitled "First and Last," is "without a spark of poetic genius."

Thomas Jefferson did excellent service for the cause of medical education in this country when, through his agent, Francis W. Gilmer, he induced Robley Dunglison to accept a chair in the University of Virginia. It was a *declaration of dependence* which proved its author to be well aware of the fact that, amid all the discussions of politics, the republic of science is one and indivisible.

Of Robley Dunglison (1798-1869), Prof. S. D. Gross, writing in 1869, said: "No physician on this continent has surpassed him in the extent of his erudition, in the variety of his information, or in the magnitude of his labors," and the writer sees no reason to modify this opinion. He is best known at the present day by his

Dictionary of Medical Science, of which the twenty-first edition, thoroughly revised and greatly enlarged by his son, Richard J. Dunglison, was published by Lea Bros. & Co. in 1893. Fifty-five thousand copies of this work were issued during the lifetime of its author, and "of all his works, 125,000 copies, equal to between 150,000 and 160,000 volumes." His industry was amazing and its products of the highest order. He spent nine years (1825-1833 inclusive) at the University of Virginia, and while, in virtue of his contract with that institution, he was teaching anatomy, physiology, surgery, materia medica, pharmacy and the history of medicine (*mirabile dictu!*), he brought out his Human Physiology in two large octavo volumes, and his Dictionary. The former passed through eight editions and the latter, now in its twenty-first, bids fair to maintain its place for an indefinite period. From the autumn of 1833 to that of 1836, he belonged to the Faculty of the University of Maryland and taught materia medica, therapeutics, hygiene and medical jurisprudence. During this period, he composed his admirable work on General Therapeutics and Materia Medica, and his elements of Hygiene, of which the former reached six editions and the latter two. The Medical Student, or Aids to the Study of Medicine, appeared in 1837, and a second and much larger edition in 1844. New Remedies was published in 1839. This work first appeared as a part of the American Medical Library, but was subsequently published separately. It passed through seven editions, the last, an octavo of 750 closely printed pages, in 1856. The Practice of Medicine, in two volumes, was issued in 1842. In the course of six years it passed through three editions, of which the last contained nearly 1,500 pages. This is but a tithe of the work of this literary giant. In 1837 he founded a monthly periodical, the American Medical Library and Intelligencer, which was "devoted to the republication of foreign medical and surgical works and the dissemination of medical news." It survived only five years, but during that period the portion contributed by Dunglison, as collator and editor, amounted to five volumes. In association with Mr. W. Chapin, he brought out a Dictionary for the Blind in raised type, in three folio volumes, and edited, with valuable notes and additions,

Roget's Physiology, Traill's Lectures on Medical Jurisprudence, and Forbes's Cyclopædia of Practical Medicine. The rest of his literary work is made up of addresses, introductory and valedictory, biographical memoirs of distinguished men, and a large number of articles on non-medical subjects, which appeared in the Virginia Literary Museum, of which he was a founder and an editor, and in other periodicals. One of these articles, it may be mentioned, was on the Sanscrit Language. It is humbly hoped that this brief notice may help to keep green the memory of this remarkable man, who was no mere accumulator of words and phrases, but a finished scholar and a master of English prose. To repeat the quotation employed by his distinguished biographer: *Nihil tetigit quod non arnavit.*

Samuel David Gross (1805-1884) was as eminent in surgical, as was Dunglison in medical, literature; but unlike the latter, Gross displayed his activity in many other fields than those of literature. He was, undoubtedly, the foremost surgeon of his day, and has been recognized as such by the medical profession. There may have been more brilliant operators and more thorough anatomists, but as scholar, teacher, writer and surgeon combined, Gross stands unrivaled. He began his literary career very early in life. Graduating in 1828, he published in 1830 a work of 389 pp., 8vo, on the Anatomy, Physiology and Diseases of the Bones and Joints. In 1839 he published his celebrated Elements of Pathological Anatomy, which passed through three editions. The first edition of this work was in two volumes of more than five hundred pages each; the last two editions were issued in a single volume. This book was a favorite with Professor Virchow and was heartily commended by him upon a memorable occasion. At a dinner given by Virchow in honor of his American confrère, the former took the opportunity of alluding to the work in a manner and in terms that were most grateful to his distinguished guest. The interesting event is thus related by Professor Gross in his Autobiography:

"After the viands were pretty well disposed of, Virchow, availing himself of a lull in the conversation, drew forth a large volume from under the table, and, rising, he took me by the hand and made

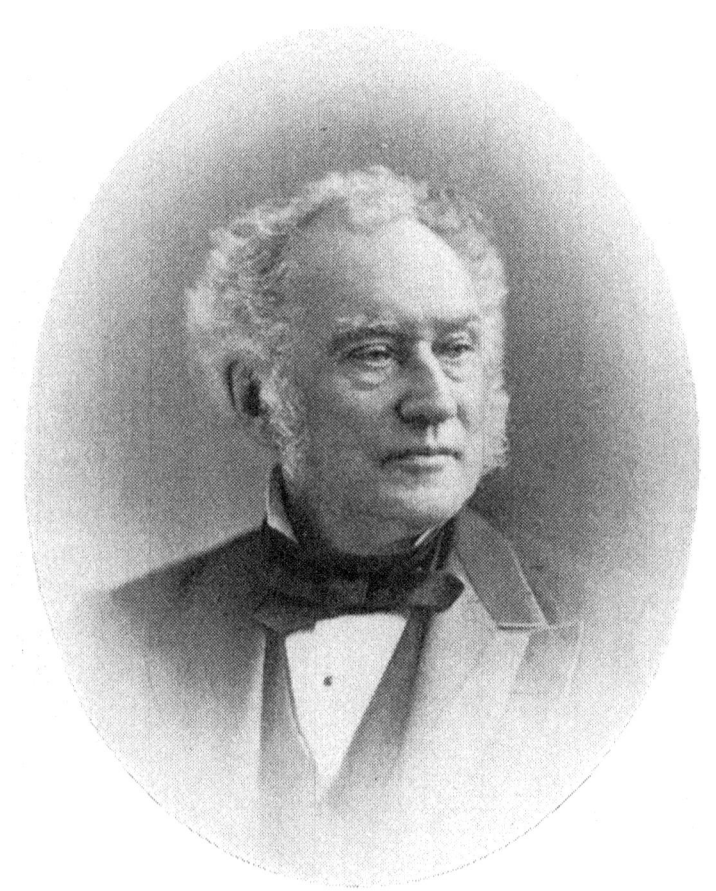
SAMUEL D. GROSS.

me an address in German, complimenting me upon my labors as a pathological anatomist and referring to the work, which happened to be the second edition of my Elements of Pathological Anatomy, as one from the study of which he had derived much useful instruction, and one which he always consulted with much pleasure. I need not say how deeply flattered I felt by this great honor, so unexpectedly and so handsomely bestowed upon me by this renowned man. I felt that I had not labored in vain and that the compliment was more than an equivalent for all the toil and anxiety which the work had cost me." This happened in Berlin in the summer of 1868, and among the witnesses of a scene which should be portrayed, not only in words, but by the brush of a great artist, were von Langenbeck, von Graefe, Donders and Gurlt.

In 1843, Dr. Gross published An Experimental and Critical Inquiry Into the Nature and Treatment of Wounds of the Intestine, of which the third edition was edited by his son, the late Professor Samuel W. Gross. The enormous advances in abdominal surgery that have lately been made, have relegated this treatise to the limbo of obsolete publications. In the time of Gross, the greatest triumph of abdominal surgery was the formation of an artificial anus.

In 1851, appeared a Practical Treatise on the Diseases, Injuries and Malformations of the Urinary Bladder, the Prostate Gland, and the Urethra, of which a third edition, in 1876, was also edited by the late Professor S. W. Gross.

A Practical Treatise on Foreign Bodies in the Air Passages appeared in 1854.

The work by which Professor Gross was most widely and popularly known was his System of Surgery, Pathological, Diagnostic, Therapeutique and Operative. This colossal work was contained in two large octavo volumes, each of nearly 1,200 pages. The first edition was issued in 1859 and the sixth in 1882. In 1863 it was translated into the Dutch language. The labor involved in the composition of this book and in the revision of its successive editions, was immense. "Rising early, working late, writing with an assiduity that only a man of his wonderful physique could have kept up, he generally gave from five to eight hours a day to the cherished project, no matter what the interruptions or whatever else he had (h) to do." In 1861, Dr. Gross was editor of, and principal contributor to, a volume entitled Lives of Eminent American Physicians and Surgeons of the Nineteenth Century, and in 1876 he contributed to the literature of the Centennial year, a learned and voluminous History of American Surgery from 1776 to 1876.

His autobiography in two large octavo volumes was published in 1887, three years after his death, under the editorship of his sons. The passage quoted above may be regarded as a specimen of the interesting reminiscences contained in this work, of which the last two hundred pages are devoted to biographical sketches of distinguished contemporaries of its more distinguished author. In addition, Dr. Gross published addresses, introductory and valedictory, and biographical memoirs which, while they fall into the rank of *opera minora*, would have sufficed to perpetuate his literary reputation.

One rises from a study of the life work of Samuel D. Gross with a profound sense of the magnitude of his self-imposed tasks. They were, however, labors of love. His whole soul was devoted to his profession and he sustained the heaviest burdens with that lightness and grace which are the expression of a superb mental and physical endowment.

Joseph Pancoast (1805-1882), the brilliant colleague of Gross, is remembered as a most dexterous operator and an admirable teacher, and this memory will be transformed into a tradition by future generations. He contributed very little to medical literature. Early in life, he translated Lobstein's Treatise, "De nervi sympathici humani fabrica et morbis," Paris, 1823. It is no injustice to Pancoast to say that he was not fully aware of the value of the little book which he took the trouble to translate. The first case of Addison's disease on record is to be found in Lobstein's book, but Addison's disease was not recognized as a distinct morbid entity until the publication, in 1855, of Addison's classical work "On the

---

(h) Biographical sketch of Prof. Samuel D. Gross, by J. M. Da Costa, M. D., LL. D.

Constitutional and Local Effects of Disease of the Supra-renal Capsules."

The remaining principal publication of Professor Pancoast is his Treatise on Operative Surgery, a work of 380 pages, with 80 plates, which was issued in 1844 and reached a third edition in 1852.

George W. Norris (1808-1875) was not a voluminous writer. His papers, devoted exclusively to surgical subjects, and dealing especially with the statistics of operations, appeared, for the most part, in the American Journal of the Medical Sciences. The first of these valuable contributions to surgical literature is the report of a case of dislocation and fracture of the astragalus, which appeared in the above-named journal in August, 1837, just one year after Norris was elected surgeon to the Pennsylvania Hospital. In 1873 he collected his principal writings and issued them in a single volume, entitled Contributions to Practical Surgery. In publishing this work, Dr. Norris conferred a favor upon his surgical contemporaries, to whom he thus made readily accessible a series of observations that had previously been widely scattered. Many of the papers were classical, and, to use the words of Ashhurst, were "quoted in all parts of the civilized world where the English language is either read or spoken." The essay upon the "Occurrence of Non-Union After Fractures" was described by William Hunt as "an exhaustive masterpiece," and by Frank Hastings Hamilton as "the most complete and reliable monograph upon this subject contained in any language."

After the death of Dr. Norris, in March, 1875, there was found, among his papers, the manuscript of an Early History of Medicine in Philadelphia. "The notes and memoranda which accompany the manuscript show that it was for the most part written in 1845, but laid aside for a time, owing to press of active work as a surgeon, while in later years failure of health prevented the finishing touches necessary to its completion" (i). The manuscript was printed and published, in 1886, for private distribution, by Dr. William F. Norris, the son of its distinguished author. The edition was limited to

---

(i) From the preface by Dr. Wm. F. Norris.

one hundred and twenty-five copies, and has been distributed among those who, on account of their friendship for its author, their general culture, or their devotion to historical studies, are most capable of appreciating it. It is certainly the most interesting and valuable record of medical annals that has ever appeared in this country, and the work is numbered by its fortunate possessors among their greatest treasures. The book is a veritable *edition de luxe,* and is a fit setting for the literary gems with which it sparkles.

Joseph Carson (1808-1876), who occupied the chair of Materia Medica and Therapeutics from 1850 to 1876, published numerous articles relating to the subjects he taught, the majority of which appeared in the American Journal of Pharmacy. His chief contribution to strictly medical literature is an article on Puerperal Eclampsia, which occupies thirty-three pages of the American Journal of the Medical Sciences for April, 1871. The writer ventures the opinion that the obstetricians of the present day are not sufficiently acquainted with this admirable paper, which, at the time of its publication, attracted great attenion. It appeared in the form of a review of more than a dozen separate works upon eclampsia and allied subjects, and is apt to be overlooked by those who are not aware that, formerly, it was the custom of the ablest writers in Philadelphia to publish a goodly proportion of their best work in the form of reviews. This was notably the case with Professor Joseph Carson.

Washington L. Atlee (1808-1878) did more than any one in the world to establish ovariotomy as a legitimate operation, and he accomplished this herculean feat, not so much by words as by deeds. His contributions to literature were but scanty, and consist for the most part of reports of operations performed by himself and others. In 1845, by dint of indefatigable research, he collected the statistics of one hundred and one ovariotomies, and published them in the American Journal of the Medical Sciences for April of the same year. He was led to undertake this investigation by his interest in a case of ovarian tumor on which his brother, Dr. John L. Atlee of Lancaster, operated successfully, on the 29th of June, 1843. By 1851 he had collected the records of two hundred and twenty-two cases of ovariotomy and published them, in abstract, in the Transactions of the American Medical Association for that year. His first operation was performed on March 29, 1844, and his three hundred and eighty-seventh on May 31, 1878. Dr. Atlee was a pioneer in a field of surgery that, up to his time, had been almost completely neglected. In spite of his brilliant success, perhaps rather because of it, he was the victim of such misrepresentation and abuse as would have caused an ordinary man to sink broken-hearted into an untimely grave. It is impossible, at the present day, to understand the attitude assumed by some of Atlee's most distinguished contemporaries. They vilified him publicly before their students, and endeavored, privately, to dissuade his patients from submitting to operations which he had recommended. In short, he suffered, to the fullest extent, the penalty of being in advance of his time. Fortunately, his life was sufficiently prolonged for him to witness the triumph of his opinions, and to enjoy the rewards of his courage and skill. His paper on the Treatment of Fibroid Tumors of the Uterus, read before the International Medical Congress in September, 1876, was warmly applauded by the most eminent gynecologists of the day.

William Wood Gerhard (1809-1872) is justly regarded as the greatest of Philadelphia clinicians. His chief claim to distinction is derived from his studies of typhoid and typhus fevers, by which he was led to establish the separate natures of these diseases. His best work was done early in life. Graduated from the University of Pennsylvania in 1832, he immediately proceeded to Paris, at that time the medical center of the world, and diligently followed the teachings of Chomel, Andral and Louis. Of these three distinguished men, the last-named is the one from whom Gerhard, in common with the medical world at large, derived the most valuable instruction. While "walking the hospitals" of Paris, Gerhard was diligently collecting the materials of his earlier publications, and his methods were identical with those of Sydenham, who declared, with the voice of authority, that "all diseases should be described as objects of natural history." It is related of Sydenham that he advised a young man who asked him to prescribe a course of medical reading, to read Don Quixote; in other words, to eschew the works of hair-splitting theorists, and study disease, not in the library, but at the bedside. This was the method of Gerhard, to whom his friends, on hearing the story above referred to, might well have said, in the words of Horace: *Mutato nomine de te fabula narratur.* "Such was his desire for impartial observation that he not only avoided, as he tells us, the examination of books, but even abstained from the comparison of his own observations with each other, until the series was completed and he was prepared to analyze them and then compare the results with what has been related by others" (j).

The first fruit of this conscientious study was the publication, in association with his friend and fellow-student, Dr. Caspar Wistar Pennock, of Observations on the Cholera as it appeared in Paris in 1832. He then turned his attention almost exclusively to the study of the diseases of children, for which, at that time, unusual facilities were afforded in Paris. The hospital in which Gerhard pursued his investigations, contained 500 beds, the age of the patients ranging from two to sixteen years. It needs but a slight exercise of the imagination, especially on the part of those who remember the man and his methods, to depict the young student pondering over the specimens of this rich collection, interpreting their signs, classifying their symptoms and correlating both symptoms and signs with the post-mortem lesions. One of the first results of his investigations in this field was the observation that inflammation of the glands of Peyer, to which Louis had directed attention as the specific lesion of typhoid fever, is by no means rare in other diseases of childhood. He next turned his attention to the cerebral affections of children, and soon demonstrated the association of the most frequent variety of meningitis with the deposit of tubercles in the pia mater. Cases of the kind referred to had been previously classified under the generic title of hydrocephalus, but are now correctly described as tubercular meningitis. His studies of the pneumonia of childhood are of equal interest and value. He pointed out with great accuracy the differences in the signs and symptoms, the clinical course, and the post-mortem appearance of the so-called

(j) Stewardson's Memoir of Gerhard.

pneumonia of children, and led to its classification under the title of lobular pneumonia. Our views of pneumonia in childhood have naturally undergone considerable modification since the time of Gerhard's first studies of this disease. Genuine lobar pneumonia, identical in all respects with the pneumonia of adults, may attack the infant at the breast, but its lesions are rarely observed, because it is a comparatively benign affection. It is also held at the present day that many of the cases of so-called lobular pneumonia, catarrhal pneumonia, broncho-pneumonia, are of tubercular origin. This statement, it is scarcely necessary to say, is not intended to detract, in the slightest degree, from the value of Gerhard's work. On the contrary, the writer is firmly of the opinion that the path to our present knowledge of these affections was made smooth by his pioneer researches. These admirable contributions to pædiatrics are but little known to the physicians of to-day. This is partly due to the fact that Gerhard is chiefly remembered for his work on the continued fevers, and partly because he was the least self-assertive of men. Returning to Philadelphia in the autumn of 1833, he entered the Pennsylvania Hospital as resident physician in the spring of 1834, and soon demonstrated that the symptoms and lesions of the common continued fever of the United States were identical with those of the typhoid which he had studied in the wards of Louis. This was the first step toward his great discovery. In the spring and summer of 1836 an epidemic of typhus fever prevailed in Philadelphia, and was so extensive that Gerhard had the opportunity of studying two hundred cases of the disease. He had previously seen cases of typhus during a visit to Edinburgh, and he was thus enabled to determine the identity of the epidemic fever of Philadelphia with the typhus of Great Britain, and the dissimilarity of both from typhoid.

This, very briefly stated, is the method by which Gerhard demonstrated the fact that typhus and typhoid fevers are distinct diseases. The physician of to-day who is not familiar with the state of medical science in the early part of this century may be surprised that the distinction between the two diseases was not sooner recognized. A study of medical history will, however, soon convince him of the difficulties in the way of their differential diagnosis, and, at the same time, excite his admiration for Gerhard's brilliant work. Up to the time of Louis, the pathology of the continued fevers had not been accurately studied, and there can be little doubt that if this great clinician had had the opportunity of observing both typhus and typhoid fevers, he would have recognized their separate natures. The fever studied by Louis was typhoid, the prevailing fever of France, and he investigated it from every standpoint except that of bacteriology (a science then unknown), with a thoroughness that left little to be done by later students of the disease. When Gerhard returned to Philadelphia he was thoroughly familiar with the symptoms, the clinical course, and, above all, with the pathological anatomy of typhoid fever. Soon after his arrival, he had the good fortune to have under his care a large number of cases of typhus, a disease hitherto confounded with typhoid—but let him tell the story of his discovery in his own words:

"There is another disease which, in many respects, bears a certain relation to typhoid fever. Of this I have shown numerous examples to the class during the twenty-three years of my attendance at this hospital. It is the English or Irish typhus, as it was formerly called. This disease was first studied at Philadelphia by my late lamented colleague, Dr. Pennock, and myself, at the Almshouse Hospital. The results of our observations I published at that time in the American Journal of the Medical Sciences. It differed totally from typhoid fever in the character of the lesions, there being no distinctive anatomical lesion at all existing in the disease, excepting the condition of the blood, which was evidently somewhat altered from its normal condition, the intestines and mesenteric glands remaining in a state of perfect integrity. This disorder we were enabled to prove was totally different from the typhoid fever of France, described so minutely by Dr. Louis, with which we had been familiar for many years" (k).

This is not the place in which to enter into an elaborate argument in favor of Gerhard's priority in distinguishing between

---

(k) Pennsylvania Hospital Reports, 1868.

typhus and typhoid fevers. Murchison divides the honor of the discovery between Perry of Glasgow (1836), H. C. Lombard of Geneva (1836), Gerhard and Pennock of Philadelphia (1836), Shattuck of Boston (1839), and others; but there can be no doubt that, in the words of Osler, Gerhard's papers in the American Journal of the Medical Sciences, 1837, are "the first in any language which give a full and satisfactory account of the clinical and anatomical distinctions we now recognize."

Gerhard's chief remaining works are a treatise on the Diagnosis of Diseases of the Chest, based upon the comparison of their physical and general signs, 1836, and Lectures on the Diagnosis, Pathology and Treatment of the Diseases of the Chest, 1842.

The first edition of the latter work contained 157 pp., the fourth edition, issued in 1860, contained 448 pp., and was a standard authority upon the subject of which it treats.

William Pepper (1810-1864) was one of the most brilliant contemporaries of Gerhard, and, like the latter, after graduation from the University, pursued his studies in Paris under Louis and Dupuytren. He was renowned for his skill in diagnosis, and, as a natural consequence, was in great demand as a consultant. His literary work was limited to articles, which were published for the most part in the American Journal of the Medical Sciences, the Medical Examiner, the Transactions of the College of Physicians, and of the Pathological Society. They were "distinguished by brevity, clearness of expression and an eminently practical character." Dr. Thomas S. Kirkbride, in his biographical memoir of Dr. Pepper, gives a list of his principal writings, but has omitted one of the best of them. The paper referred to is on Pleuritic Effusions, and was published in the American Journal of the Medical Sciences in 1852. Nearly twenty years ago (in 1879) the writer consulted this paper and quoted it (l), and he still retains a vivid sense of the pleasure and profit he derived from its perusal. In the same volume of the "American Journal" in which Dr. Pepper's article appeared, there is another paper on Pleuritic Effusions, by Dr. Bowditch of Boston, and these two papers are among the best contributions to this

(l) See Trans. of the Path. Soc. of Philadelphia, Vol. X, p. 220.

important subject that can be found in medical literature. It would be invidious to compare them. They are both admirable, and if any deficiency may be found in the one, it is supplemented by the completeness of the other.

John Barclay Biddle (1815-1879) was the author of one of the most popular books on Materia Medica that has ever been published. The first edition of the work was issued in 1852, under the title of a "Review of the Materia Medica, for the Use of Students," and contained about three hundred pages. In 1865 a second edition was called for, and the title was changed to "Materia Medica, for the Use of Students." This name was adopted for the eight editions which subsequently appeared, of which the last was issued in 1878, and contained 462 pages. In the words of Dr. E. B. Gardette, this work "must long remain a positive help to every medical student that seeks it, and be, in the profession he adorned, a monument to the memory of its author's ability." Dr. Biddle was not only an author, but a journalist of distinction. In 1838, when but twenty-three years of age, he founded, in association with Dr. Meredith Clymer, the Medical Examiner, which became almost immediately successful. It was at first a fortnightly journal, but later was issued weekly. In a few months after it was started, Dr. W. W. Gerhard was added to its editorial staff, and shortly afterward, Dr. Francis Gurney Smith. "In examining the early numbers, one cannot fail to be struck with the high professional tone, the wide grasp and the good sense which characterized the editorials, as well as the admirable bibliographical notices with which the pages of the Medical Examiner were enriched. The editors, youthful as they were, gave evidence of being trained writers, and brought to the journal professional knowledge and vigor of intellect not often united in men of their age and supposed inexperience" (Gardette).

Thomas Dent Mütter (1811-1859) was one of the first American surgeons to give special attention to plastic operations and operations for club-foot. His bent in this direction was doubtless chiefly derived from his studies under Dieffenbach and Liston. His first publication was a brochure on "The Salt Sulphur Springs of Monroe County, Virginia," in 1840. Shortly after this, he published a pamphlet on club-feet. "In 1846 he edited, with numerous and extensive additions, Lectures on the Operations of Surgery, by Robert Liston, Esq., F. R. S. These works, with the exception of a syllabus to his Course on Surgery, and some short essays and addresses, are unfortunately all that he was enabled to accomplish" (m).

Among the contributors to surgical literature, Henry Hollingsworth Smith (1815-1890) is prominent. His Minor Surgery, which appeared in 1844, went through four editions, as did also his System of Operative Surgery, which was first published in 1852. The latter is characterized by the number and beauty of its illustrations, and, therefore, even at the present day, it may be consulted with great profit by the undergraduate or practitioner who wishes either to learn, or review, the mere mechanical technique of any given operation. Both of these works were published before Dr. Smith was elected to the chair of Surgery in the University of Pennsylvania, and, doubtless, were of influence in securing his appointment to that position. In addition, Professor Smith contributed numerous papers on surgical subjects to the medical journals, especially the American Journal of the Medical Sciences and the Medical Examiner, and signalized the first year of his medical career (1838) by translating Civiale's Treatise on the Prophylactic Treatment of Stone and Gravel.

D. Hayes Agnew (1818-1892) found time, amid the incessant interruptions of an extensive practice, to contribute bountifully to surgical literature. He was a man who never disappointed expectation, and it seemed but natural to those who knew him that the treasures of his mind should be lavishly bestowed. His earlier writings were on various subjects of a surgical nature, and at one time he seemed to have a decided predilection for gynecology: witness his admirable paper on Laceration of the Perineum, in the first volume of the Pennsylvania Hospital Reports; also his articles on Vesico-Vaginal Fistula. His life-work, however, is comprised in his Treatise on the Principles and Practice of Surgery, in three volumes, dated, respectively, 1878, 1881 and 1883. Concerning this

(m) Memoir of Thomas D. Mütter, by R. J. Levis, M. D.

work, the friend and biographer of Agnew, Professor J. William White, remarks: "It is safe to say that this magnificent monument to the learning, skill and industry of one man will remain unrivaled in surgical literature. It is not likely that there will ever again be anyone who will combine the enormous experience, embracing every department of surgery, the clear judicial intellect and the patient, untiring energy which enabled him, in hours stolen from his family, from social pleasures and from much-needed rest, to produce this remarkable exposition of his work and views." After speaking of the necessity of revision to keep the work abreast of the march of progress, Dr. White continues: "And yet there are portions, and large portions of the book, which, it seems to me, can never grow surgically old or useless. Our successors may be too hurried to read the abstracts of the history of important surgical procedures, which, with infinite labor and painstaking, he had conscientiously compiled; his pathology may become antiquated, and his therapeutic measures come to be looked upon as are those of Paré or Wiseman, but his admirable clinical descriptions, his comprehensive and well-balanced consideration of diagnostic points, his clear explanation of the surgical anatomy of disease, injury and operation, must always remain, as at present, a mine of information for the busy practitioner."

The book, which reached a second edition in 1889, is the property of the trustees of the University of Pennsylvania.

The reputation of J. Forsyth Meigs (1818-1882) rests chiefly upon his work on the Diseases of Children, and it would be hard to find a better pedestal for a literary monument. The first edition of this book appeared in 1858 as one of the Medical Practitioners' and Students' Library, and, after passing through three editions, was allowed to go out of print. In a letter to Dr. Arthur V. Meigs, Dr. Alfred Stillé speaks of Meigs on Diseases of Children in the following terms: "More than once in later years and before he reached middle life, he has lamented to me that he was too much hemmed in by pædiatry. Yet in this he laid the strong foundations of his professional success. All the while, he was collecting the material for the work upon which his reputation must chiefly rest. Every case was recorded, and by degrees a mass of material accumulated that formed a mine out of which at last was built up his work upon diseases of children. From time to time he conversed with me about these papers, read them to me for criticism, and finally, taking Rilliet and Barthez as his model, he produced the best and most original work upon the subject in the English language."

In 1869, Dr. Meigs decided to reissue the work, and with this object in view, he secured the valuable assistance of Dr. William Pepper. The fourth edition appeared in 1870, and this and the three subsequent editions have been known as Meigs and Pepper on Diseases of Children. The book, under this joint authorship, was entirely remodeled, many of the original articles being rearranged or rewritten, and many new ones added. The fourth edition (the first under the joint authorship) contained more than two hundred pages of new matter. The seventh was issued in 1882, less than a year before the death of Dr. Meigs. There can be no question that this book, in its first edition, fully deserved the encomiums of Dr. Stillé, and that, through the able collaboration of Dr. Pepper, it maintained its place in the first rank of works upon diseases of children. It superseded the contemporaneous work of Dr. D. Francis Condie upon the same subject, although the latter also had a large sale, going through six editions, the first in 1844, the sixth in 1868.

In addition to his great work on the Diseases of Children, Dr. Meigs contributed numerous articles to various medical journals, all of which displayed the signs of acute clinical observation. Among them were "Remarks on Atelectasis Pulmonum," etc., "Heart-clot as a Cause of Death in Diphtheria," the "Morphological Changes in the Blood in Malarial Fever," and a report of a remarkable case of pneumopericardium. He also wrote a most interesting memoir of his distinguished father, Professor Charles D. Meigs, and a "History of the First Quarter of the Second Century of the Pennsylvania Hospital." The last-mentioned paper was read before the Board of Managers of the Pennsylvania Hospital, at their stated meeting of September 25, 1876.

The only original work of Francis Gurney Smith (1818-1878)

is a pamphlet embodying the results of a series of experiments on digestion; or rather on *the* digestion of a single individual—Alexis St. Martin. They were performed in the year 1853, while he was incumbent of the chair of Physiology in the Pennsylvania Medical College, and they led him and his colleague, Professor R. E. Rogers, to the erroneous conclusion that lactic acid is the acid of the gastric juice in man. In addition, he translated and made additions to Barth and Rogers' Manual of Auscultation and Percussion, and was one of the authors of Neill and Smith's Compendium for Students, which passed through many editions. For five years, he was one of the editors of the Philadelphia Medical Examiner, and was co-editor of Drake's Diseases of the Mississippi Valley. He also edited Carpenter's works on Physiology and on the Microscope, and Marshall's Outlines of Physiology, Human and Comparative.

John Neill (1819-1880), the first incumbent of the chair of Clinical Surgery in the University of Pennsylvania, contributed a number of valuable articles to the Medical Examiner, while it was edited by his brother-in-law, the late Dr. Samuel Hollingsworth, and to the American Journal of the Medical Sciences. Two of the articles published in the Examiner, namely, those on the Treatment of Fracture of the Patella and on Extension and Counter-Extension of the Leg, have a permanent place in surgical literature. The various articles in the "American Journal," seven in number, are, in the words of his biographer, Dr. Edward Shippen, "of more than common interest." Early in his career, he published three treatises on the Veins, Arteries and Nerves, which had an extensive circulation. One of their chief merits was their illustrations from original drawings containing the names "placed upon the parts, instead of being referred to by numbers—rather a novelty then and a great relief to the student." In association with Dr. Francis Gurney Smith, Dr. Neill compiled the Compendium of Medical Sciences, to which Dr. Rees contributed the sections upon Materia Medica and Chemistry. This work, as previously stated, enjoyed a phenomenal success, but, according to Shippen, Dr. Neill, "in after years, frequently was heard to regret that he had ever been connected with a publication, however successful, which contributed so largely to make medical education superficial." This reflection may have been suggested by the avalanche of "quiz compends" which began to descend during the latter years of Neill's life, and of which the Compendium was the forerunner.

Henry Hartshorne (1823-1897) was the author of two popular text-books—The Essentials of the Principles and Practice of Medicine, and the Conspectus of the Medical Sciences. The first is, as its name implies, "a Handbook for Students and Practitioners, while the second is an elaborate *quiz compend*, "comprising manuals on anatomy, physiology, chemistry, materia medica, practice of medicine, surgery and obstetrics." The "Essentials" was first issued in 1867, and reached its fifth edition in 1881. The "Conspectus" was published in 1869, and reached its second edition in 1874. Dr. Hartshorne also wrote small monographs on Glycerine and its Uses (1865), and on Cholera (1866), and edited the American edition of Reynolds' System of Medicine (1880), with valuable additions, notably the article on Progressive Pernicious Anæmia. In 1872, he edited the fifth edition of Watson's Lectures on the Principles and Practice of Physic, a work which had previously been edited by Dr. D. Francis Condie in 1858.

Dr. William Hunt (1825-1896), who, for thirty years, was on the surgical staff of the Pennsylvania Hospital, contributed numerous articles to medical journals, hospital reports, transactions of societies, etc., nearly all of which retain the interest attached to them at the time of their publication. Dr. Thomas G. Morton has appended to his interesting memoir of his hospital colleague, Dr. Hunt, a list of the writings of the latter, and, on reading it, anyone would be impressed by the practical character of the subjects he chose for discussion. To those who knew him, however, and their name is legion, the subjects of these papers are eminently in keeping with the character of their author, who was, in the best sense of the word, a "practical" man. This epithet undoubtedly conveys to the mind of many persons the idea that the individual to whom it is applied is necessarily deficient in culture; or, rather, and conversely, it seems to be taken for granted that the possession of high scientific attainments is incompatible with the exercise of keen observation and discriminating judgment. The career of Dr. Hunt, in common with that of many of the most eminent physicians and surgeons of Philadelphia, demonstrates the fallacy of this popular impression. Dr. Hunt was widely known as a thorough anatomist, and his opinion of difficult surgical cases was highly esteemed by his surgical colleagues. At the same time he was an active member of the Academy of Natural Sciences, an excellent botanist, a student of modern languages, and, above all, a lover of English, pure and undefiled.

One of the last articles written by Dr. Hunt, and one of his best, appeared in 1888. Its subject was Diabetic Gangrene, and, strange to say, it was the only article upon that affection which, up to that date, had been published in America. This, at least, is stated to be the case by Dr. John S. Billings, who, in acknowledging a copy of the paper that had been sent to the Surgeon-General's office, wrote: "I have read the paper with much interest. I know of no other American paper on the subject."

In 1881, Dr. Hunt wrote several articles in defense of American Surgery, which were widely published. They were elicited by the criticisms of Professor Esmarch upon the management of the case of President Garfield, and were prompted by friendship for Professor D. Hayes Agnew, who was one of the surgeons in charge of the distinguished patient. This motive was in keeping with the loyal character of Hunt, but it is open to question whether one should ever condescend to notice criticisms based upon such imperfect knowledge as must have been possessed by Esmarch with reference to the case of Garfield. Besides, American Surgery, as represented by Agnew, needed no defender.

Richard J. Levis (1827-1890) was known throughout the United States, both as a surgeon of great dexterity and an excellent clinical teacher. In the latter capacity, at the Pennsylvania Hospital, of which he was one of the surgical staff from 1871 to 1885, and at the Jefferson Medical College Hospital, he exercised a wide influence. His contributions to surgical literature are, however, limited to a few short articles, among which may be mentioned the "New Operation for Coloring Corneal Opacities," "Skin Grafting," "Ethylization, the Anæsthetic Use of the Bromide of Ethyl," and the "Treatment of Hydrocele by Excision of Redundant Scrotum."

James E. Garretson (1828-1895) was widely and favorably known to the laity under the *nom de plume* of John Darby. With his non-medical works, however, with perhaps the exception of the "Odd Hours of a Physician," we are not here concerned. He was one of the earliest in this city to adopt the specialty of Oral Surgery, for which, having studied dentistry before he took his medical degree, he was thoroughly equipped. He has left a magnificent monument to his memory in his System of Oral Surgery, a profusely illustrated work of 1,084 pages, which reached a sixth edition in 1895. He also wrote an excellent treatise on the Diseases and Surgery of the Mouth and Jaws.

For an elaborate analysis of the works of William Goodell (1829-1894) a volume would be necessary, as well as an amount of special knowledge such as few possess. Even a mere enumeration of the titles of his publications would cover several pages. The list of his works appended to Professor Parvin's excellent memoir numbers one hundred and thirteen. Although a voluminous writer, his works, whether in the form of clinical lectures, reports of cases, addresses or monographs, are models of literary style. The same faculty of lucid expression was manifest in his impromptu speech and added greatly to his powers as a teacher.

Although Dr. Goodell wrote but one book, his celebrated Lessons in Gynecology, he contributed an elaborate monograph on the Diseases of the Ovaries and Oviducts to the System of Practical Medicine, edited by Dr. William Pepper, and another on the Treatment of Ovarian and Extra-Ovarian Tumors, to the American System of Gynecology. The first edition of the Lessons in Gynecology appeared in 1879; the second in 1880, and the third in 1887. For a period of six years (from 1882 to 1887, inclusive) he published annually a summary of his year's work in ovariotomy. These articles appeared in the Medical News, and were held in the highest estimation by gynecologists throughout the world. A large percentage of Dr. Goodell's publications is in the form of lectures, either clinical or didactic. In the list above referred to, there are forty-three lectures, several of which were published in the International Clinics. Among these numerous papers the most original and, in some respects, the most valuable, is the one entitled "What I Have Learned to Unlearn in Gynecology." In it, Dr. Goodell describes the mistakes arising from a blind adherence to old wives' fables concerning the catamenia, the menopause, mammary abscesses, leucorrhœa, etc., and shows the important part played by neurasthenia in the production of uterine symptoms. In short, he virtually acknowledges that he, in common with the vast majority of his colleagues, had, for years, in many cases, been putting the cart before the horse.

Albert H. Smith (1835-1885) one of the founders of the Philadelphia Obstetrical Society, and also of the American Gynecological Society, was an excellent teacher of Obstetrics, and a ready debater, but left few evidences of his ability as a writer. His contributions to medical literature, though few in number, are well described by his biographer, Dr. James Tyson, as "brief, clear, fearless and forcible." They deal mostly with the mechanical aspects of obstetrics and gynecology, as is indicated by the following selection from the list of nineteen articles appended to Tyson's memoir: An Improved Speculum (1869), the Use of Pessaries in the Early Months of Pregnancy (1875), A Vulsellum for Using with the Écraseur (1875), Use of Catgut in Gynecological Surgery (1878), Application of the Rotating Burr for Denuding Tissues in the Restorative Surgery of the Female Pelvis (1878), Pendulum Leverage of the Obstetric Forceps (1879), On the Use of Intrauterine Stem Pessaries (Proceedings Phila. Co. Med. Soc., 1879-80), Axis Traction with the Obstetric Forceps (1882), etc.

Dr. Albert H. Smith was a man who, partly in virtue of an impressive personality, exerted a great influence upon the men of his generation. His writings, though few in number, are of great value, as they embody the results of an enormous experience in his chosen field of labor.

James Howell Hutchinson (1834-1889), at the time of his death Vice-President of the College of Physicians, was one of the most valuable contributors to Transactions of the Pathological Society of Philadelphia, of which he was elected President in 1871 and 1872; to the Pennsylvania Hospital Reports, to the American Journal of the Medical Sciences, and other journals; the Transactions of the Association of American Physicians, etc. He also contributed valuable articles on typhus, typhoid and simple continued fevers, to the System of Medicine, edited by Drs. William Pepper and Louis Starr, and edited two American editions of Bristowe's Practice of Medicine. The latter undertaking was performed to the entire satisfaction of the distinguished author of the book, who wrote to Dr. Hutchinson when the second American edition was announced: "I am gratified to hear that you will undertake to edit my work. . . . . I could not wish that it should be in better hands," meaning, undoubtedly, by this ambiguous expression, that it could not be in better hands. One of Dr. Hutchinson's best papers, and also one of his latest, is on "The Management of the Stage of Convalescence in Typhoid Fever," and is contained in the Transactions of the Association of American Physicians, Vol. III.

Dr. Hutchinson was eminently conservative. There are those who appropriate this epithet to themselves on the ground that they reject everything that is new. Hutchinson was not of this type. While not "carried away by every wind of doctrine," he was a diligent student of the medical literature of the day, and adopted such methods of diagnosis and treatment as stood the test of clinical experience; for, like Gerhard, whom he succeeded at the Pennsylvania Hospital, he was, above all things, a clinician. "As a writer," to quote the words of Professor John Ashhurst, "Dr. Hutchinson was noted for the correctness and dignity of his style, saying just what he meant in few but well chosen words, and rigidly avoiding all flowing excrescences and ambiguities of language."

Samuel Weissel Gross (1837-1889), late Professor of Surgery in the Jefferson Medical College, was a man of great learning, so far as surgical literature is concerned, of acute powers of diagnosis, and with a large field in which to exercise them. In addition, he was an able writer and a teacher whose words, always well chosen and to the point, were enforced by a commanding presence and a graceful delivery. His writings are distinguished by their exactness of observation and induction, and, consequently, abound in valuable statistics. In 1859, when twenty-two years of age, he reported in the North American Medico-Chirurgical Review "A case of aneurism of the right femoral artery cured by digital compression, with remarks and a statistical report of twenty-two other cases treated by this method." In the American Journal of the Medical Sciences for January and April, 1867, he published an article on "Wounds of the Internal Jugular Vein and Their Treatment." To the same journal for October of the same year (1867), he contributed a review of sixty pages on eleven French and German works on Military Surgery, and gave statistics of 13,514 amputations for gunshot injuries, which he afterward enlarged to 20,933. The study of tumors and malignant growths especially attracted him, and he had a thorough, practical knowledge of their minute anatomy. Some of the results of these researches are to be seen in his paper on Sarcoma of the Long Bones, in the American Journal of the Medical Sciences for July and October, 1879. This paper, as well as his classical monograph on Tumors of the Mammary Gland, are partly the outcome of his course of Mütter lectures on the Surgical Pathology of Tumors, before the College of Physicians. In 1881 he published a Practical Treatise on Impotence, Sterility and Disorders of the Male Sexual Organs. He was also a frequent contributor to the Transactions of the American Surgical Association, and wrote an elaborate article on Tumors of the Breast, for the American System of Gynecology, edited by Mann. Many of Dr. Gross' writings appeared anonymously in the form of editorials in the Medical News, and were characterized by "learned research, surgical acumen, clearness of expression and practical application." Dr. Gross was carried off in the prime of life by an acute illness. Had he lived, he would probably have added greatly to the amount of his literary work, the value of which was steadily increasing. At his death there was found on his desk the MS. of a paper on Stone in Children, which he was preparing for a Cyclopœdia on Diseases of Children.

H. Lenox Hodge (1836-1881), who was, at the time of his death, Demonstrator of Anatomy at the University of Pennsylvania, was of great assistance to his father in his preparation of his "Principles and Practice of Obstetrics." In the preface to that celebrated work Professor Hugh L. Hodge remarks: "The superintendence of the illustrations and the laborious duties of editor have chiefly devolved on the author's son, H. Lenox Hodge, M. D., without whose assistance this work would probably never have been completed." Dr. Hodge's writings were in the form of contributions to journals and "Transactions," and dealt with subjects of obstetrical, gynecological, and general surgical interest. Among them were papers on Excision of the Knee, Excision of the Hip, Subcutaneous Osteotomy, Kolpo-Cystotomy, Metallic Sutures, Tracheotomy for Pseudo-membraneous Croup, and the Drainage of Abscesses and Wounds by Solid Metallic Probes. He was the inventor of a canula for tapping ovarian cysts.

Joseph Gibbons Richardson (1836-1886) was the author of the well-known Handbook of Medical Microscopy, and of numerous articles on the same subject. His report on the Structure of the White Blood Corpuscles (Trans. Am. Med. Ass., Vol. 23) is a careful study of the anatomy of those bodies. He describes the granules which they contain, and their vibratory movement; but, it is scarcely necessary to say, did not employ any of the staining methods by means of which these minute particles have acquired so great a clinical interest. His main object, in the paper referred to, was to prove the identity of the white blood cells with the so-called salivary corpuscles. Richardson was also a worker with the micro-spectroscope, and wrote a paper on the method of applying that instrument to the detection of blood-stains. In 1879, he issued a work, which appeared as one of the American Health Primer Series, under the title of "Long Life and How to Reach It." This was translated into French by P. Barrué, and from the French into Greek by S. Kastoriadou.

Edward Rhoads (1841-1871) assisted Dr. J. Forsyth Meigs in the preparation of his elaborate paper on the Morphological Changes of the Blood in Malarial Fever, already referred to; and, in association with Dr. William Pepper, published, in the first volume of the Pennsylvania Hospital Reports, the results of an experimental investigation into the Fluorescence of the Tissues of the Body. He was elected editor of the Philadelphia Medical Times, when that journal was founded, but was only able to make the preliminary arrangements for its publication, being compelled to resign the position on account of his failing health.

George Pepper (1841-1872) was one of the founders of the Philadelphia Obstetrical Society; in fact, as Goodell says of him (Trans. Phila. Obstet. Soc., Vol. 1-2), he was "more than that—he was one of its prime originators." To the first volume of the Pennsylvania Hospital Reports he contributed an excellent paper upon a case of "Retroversion of the Womb, Complicated by a Large Fibroid," and to the Transactions of the Philadelphia Obstetrical Society two papers, the one entitled Adipose Deposits on the Omentum and Abdominal Walls as a Source of Error in Diagnosis; the other on the Mechanical Treatment of Uterine Displacements.

Drs. Rhoads and Pepper are mentioned, not so much for what they did, as for what, one is pleased to think, they would have accomplished had their lives been prolonged. They are well remembered as two of the most promising young men who ever entered upon the practice of Medicine in Philadelphia.

Elliott Richardson (1842-1887) was the first in this country to perform successfully Cæsarean Section, with removal of uterus and ovaries after the Poro-Müller method. The case is fully reported in the American Journal of the Medical Sciences, 1881. He also published an excellent paper upon the Use of the Obstetric Forceps.

John S. Parry (1843-1876) was one of the most valuable contributors to Philadelphia medical literature. It is not an object of this article to institute comparisons, but the writer cannot refrain from stating that he cannot recall to mind any physician who has accomplished such valuable clinical work within ten years from the time of taking his medical degree as was recorded by Parry during that period of his career. In October, 1870, he published his first paper, entitled Observations on Relapsing Fever, as it occurred in Philadelphia in the winter of 1869-70. It appeared in the American Journal of the Medical Sciences for October, 1870, and attracted universal attention. It has been quoted, both in this country and abroad, by all writers on "Spirillum Fever."

Of the numerous papers which he contributed to medical journals, transactions of societies, etc., three, in addition to that on relapsing fever, attracted special attention, and "would alone have given to Dr. Parry a prominent and permanent place among the medical writers in this country" (n). Two of these papers were on Rachitis, and were designated by Dr. R. W. Taylor of New York as "the best and most comprehensive articles in any language upon the subject." The other article referred to was on Inherited Syphilis.

In his papers on Rachitis, Parry was the first to advance the opinion, subsequently confirmed by others, that Rachitis is "scarcely less frequent in Philadelphia than it is in the large cities of Great Britain and the Continent of Europe." Previous to Parry's time, it was supposed that this disease was comparatively rare in the United States. In the American Journal of Obstetrics, 1883, Vol. V, he published an article on the Comparative Merits of Craniotomy and Cæsarean Section, in Small Pelves with Conjugate Diameter of two and-one half inches or less. This paper occupied forty-three pages of the Journal. Parry's principal work was a Treatise on "Extra-uterine Pregnancy; Its Causes, Species, Pathological Anatomy, Diagnosis, Prognosis and Treatment, 8vo, pp. 275, Philadelphia, 1875. An elaborate review of this work in the American Journal of the Medical Sciences for April, 1876, concludes with the following words: "Dr. Parry's book, therefore, is destined to be long consulted, and deservedly, too, as the highest authority on this obscure and difficult class of cases." Parry edited the second and third American editions of Leishmann's System of Midwifery, and made additions to the work, "the most valuable of which are contained in the chapters on the Forceps and in the new chapter . . . . on Diphtheritic Wounds of the Vagina."

Henry F. Formad (1847-1892) was one of the most active workers in the Pathological Society, of which he was elected a member in 1878 and its president in 1889 and 1890. His position as coroner's

---

(n) Memoir of Dr. John S. Parry, by James V. Ingham, M. D., Trans. Coll. Phys., 1876.

physician, during the latter years of his life, gave him abundant opportunities for securing interesting specimens of disease, and he fully availed himself of them. His best work was in the line of pathological research. Formad was the first in this city to insist on ectopic pregnancy as a frequent cause of sudden death, and to prove that many cases in which certificates of death from "peritoneal hemorrhage from causes unknown," or from "probably injury of abdomen," or "rupture of abdominal vessels," "hæmatoceles and varicoceles of tubes," etc., were, in all probability, cases of extrauterine fœtation. He admits having made such mistakes in the early part of his career as coroner's physician, but he soon discovered his error and collected thirty-five cases in which he traced a fatal peritoneal hemorrhage to its true source—an extra-uterine ovum.

It is impossible to give a complete list of Formad's writings. One volume of the Transactions of the Pathological Society (Vol. XV) contains thirty-five of his communications to that body, besides numerous discussions of the papers of other members. Outside of these "Transactions," which contain his best work, he published "Comparative Studies of Mammalian Blood, with Special Reference to the Differential Diagnosis of Bloodstains in Criminal Cases" (1888, p. 61); the Distribution of Nerves in the Iris (Am. Jour. Med. Sci., Jan., 1878); the Etiology of Tumors (1881, p. 53); the Pig-backed or Alcoholic Kidney of Drunkards, a Contribution to the Post-mortem Diagnosis of Alcoholism (1886); and a special edition of 74 plates, illustrating the Etiology of Tumors (1883). In 1884, in association with Prof. H. C. Wood, he wrote a Memoir on the Nature of Diphtheria, and, in 1889, he contributed to Vol. IV of the Transactions of the Association of American Physicians, an elaborate paper on the Anatomical Relations of Lesions of the Heart and the Kidneys in Bright's Disease, from the Study of Three Hundred Cases. An abstract of each of the three hundred cases is appended to this paper.

Edward Tunis Bruen (1851-1889) was rapidly adding to his well-earned reputation as writer, teacher and clinician, up to the time of his death, at the age of thirty-eight. Like Formad, he was an active worker in the Pathological Society, as has been nearly every physician of the present day who has attained distinction in Philadelphia. His principal works are the following: Anasarca as a Symptom of Deficient Vaso-motor Tonus (Med. Times, 1879); A Pocketbook of Physical Diagnosis, 1881, pp. 256. This was an excellent manual for the student and practitioner, and, had the author lived, would doubtless have continued to maintain a high rank among the numerous works of its class. It reached a second edition in 1883. In 1884, Dr. Bruen wrote, in collaboration with Professor J. William White, a contribution to the Operative Treatment of Purulent Pleural Effusions. In 1887, he published his second Monograph, entitled, Outlines for the Management of Diet, or the Regulation of Food to the Requirements of Health and the Treatment of Disease; and in 1888, a paper on the Relative Importance of Different Climatic Elements in the Treatment of Phthisis (Med. News, Oct. 13, 1888). He also contributed to Wood's Reference Handbook of the Medical Sciences (edited by Dr. Albert H. Buck of New York) an excellent article on Pericarditis.

Dr. John M. Keating (1852-1894) is most widely known as the editor of the Cyclopædia of the Diseases of Children, and the founder of the *International Clinics*. He was also the founder of *The Climatologist* and editor of the *Archives of Pediatrics*. The fact that he was so intimately associated with these successful enterprises, shows him to have been a man of marked executive ability. In addition, however, he was a well-known writer, especially upon the Diseases of Children. His principal contributions to Pediatrics are the following: "The Mothers' Guide to the Management and Feeding of Infants;" "Diseases of the Heart and Circulation in Children;" "Maternity—Infancy—Childhood;" and "Mother and Child." Outside of Pediatrics, his work was also extensive. For several years before removing to Colorado (in 1890), Dr. Keating had been Medical Director of the Penn Mutual Life Insurance Company, and was, therefore, eminently qualified to write upon "How to Examine for Life Insurance." His work bearing that title is a recognized authority among medical examiners for life insurance companies. In 1879, Dr. Keating was one of the parties that accompanied General Grant to India, Burmah, Siam and China, and on his return he published an interesting record of the voyage, entitled "With General Grant in the East." Besides the above works, and in spite of feeble health, Dr. Keating compiled "A New Pronouncing Dictionary of Medicine," and contributed articles to Pepper's System of Medicine, Sajous's Annual, Buck's Reference Hand-Book, etc.

Nathaniel Archer Randolph (1858-1887) wrote a number of excellent papers on digestion and food substances, and on the action of drugs, such as hydrobromic acid and nicotine. In collaboration with Dr. Samuel Dixon, he published Notes from the Physiological Laboratory of the University of Pennsylvania; and, with Dr. A. E. Roussel, he issued A Study of the Nutritive Value of Branny Foods. The latter was published in the Transactions of the College of Physicians, third series, Vol. VII.

In writing this chapter, the impression of the inestimable value of Philadelphia's contributions to medical literature has steadily deepened in the mind of the writer. From the list of authors, many distinguished names will undoubtedly be missed, but it will be found, as a rule, that they belong to those who have written little or nothing of permanent value, or to those who have won renown for their researches in departments that cannot strictly be called medical. Among the latter are Bartram, Harlan, Godman, Barton, Hare, Rogers, S. G. Morton, Seybert, Ruschenberger, J. Gibbons Hunt, Aitkin Meigs, Le Conte, Wormley, George A. Rex, and last and greatest of all, Joseph Leidy.

There is another to whom a tribute of gratitude is due from every medical author of Philadelphia. Reference is made to Dr. Samuel Lewis, the munificent founder of the Lewis Library of the College of Physicians.

Living writers have not been mentioned, first, because this work is a history, not a record of current events; and, secondly, because their works are known and read by all. Suffice it to say that they have kept up the tradition of their fathers and that Philadelphia, so far as concerns her medical literature, might truly adopt as her motto: "*Nulla vestigia retrorsum.*"

MEDICAL JOURNALS OF PHILADELPHIA.

1. The Philadelphia Medical and Physical Journal. Quarterly. Collected and arranged by Benjamin Smith Barton. Vols. I-III, 1804-09, 8vo, with a fourth volume containing three supplements, 1806-1809.

2. The Philadelphia Medical Museum. Quarterly. Conducted by John Redman Coxe. Seven volumes, 1805-1811, 8vo, completed. After Vol. II, a portion of each volume, entitled Medical and Philosophical Register, is paged separately in Roman numerals.

3. The Eclectic Repertory and Analytical Review. Medical and Philosophical. Edited by a Society of Physicians. Quarterly. Vols. I-X, 1811-1820, 8vo. Continued as the Journal of Foreign Medical Science and Literature. Quarterly. Conducted by Samuel Emlen, Jr., and William Price. 1821-1824, 8vo. The first two volumes were conducted by Price and Emlen, the third by Samuel Emlen, the fourth by John D. Godman.

4. The American Medical Recorder. Vols. I-XV, 1818-1829. "Conducted by several respectable physicians of Philadelphia." Quarterly. The title of Vols. VII-XII inclusive was changed to Medical Recorder of Original Papers and Intelligence in Medicine and Surgery. Vols. XIII-XV have the original title. Vol. II was conducted by John Eberle; Vols. III and IV by John Eberle, Granville Sharp Pattison, of the University of Maryland, Henry William Ducachet, of New York, and John Revere, of Baltimore; Vol. V by Eberle and Ducachet; Vol. VI conducted by an association of physicians in Philadelphia, Baltimore and Norfolk; Vols. VII, VIII, IX and X conducted by Samuel Colhoun; Vols. XI, XII, XIII and XIV by James Webster, Caleb B. Matthews and Isaac Remington. Merged in the American Journal of the Medical Sciences after No. 2, Vol. XV, April, 1829.

5. The Philadelphia Journal of the Medical and Physical Sciences, supported by an association of physicians and edited by N. Chapman. With Vol. X begins a new series edited by N. Chapman, W. P. Dewees, and John D. Godman. Vol. XIV edited by the

same, with the addition of Isaac Hays. Continued as the American Journal of the Medical Sciences.

6. The American Journal of Medical Sciences. Quarterly until 1888 (Vol. 95), when it became a monthly. Edited solely by Isaac Hays until 1869 (Vol. 58). Vols. 58 to 73 inclusive edited by Isaac Hays, assisted by I. Minis Hays; Vols. 74-77, inclusive, edited by Isaac Hays and I. Minis Hays; Vols. 78-90, inclusive, edited by I. Minis Hays; Vols. 91-94, inclusive, have the additional title of the "International Journal of the Medical Sciences," and are edited by I. Minis Hays and Malcolm Morris, of London; Vols. 95-100, inclusive, are edited solely by I. Minis Hays. In January, 1891 (Vol. 101), Edward P. Davis became sole editor. From 1893 (Vol. 106) to the present time this journal has been published under the editorship of Edward P. Davis "with the coöperation in London of Hector Mackenzie."

Beginning in 1827, this remarkable journal was edited for forty-two years by one man, Dr. Isaac Hays, with steadily increasing prosperity. After the death of Dr. Hays (April 12, 1879) the high standard of the journal was maintained by his son, Dr. I. Minis Hays, and the methods which insured the success of "Hays' Journal" are still successfully pursued by its present editor, Dr. Edward P. Davis. In his obituary notice of Dr. Isaac Hays, the late Professor S. D. Gross, writing in 1879, says, with reference to the American Journal of the Medical Sciences: "What other journal, American or foreign, can boast of having furnished its readers, during the same period, upward of 50,000 octavo pages of closely printed matter, of which at least three-fourths are original? Many of the original articles will be ranked in all time to come as among the most valuable contributions to our medical literature, while not a few of its reviews will be regarded as models of English composition, equal to any that ever appeared in the United States or Great Britain." Still more emphatic is the testimony of Dr. John S. Billings concerning the value of this periodical. In his Centennial History of American Medical Literature, this eminent authority remarks: "The ninety-seven volumes of this journal need no eulogy. They contain many original papers of the highest value;

nearly all the real criticisms and reviews that we possess; and such carefully prepared summaries of the progress of medical science, and abstracts and notices of foreign works, that from this file alone, were all other productions of the press for the last fifty years destroyed, it would be possible to reproduce the great majority of the real contributions of the world to medical science during that period."

7. The Æsculapian Register. Weekly. "Edited by several physicians." Vol. I, June 17 to December 9, 1824. Ended.

8. The Medical Review and Analectic Journal. Quarterly. Conducted by John Eberle and George McClellan. Vols. 1-3, June, 1824, to August, 1826. Ended. The title of the last two volumes was changed to "The American Medical Review and Journal of Original and Selected Papers in Medicine and Surgery," and Nathan Smith and Nathan R. Smith were added as editors.

9. North American Medical and Surgical Journal, conducted by H. L. Hodge, F. Bache, C. D. Meigs, B. H. Coates and R. La Roche. Quarterly. Two volumes, annually. Vols. 1-12, January, 1826, to October, 1831, 8vo. Ended. Vols. 5-12 published by the Kappa Lambda Association of the United States.

10. The Philadelphia Monthly Journal of Medicine and Surgery. Edited by N. R. Smith. Two volumes annually. Vol I, June, 1827, to December, 1827; Vol. II, December, 1827, to February, 1828. Merged in the American Journal of the Medical Sciences.

11. The Monthly Journal of Foreign Medicine. Edited by Squire Littell. Vols. 1-3, January, 1828, to June, 1829.

12. The Cholera Gazette. Edited by Isaac Hays. Weekly. Nos. 1-16, July 11 to November 21, 1832. Ended.

13. The American Lancet. Bi-weekly. Edited by F. S. Beattie. Nos. 1-7, Vol. I, 1833.

14. American Cyclopædia of Practical Medicine and Surgery. A digest of medical literature. By Isaac Hays. Vols. 1-2, 1834-1836. Properly speaking, this is not a "journal," although included among the Medical Journals of the United States by Dr. John S. Billings.

15. The American Medical Library and Intelligencer. Edited

by G. S. Pattison and R. Dunglison, 1836. Specimen sheet. Continued as the American Medical Intelligencer.

16. The Eclectic Journal of Medicine. Monthly. Edited by John Bell. Vols. I-IV., 1836-1840.

17. The American Medical Intelligencer. A concentrated record of medical science and literature. Semi-monthly and monthly. Edited by Robley Dunglison. Five volumes, 1837-1842. Continued as the Medical News and Library.

18. Medical News and Library. Monthly. Vols. 1-37, 1843-1879. In 1880 united with the Monthly Abstract of Medical Science to form

19. The Medical News and Abstract. Monthly. Edited by I. Minis Hays. Vols. 38-39, 1880-1881. Continued as

20. The Medical News. Weekly. Beginning 1882. Edited by I. Minis Hays, until the completion of Vol. 54. Vols. 55-57, inclusive, edited by Hobart A. Hare; Vols. 58-67, inclusive, edited by George M. Gould. In January, 1896, the News began to be published in New York under the editorship of J. Riddle Goffe. Current.

21. The Medical Examiner. Bi-weekly and monthly. Vols. 1-3 edited by J. B. Biddle, M. Clymer and W. W. Gerhard; Vol. 4 by J. B. Biddle, W. W. Gerhard and W. Poyntell Johnston; Vol. 5 by J. B. Biddle and W. W. Gerhard; Vol. 6 by Meredith Clymer; Vol. 7 by Robert M. Huston. In 1845 this journal entered upon a "new series" under the title of the Medical Examiner and Record of Medical Science. The first four volumes of the new series were edited by Robert M. Huston; Vol. 5 by Francis G. Smith and David H. Tucker; Vol. 6 by Francis Gurney Smith; Vols. 7, 8 and 9 by Francis Gurney Smith and J. B. Biddle; Vols. 10, 11, 12 (1856) by Samuel L. Hollingsworth. In 1857, this journal was united with the Louisville Review to form the North American Medico-Chirurgical Review.

22. The Bulletin of Medical Sciences. Monthly. Edited by John Bell. Four volumes, 1843-46, 8vo. Completed.

23. Nordamerikanischer Monatsbericht für Natur and Heilkunde. Four volumes, 1850-52, 8vo.

24. The Philadelphia Medical and Surgical Journal. Semi-monthly. Edited by James Bryan. Vols. 1-6, 1853-58, 8vo.

25. The North American Medico-Chirurgical Review. Edited by S. D. Gross and T. G. Richardson. Bi-monthly. Vols. I-V, 1857-61, 8vo. Completed. Founded by consolidation of the Medical Examiner and the Louisville Review.

26. The Medical and Surgical Reporter. A weekly journal edited by S. W. Butler and R. J. Levis. Two volumes annually. Vol. I, 1859; Vol. 7, L. C. Butler added to the editorial staff; Vol. 8, L. C. Butler retired; Vol. 9, Levis retired; Vol. 16, D. G. Brinton added. S. W. Butler died January 6, 1874. In 1882, J. F. Edwards added. In May, 1887, N. A. Randolph and Charles W. Dulles became editors. January, 1888, to April 26, 1891, Charles W. Dulles, sole editor. April 26, 1891, to June, 1892, Edward T. Reichert, sole editor. July, 1892, to the present time, Harold H. Kynett, sole editor.

27. Half Yearly Compendium of Medical Science. Edited by S. W. Butler, D. G. Brinton and G. H. Napheys, 1868-82, 8vo. 1875-77, Dr. Brinton sole editor; in 1878, C. C. Vanderbeck, co-editor. In 1883, continued as Quarterly Compendium of Medical Science, under the same editorial management as that of the Medical and Surgical Reporter. Ended in 1889.

28. The Photographic Review of Medicine and Surgery. A bi-monthly illustration of interesting cases, accompanied by notes. Edited by F. F. Maury and L. A. Duhring. Two volumes, 1870-72, 8vo. Completed.

29. The Philadelphia Medical Times. A semi-monthly journal of medical and surgical science. The title of Vol. I, 1870-71, was The Medical Times, and the names of Dr. James H. Hutchinson, editor, and Dr. James Tyson, assistant editor, appear on the title page. Vols. 3-5 (1872-75) were published weekly. With, and subsequently to, Vol. 6 (1875-76), it became a fortnightly journal, with Horatio C. Wood as editor. With Vol. 14 (1883-84) Frank Woodbury became editor. With Vol. 18 (1887-88) W. F. Waugh became editor. Vol. 19, completed.

Owing to the fact that the names of the editors of this journal rarely appear on the title page (they are on the title page of Vol. I and are not printed again until the issue of Vol. XV), its editorial history is somewhat obscure. As previously stated, Dr. Edward Rhoads was chosen as editor when the Medical Times was founded, but, owing to failing health, was only able to make the preliminary arrangements for its publication. For the first few months of its publication, the "Times" was edited anonymously by Dr. William Pepper. Drs. Hutchinson and Tyson were succeeded by Dr. John H. Packard and by Dr. Horatio C. Wood.

30. The Medical Cosmos. A monthly abstract of medical science and art. G. J. Zeigler, editor. Vol. I, Nos. 1-5. Vol. II, 1871-1872, 8vo.

31. The Obstetrical Journal of Great Britain and Ireland, etc. Monthly. Edited by J. H. Aveling and A. Wiltshire, with an American supplement edited by Wm. F. Jenks, Philadelphia. Vols. I-VIII, 1873-80, 8vo. Ended. Vols. IV-VII of the American supplement edited by J. V. Ingham. The supplement discontinued after end of Vol. VII, January, 1880.

32. The Monthly Abstract of Medical Science. A digest of the purposes of medicine and the collateral sciences; being a supplement to the Medical News and Library. Vols. 1-6, July, 1874, to December, 1879. After 1879 united with the Medical News and Library, forming the Medical News and Abstract.

33. The Medical Bulletin. A bi-monthly journal for physicians and students. Editorial committee for 1879: J. V. Shoemaker, H. Leffmann and J. T. Eskridge. In 1880, Dr. Shoemaker became sole editor. In May, 1880, became a monthly. Current.

34. The College and Clinical Record. A monthly medical journal conducted especially in the interest of the graduates and students of Jefferson Medical College. Edited by Richard J. Dunglison and Frank Woodbury. After Vol. 5, 1884, Dr. Dunglison became sole editor. In 1896, title changed to Dunglison's College and Clinical Record. Current.

35. The Polyclinic. A monthly journal of medicine and surgery conducted by the faculty of the Philadelphia Polyclinic and College for Graduates in Medicine. Henry Leffmann, editor-in-chief, 1883-1889.

(No. 2.) The Philadelphia Polyclinic, March, 1892. A journal of practical scientific medicine, edited by a committee of the faculty. Began as a quarterly; continued from January, 1893, as a monthly. Vol. III, 1894, weekly, and continued as such. Current.

36. The Medical World. C. F. Taylor, editor and publisher. Began September, 1883 (monthly). In Vol. 3, L. Lewis added as associate editor; Vol. 6, C. F. Taylor, Louis Lewis and J. J. Taylor, editors; Vol. 8, W. H. Walling added; Vol. 10, C. F. Taylor and J. J. Taylor, editors; 1897, C. F. Taylor, editor. Current.

37. Annals of Surgery. Monthly. Commenced January, 1885. Published in St. Louis. Place of publication changed to Philadelphia, January, 1892. In 1892, Lewis S. Pilcher, J. William White and Frederick Treves, editors. July, 1892, William Macewen added. January, 1896, Treves retired and W. H. A. Jacobson added.

38. Medical Register. Weekly. Commenced February 12, 1887. Followed by Times and Register. Weekly, May 4, 1889. The latter merged into Medical Times and Register. Bi-weekly, January 4, 1896. Current. Editors, J. V. Shoemaker and W. C. Wile. Vol. II, J. V. Shoemaker; Vols. III and IV, J. V. Shoemaker and William H. Pancoast; Vol. V, William F. Waugh. Times and Register, 1889, May to December, editor William F. Waugh; 1890, William F. Waugh, managing editor; January, 1894, Frank S. Parsons, manager and editor; 1895, July, Frank S. Parsons, editor, Joseph R. Clausen, manager. Medical Times and Register, January, 1896, Frank S. Parsons, editor; Joseph R. Clausen, business manager. Current.

39. Annual of the Universal Medical Sciences. A yearly report of the progress of the general sanitary sciences throughout the world. Edited by Charles E. Sajous and seventy associate editors. Five volumes yearly. Began in 1888. Current.

40. Satellite of the Annual of the Universal Medical Sciences. Quarterly. Commenced August, 1887. January, 1890, became a monthly. New series, Vol. I, 1893, title Universal Medical Journal. Monthly. Current. Vols. I and II of Satellite edited by Charles E. Sajous; Vol. III, 1889-1890, edited by Charles E. Sajous, assisted by

C. Sumner Witherstine. Universal Medical Journal, Vols. I and II edited by Charles E. Sajous; Vol. III, 1895, by Charles E. Sajous and Eugene Devereux, assistant editor. Current.

41. University Medical Magazine. Monthly. Commenced October, 1888. Edited under the auspices of the Alumni and Faculty of Medicine of the University of Pennsylvania. Vol. IV, editorial committee, J. Howe Adams and Alfred C. Wood; Vol. V, Alfred C. Wood and A. A. Stevens. Current.

42. International Clinics. Quarterly. Commenced April, 1891. Editors, John M. Keating, J. P. Crozer Griffith, J. Mitchell Bruce and David W. Finlay; Vol. I, 1892, editors, John M. Keating, Judson Daland, J. Mitchell Bruce and David W. Finlay; Vol. IV, 1894, and subsequently, Drs. Daland, Bruce and Finlay, editors. Current.

43. International Medical Magazine. Monthly. Commenced February, 1892. Editor, Judson Daland. June, 1893, to January, 1894, editor, Joseph P. Tunis; February, 1894, and subsequently, edited under the supervision of John Ashhurst, Jr., James Whittaker and Henry W. Cattell. Current.

44. Public Health. Quarterly. W. B. Atkinson, editor. Commenced January, 1896. Current.

45. The Medical Council. Monthly. Began March, 1896. Edited by J. J. Taylor; A. H. P. Leuf, associate editor. Current.

www.ingramcontent.com/pod-product-compliance
Lightning Source LLC
Chambersburg PA
CBHW030102010526
44116CB00005B/62